Pediatric Liver Disease

Editor

PHILIP ROSENTHAL

CLINICS IN
LIVER DISEASE

www.liver.theclinics.com

Consulting Editor
NORMAN GITLIN

August 2022 • Volume 26 • Number 3

ELSEVIER

1600 John F. Kennedy Boulevard • Suite 1800 • Philadelphia, Pennsylvania, 19103-2899

http://www.theclinics.com

CLINICS IN LIVER DISEASE Volume 26, Number 3
August 2022 ISSN 1089-3261, ISBN-13: 978-0-323-89754-9

Editor: Kerry Holland
Developmental Editor: Ann Gielou M. Posedio

Clinics in Liver Disease (ISSN 1089-3261) is published quarterly by Elsevier Inc., 360 Park Avenue South, New York, NY 10010-1710. Months of issue are February, May, August, and November. Business and Editorial Offices: 1600 John F. Kennedy Blvd., Ste. 1800, Philadelphia, PA 19103-2899. Customer Service Office: 3251 Riverport Lane, Maryland Heights, MO 63043. Periodicals postage paid at New York, NY and additional mailing offices. Subscription prices are $329.00 per year (U.S. individuals), $100.00 per year (U.S. student/resident), $782.00 per year (U.S. institutions), $421.00 per year (international individuals), $200.00 per year (international student/resident), $813.00 per year (international instituitions), $382.00 per year (Canadian individuals), $100.00 per year (Canadian student/resident), and $813.00 per year (Canadian institutions). Foreign air speed delivery is included in all *Clinics* subscription prices. All prices are subject to change without notice. **POSTMASTER:** Send address changes to *Clinics in Liver Disease*, Elsevier Health Sciences Division, Subscription Customer Service, 3251 Riverport Lane, Maryland Heights, MO 63043. **Customer Service: Telephone: 1-800-654-2452 (U.S. and Canada); 314-447-8871 (outside U.S. and Canada). Fax: 314-447-8029. E-mail: journalscustomer service-usa@elsevier.com (for print support); journalsonlinesupport-usa@elsevier.com (for online support).**

Reprints. For copies of 100 or more of articles in this publication, please contact the Commercial Reprints Department, Elsevier Inc., 360 Park Avenue South, New York, NY 10010-1710. Tel.: 212-633-3874; Fax: 212-633-3820; E-mail: reprints@elsevier.com.

Clinics in Liver Disease is covered in *MEDLINE/PubMed (Index Medicus)*, Science Citation Index Expanded, Journal Citation Reports/Science Edition, and Current Contents/Clinical Medicine.

Contributors

CONSULTING EDITOR

NORMAN GITLIN, MD, FRCP (LONDON), FRCPE (EDINBURGH), FAASLD, FACP, FACG
Head of Hepatology, Southern California Liver Centers, San Clemente, California, USA

EDITOR

PHILIP ROSENTHAL, MD
Professor of Pediatrics and Surgery, Departments of Pediatrics and Surgery, Benioff Children's Hospital, University of California, San Francisco, San Francisco, California, USA

AUTHORS

ESTELLA M. ALONSO, MD
Vice Chair, Department of Pediatrics, Associate Chair for Clinical Services, Department of Pediatrics, Sally Burnett Searle Professor of Pediatric Transplantation, Professor, Departments of Pediatrics and Medical Social Sciences, Ann and Robert H. Lurie Children's Hospital of Chicago, Northwestern University Feinberg School of Medicine, Chicago, Illinois, USA

SWATI ANTALA, MD
Division of Pediatric Gastroenterology, Hepatology, and Nutrition, Department of Pediatrics, Ann and Robert H. Lurie Children's Hospital of Chicago, Chicago, Illinois, USA

MARY AYERS, MD
University of Pittsburgh School of Medicine, Children's Hospital of Pittsburgh of UPMC, Pittsburgh, Pennsylvania, USA

MOHAMMED D. AYOUB, MD, FRCPC
Pediatric Hepatology and Liver Transplantation Fellow, Division of Gastroenterology, Hepatology, and Nutrition, The Hospital for Sick Children, University of Toronto, Toronto, Ontario, Canada; Pediatric Gastroenterology Teaching Assistant, Department of Pediatrics, Faculty of Medicine, Rabigh Branch, King Abdulaziz University, Jeddah, Saudi Arabia

AARON BENNETT, MD
The Children's Hospital of Philadelphia, Perelman School of Medicine, University of Pennsylvania, Philadelphia, Pennsylvania, USA

CATHERINE A. CHAPIN, MD, MS
Assistant Professor, Department of Pediatrics, Ann and Robert H. Lurie Children's Hospital of Chicago, Northwestern University Feinberg School of Medicine, Chicago, Illinois, USA

ANNA MARÍA GÓMEZ, MD, PhD
Assistant Professor of Pathology, University of Pittsburgh School of Medicine, Children's Hospital of Pittsburgh of UPMC, Pittsburgh, Pennsylvania, USA

NITIKA A. GUPTA, MD, DCH, DNB, MRCPCH
Professor of Pediatrics, Division of Gastroenterology, Hepatology and Nutrition, Emory University School of Medicine, Transplant Services, Children's Healthcare of Atlanta, Atlanta, Georgia, USA

SARA HASSAN, MD
Assistant Professor, Department of Pediatrics, Division of Gastroenterology, Hepatology and Nutrition, Mayo Clinic, Rochester, Minnesota, USA

PAULA HERTEL, MD
Associate Professor, Department of Pediatrics, Division of Gastroenterology, Hepatology and Nutrition, Baylor College of Medicine, Texas Children's Hospital, Houston, Texas, USA

JAMES E. HEUBI, MD
Division of Gastroenterology, Hepatology and Nutrition, Professor of Pediatrics, Associate Dean for Clinical and Translational Research, Director, Center for Clinical and Translational Science and Training, University of Cincinnati/Cincinnati Children's Hospital Medical Center, Cincinnati, Ohio, USA

SIMON P. HORSLEN, MB,ChB, FRCPCH
Professor of Pediatrics, Director of Hepatology, University of Pittsburgh School of Medicine, Children's Hospital of Pittsburgh of UPMC, Pittsburgh, Pennsylvania, USA

BINITA M. KAMATH, MBBChir, MRCP, MTR
Professor, Division of Gastroenterology, Hepatology, and Nutrition, The Hospital for Sick Children, Professor of Pediatrics, University of Toronto, Toronto, Ontario, Canada

SAUL J. KARPEN, MD, PhD, FAASLD
Raymond F. Schinazi Distinguished Biomedical Chair, Professor of Pediatrics, Division Chief, Pediatric Gastroenterology, Hepatology and Nutrition, Emory University School of Medicine, Children's Healthcare of Atlanta, Atlanta, Georgia, USA

NANDA KERKAR, MD, MRCPCH, FAASLD
Professor of Pediatrics, University of Rochester Medical Center, Director, Pediatric Liver Disease and Liver Transplant Program, Golisano Children's Hospital, Rochester, New York, USA

SAKIL KULKARNI, MD
Assistant Professor, Department of Pediatrics, St. Louis Children's Hospital, Washington University School of Medicine, St Louis, Missouri, USA

TAMIR MILOH, MD
Professor of Clinical Pediatrics, Department of Pediatric Gastroenterology, Hepatology, and Nutrition, University of Miami, Miami, Florida, USA

DHIREN PATEL, MBBS, MD
Associate Professor, Division of Pediatric Gastroenetrology, Hepatology and Nutrition, Department of Pediatrics, Saint Louis University School of Medicine, St Louis, Missouri, USA

AJAY RANA, MD, MTR
Associate Professor of Pediatrics, University of Rochester Medical Center, Golisano Children's Hospital, Rochester, New York, USA

DAVID A. RUDNICK, MD, PhD
Associate Professor, Departments of Pediatrics and Developmental Biology, St. Louis Children's Hospital, Washington University School of Medicine, St Louis, Missouri, USA

BENJAMIN L. SHNEIDER, MD, FAASLD
George Peterkin Endowed Chair, Section Head, Gastroenterology, Hepatology and Nutrition, Professor of Pediatrics, Baylor College of Medicine, Texas Children's Hospital

SARA KATHRYN SMITH, MD
Professor of Pediatrics, Department of Pediatric Gastroenterology, Hepatology, and Nutrition, Johns Hopkins University, Baltimore, Florida, USA

RONALD J. SOKOL, MD, FAASLD
Chief, Section of Pediatric Gastroenterology, Hepatology and Nutrition, Arnold Silverman MD Endowed Chair in Digestive Health, Professor and Vice Chair of Pediatrics, Director, Colorado Clinical and Translational Sciences Institute, Assistant Vice Chancellor for Clinical and Translational Science, University of Colorado Denver, University of Colorado School of Medicine, Children's Hospital Colorado, Aurora, Colorado, USA

A. BAILEY SPERRY
Lewis Katz School of Medicine at Temple University, Philadelphia, Pennsylvania, USA

JAMES E. SQUIRES, MD, MS
Associate Professor of Pediatrics, Associate Director of Hepatology, University of Pittsburgh School of Medicine, Children's Hospital of Pittsburgh of UPMC, Pittsburgh, Pennsylvania, USA

JAMES P. STEVENS, MD
Department of Pediatrics, Emory University School of Medicine, Transplant Services, Children's Healthcare of Atlanta, Atlanta, Georgia, USA

SHIKHA S. SUNDARAM, MD, MSCI, FAASLD
Associate Professor of Pediatrics, Medical Director, Pediatric Liver Transplant Program, Section of Pediatric Gastroenterology, Hepatology and Nutrition, The Digestive Health Institute, University of Colorado School of Medicine, Children's Hospital Colorado, Aurora, Colorado, USA

ANANDINI SURI, MD
Fellow, Pediatric Gastroenterology; Saint Louis University School of Medicine, St Louis, Missouri, USA

SARAH A. TAYLOR, MD
Division of Pediatric Gastroenterology, Hepatology, and Nutrition, Department of Pediatrics, Ann and Robert H. Lurie Children's Hospital of Chicago, Chicago, Illinois, USA

JEFFREY H. TECKMAN, MD
Professor of Pediatrics and Biochemistry, Division of Pediatric Gastroenetrology, Hepatology and Nutrition, Department of Pediatrics, Saint Louis University School of Medicine, St Louis, Missouri, USA

JESSICA WEN, MD
Associate Professor of Clinical Pediatrics, The Children's Hospital of Philadelphia, Perelman School of Medicine, University of Pennsylvania, Philadelphia, Pennsylvania, USA

STAVRA A. XANTHAKOS, MD, MS
Medical Director, Surgical Weight Loss Program for Teens, Division of Gastroenterology, Hepatology and Nutrition, Cincinnati Children's, Professor, Department of Pediatrics, Director, Nonalcoholic Steatohepatitis Center, University of Cincinnati College of Medicine, Cincinnati, Ohio, USA

Contents

Biliary atresia is a rare disease but remains the most common indication for pediatric liver transplantation as there are no effective medical therapies to slow progression after diagnosis. Variable contribution of genetic, immune, and environmental factors contributes to disease heterogeneity among patients with biliary atresia. Gaining a deeper understanding of the disease mechanism will help to develop targeted medical therapies and improve patient outcomes.

Alagille syndrome (ALGS) is a complex heterogenous disease with a wide array of clinical manifestations in association with cholestatic liver disease. Major clinical and genetic advancements have taken place since its first description in 1969. However, clinicians continue to face considerable challenges in the management of ALGS, particularly in the absence of targeted molecular therapies. In this article, we provide an overview of the broad ALGS phenotype, current approaches to diagnosis and with particular focus on key clinical challenges encountered in the management of these patients.

Bile acid transport and secretion is a complex physiologic process, of which disruption at any step can lead to progressive intrahepatic cholestasis (PFIC). The first described PFIC disorders were originally named as such before identification of a genetic cause. However, advances in clinical molecular genetics have led to the identification of several disorders that can cause these monogenic inherited cholestasis syndromes, and they are now increasingly referred to by the affected protein causing disease. The list of PFIC disorders is expected to grow as more causative genes are discovered. Here forth, we present a comprehensive overview of known PFIC disorders.

Liver disease in homozygous ZZ alpha-1 antitrypsin (AAT) deficiency occurs due to the accumulation of large quantities of AAT mutant Z protein polymers in the liver. The mutant Z protein folds improperly during biogenesis and is retained within the hepatocytes rather than appropriately secreted. These intracellular polymers trigger an injury cascade, which leads to liver injury. However, the clinical liver disease is highly variable and not all patients with this same homozygous ZZ genotype develop liver disease. Evidence suggests that genetic determinants of intracellular protein processing, among other unidentified genetic and environmental factors, likely play a role in liver disease susceptibility. Advancements made in development of new treatment strategies using siRNA technology, and other novel approaches, are promising, and multiple human liver disease trials are underway.

Hepatitis B and C in Children

A. Bailey Sperry, Aaron Bennett, and Jessica Wen

Hepatitis B and hepatitis C are a global burden and underscore the impact of preventable acute and chronic diseases on personal as well as population level health. Caring for pediatric patients with hepatitis B and C requires a deep understanding of the pathophysiology of viral processes. Insight into the epidemiology, transmission, and surveillance of these infections is critical to prevention and therapy. Extensive research in recent years has created a growing number of treatments, changing the landscape of the medical field's approach to the viral hepatitis pandemic.

Mitochondrial Hepatopathy

Mary Ayers, Simon P. Horslen, Anna María Gómez, and James E. Squires

Mitochondrial hepatopathies are a subset of mitochondrial diseases defined by primary dysfunction of hepatocyte mitochondria leading to a phenotype of hepatocyte cell injury, steatosis, or liver failure. Increasingly, the diagnosis is established by new sequencing approaches that combine analysis of both nuclear DNA and mitochondrial DNA and allow for timely diagnosis in most patients. Despite advances in diagnostics, for most affected children their disorders are relentlessly progressive, and result in substantial morbidity and mortality. Treatment remains mainly supportive; however, novel therapeutics and a more definitive role for liver transplantation hold promise for affected children.

Nonalcoholic Steatohepatitis in Children

Stavra A. Xanthakos

Nonalcoholic fatty liver disease (NAFLD) is the leading cause of chronic liver disease in children. Although environmental factors are major contributors to early onset, children have both shared and unique genetic risk alleles as compared with adults with NAFLD. Treatment relies on reducing environmental risk factors, but many children have persistent disease. No medications are approved specifically for the treatment of NAFLD, but some anti-obesity or diabetes treatments may be beneficial. Pediatric NAFLD increases the risk of diabetes and other cardiovascular risk factors. Long-term prospective studies are needed to determine the long-term risk of hepatic and non-hepatic morbidity and mortality in adulthood.

Binita M. Kamath, Estella M. Alonso, James E. Heubi, Saul J. Karpen, Shikha S. Sundaram, Benjamin L. Shneider, and Ronald J. Sokol

Malnutrition in children with chronic cholestasis is a prevalent issue and a major risk factor for adverse outcomes. Fat soluble vitamin (FSV) deficiency is an integral feature of cholestatic disease in children, often occurring within the first months of life in those with neonatal cholestasis and malnutrition. This review focuses on FSVs in cholestasis, with particular emphasis on a practical approach to surveillance and supplementation that includes approaches that account for differing local resources. The overarching strategy suggested is to incorporate recognition of FSV deficiencies in cholestatic children in order to develop practical plans for close monitoring and aggressive FSV repletion. Routine attention to FSV assessment and supplementation in cholestatic infants will reduce long periods of inadequate levels and subsequent adverse clinical sequalae.

CLINICS IN LIVER DISEASE

SERIES OF RELATED INTEREST

Gastroenterology Clinics of North America
https://www.gastro.theclinics.com

THE CLINICS ARE AVAILABLE ONLINE!
Access your subscription at:
www.theclinics.com

Preface

Advances in Pediatric Liver Diseases

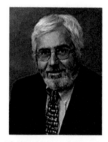

Philip Rosenthal, MD
Editor

It is truly remarkable the progress that has been made in the past few years surrounding the diagnosis, management, and treatment of so many of the liver diseases affecting children. Advances in genetic testing have recognized many previously unknown hereditary disorders. Along with this recognition has come a better understanding of the mechanism of disease and of whether potential new therapies will likely alleviate the symptoms associated with the disorder. Who could have imagined that there are now cures for children with hepatitis C infection? Or drugs to alleviate the severe itching in childhood cholestasis associated with Alagille syndrome and progressive familial intrahepatic cholestasis? The articles in this issue of *Clinics in Liver Disease* focusing on Pediatric Liver Disease are up-to-date and written by experts in the field. I hope you will enjoy reading and learning about these advances as much as I have. A huge thank you to the authors for their contributions and to the publisher and Consulting Editor Dr Gitlin for making this pediatric issue possible.

Philip Rosenthal, MD
Departments of Pediatrics & Surgery
University of California, San Francisco
Benioff Children's Hospital
550 16th Street
Mailcode 0136
San Francisco, CA 94143-0136, USA

E-mail address:
prosenth@ucsf.edu

Clin Liver Dis 26 (2022) xiii
https://doi.org/10.1016/j.cld.2022.03.012
1089-3261/22/© 2022 Published by Elsevier Inc.

Biliary Atresia in Children

Update on Disease Mechanism, Therapies, and Patient Outcomes

Swati Antala, MD, Sarah A. Taylor, MD*

KEYWORDS

- Biliary atresia • Neonatal cholestasis • Pediatric liver transplantation
- Transplant outcomes

KEY POINTS

- Biliary atresia (BA) remains the leading indication for pediatric liver transplantation as there are no established medical therapies to delay progression of liver disease after Kasai portoenterostomy.
- Despite a common clinical presentation of disease, the multifactorial nature of disease pathogenesis contributes to phenotypic heterogeneity and variable rate of disease progression.
- There remains an unmet need to develop BA-specific medical therapies and improve outcomes for patients with and without survival with their native liver.

INTRODUCTION

Biliary atresia (BA) is a progressive, obstructive cholangiopathy with neonatal onset. Although BA is a rare disease, it remains the leading indication for pediatric liver transplantation as there are no effective medical therapies to prevent or slow disease progression. The prevalence of BA varies by geographic region with an incidence of 1 in 6000 to 8000 live births in Taiwan and up to 1 in 19,000 live births in Canada with intermediate rates reported in other areas of the world.[1–3] A higher incidence of BA has been reported in patients with female versus male gender, premature infants, and in Asian and black versus white infants.[4–7] BA is most often an isolated defect but can be associated with other congenital abnormalities in up to 16% of cases of which more than half commonly have laterality defects (particularly splenic anomalies) and are referred to as syndromic BA.[8] In this article, we highlight disease biomarkers and therapies as they relate to our understanding of BA pathogenesis and outcomes.

Division of Pediatric Gastroenterology, Hepatology, and Nutrition, Department of Pediatrics, Ann and Robert H Lurie Children's Hospital of Chicago, 225 East Chicago Avenue, Box 65, Chicago, IL 60611, USA
* Corresponding author.
E-mail address: sataylor@luriechildrens.org

Clin Liver Dis 26 (2022) 341–354
https://doi.org/10.1016/j.cld.2022.03.001
1089-3261/22/© 2022 Elsevier Inc. All rights reserved.

DEFINITION AND DIAGNOSIS OF BILIARY ATRESIA

BA is the most common cause of obstructive cholestasis in the neonate in which infants develop scleral icterus, clay-colored acholic stools, and jaundice that persists beyond the first 2 weeks of life. Direct or conjugated bilirubin remains the primary screening laboratory test for BA, with elevated values shown to occur within the first 2 days of life.[9,10] The levels of gamma-glutamyl transferase (GGT) and matrix metalloproteinase-7 (MMP-7), a marker of biliary epithelial injury, also have an established role in the diagnosis of BA, and new candidate biomarkers continue to emerge (**Box 1**).[11–22] Imaging by abdominal ultrasound is considered one of the first-tier tests in a targeted investigation of BA to identify alternate anatomic etiologies of obstructive cholestasis and may also detect features supportive of BA (eg, abnormal gallbladder, absent common bile duct, vascular anomalies such as preduodenal portal vein, polysplenia or asplenia, and triangular cord sign).[9] Other imaging modalities such as hepatobiliary scintigraphy, magnetic resonance cholangiopancreatography, endoscopic retrograde cholangiopancreatography, and percutaneous transhepatic cholangiogram may also be considered with varying levels of sensitivity and specificity.[9,23]

Liver biopsy (**Fig. 1**) remains a central step in diagnosing BA, although incorporation of new biomarkers or laparoscopic evaluation may reduce the need for liver biopsy before intraoperative cholangiogram (IOC).[9,15,23–26] Once a high index of suspicion is established, IOC is performed and is considered positive if a patent extrahepatic biliary tree is not visualized. Subsequently, Kasai portoenterostomy (KPE) is performed as the primary treatment to promote biliary drainage. IOC paired with KPE also helps to define the specific anatomic variant of BA that may have prognostic implications.[27]

PATHOPHYSIOLOGY OF DISEASE ONSET AND PROGRESSION

Our understanding of early disease pathogenesis suggests that susceptible infants with possible genetic predisposition experience an in utero insult, leading to stimulation of innate and adaptive immunity, bile duct injury with impaired bile flow, accumulation of bile acids, and epithelial damage with alteration of intercellular junctions. Although the exact triggering event remains unknown, evidence supports an in utero onset of BA including the identification of prenatal gallbladder anomalies, abnormally low GGT levels in amniotic fluid, and the presence of elevated direct/conjugated bilirubin levels within 24 to 48 hours of birth.[28,29] Ongoing research suggests that there is

Box 1 Serum biomarkers in BA	
Biomarker	**Sensitivity and Specificity**
Direct or conjugated Bilirubin screening algorithm[10]	100%, 99.9%
GGT > 250 IU/L[11]	83%, 71%
GGT > 300 IU/L[12]	40%, 98%
Age 61–90 d with GGT > 303 IU/L[13]	83%, 82%
GGT/AST > 2[12]	81%, 72%
MMP-7[14,15]	96%, 91%
Candidate biomarkers:	NA
Bile acid profiles[18,19,22]	
MicroRNAs[20,21]	
Cytokines: IL-33, IL-18, IL-8[15–17]	

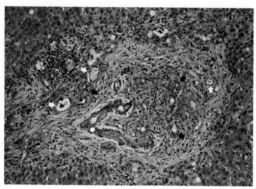

Fig. 1. Liver biopsy from an infant with BA at diagnosis that underwent liver transplant before 2 years of age. Histologic findings include expansion of the portal tract with stromal edema, prominent fibrosis, bile duct proliferation (*black arrows*), and bile plugs (*white arrows*). White star delineates a branching artery.

variable contribution among the dominant contributing factors of disease pathogenesis, thereby leading to different BA phenotypes despite a common clinical presentation.

Environmental Factors

A viral trigger causing biliary obstruction in utero has long been considered a possible etiologic factor for the development of BA. The well-established murine model of BA relies on rhesus rotavirus inoculation within the first 24 hours of life.[30] Parallel studies in humans suggest that some, but not all, cases of BA may be associated with a viral insult. Viruses implicated in BA include cytomegalovirus (CMV), reovirus, rotavirus, Epstein-Barr virus, and human papillomavirus.[31] CMV has been the most frequently analyzed virus with positive rates of detection among BA patients varying by seasonality but overall ranging from 20% to 60%.[31] A role for the gut microbiome in the pathogenesis of BA is also emerging, although further studies are needed to define how precise microbial metabolites or microbial-driven immune modulation is implicated in BA and if probiotics may be beneficial.[32]

After outbreaks of a disease similar to BA were reported in newborn lambs in Australia, a previously unknown *Dysphania* plant isoflavonoid, now named biliatresone, was hypothesized to be the suspected agent.[33] Murine extrahepatic bile ducts treated with biliatresone demonstrated the disruption of cholangiocyte apical polarity, loss of monolayer integrity, increased permeability, and luminal obstruction mediated by decreased levels of glutathione and SOX17.[34] A more recent in vivo study of mice injected with biliatresone confirmed biliary obstruction with associated inflammation and fibrosis.[35] Additionally, these BA mice demonstrated evidence for oxidative stress including altered hepatic glutathione levels similar to sequencing analysis in human tissues implicating glutathione metabolism in BA outcomes.[35,36]

Immune Factors

Various immune mechanisms have been proposed including immune dysregulation, autoimmunity, and susceptibility of the neonate's immature immune system. While the precise interplay between these processes has not been fully established, extensive research in the field has identified key components of the innate and adaptive immune responses in both the early and late stages of BA (**Fig. 2**).[37,38] Innate immunity plays a key role in the early immune response to pathogens through pathogen recognition receptors, in particular toll-like receptors (TLRs) (see **Fig. 2A**). TLRs are upregulated in BA and recognize pathogen-associated molecular patterns (PAMPs) or stimuli released from apoptotic/necrotic cells, that is, damage-associated molecular patterns (DAMPs).[39] On TLR activation, type 1 interferons are released and initiate a complex cascade of immune signaling by tumor necrosis factor alpha (TNF-α), interleukin (IL)-1, IL-6, IL-8, and IL-15.[37,38] Cholangiocytes, macrophages, and dendritic cells play a primary role in this early immune response that results in neutrophil recruitment and the activation of adaptive immunity.

Within the adaptive immune arm, the oligoclonal expansion of both T cells and B cells has been observed and various autoantibodies have been identified in infants with BA supporting a possible role in antigen-driven immune stimulation.[40–45] Most infants with BA exhibit a dominant Th1 immune response early in disease, although Th17 T-cell immunity has been demonstrated in various studies and Th2 responses may be involved in cystic BA.[46,47] Human and murine studies have also demonstrated a decrease in the frequency and function of T regulatory cells (Tregs), further supporting the premise for immune dysregulation in the setting of immature neonatal immunity.[42,48] Despite the evidence of oligoclonality and the presence of various autoantibodies, a critical antigen-independent role of B cells has also been shown.[49]

The hepatic immune response at later stages of BA commonly exhibits a Th2 immune phenotype characterized by low-level inflammation and oxidative injury, bile duct proliferation, and progressive fibrosis (see **Fig. 2B**).[38] Important at this stage of disease is the hepatocyte-derived alarmin IL-33 that triggers IL-13-driven activation of hepatic stellate cells and progressive hepatic fibrosis.[38,50] Macrophages mediate both the pro-restorative and maladaptive responses in cholestatic liver disease, and the distinct transcriptional subsets have been identified in pediatric cholestatic liver disease at the time of transplant.[38,51] Further delineating the role of profibrotic macrophages and the IL-33/IL-13 axis will help to identify therapeutic targets and prevent progression to cirrhosis.

Genetic Susceptibility

Although BA does not follow a mendelian pattern of inheritance and a single genetic variant has not been identified, various studies suggest a role for genetic susceptibility variants. Additionally, human leukocyte antigen (HLA) associations are not present within BA, supporting alternate genetic influencers of immune function.[52] Of interest in syndromic BA is the identification of variants of *PKD1L1*, a gene associated with ciliary development and laterality determination.[53] Additional ciliary gene defects have been implicated in both syndromic and nonsyndromic BA.[54] A summary of genes that may be associated with BA is shown in **Box 2**.[55,56]

Much work has also focused on defining transcriptional phenotypes that relate to patient outcomes. Moyer and colleagues[57] characterized BA patients into inflammatory or fibrotic groups by molecular profiling and found the fibrotic gene signature to be associated with reduced transplant-free survival. Similarly, Luo and colleagues[36] identified a 14-gene signature that predicted 2-year transplant-free survival in which patients with poor outcome had enrichment for genes involved in fibrosis, whereas those with good outcome expressed higher levels of genes involved in glutathione metabolism. Overall, these studies suggest that while there is no established causal gene in BA, various susceptibility genes and specific gene pathways may be involved in pathogenesis and outcome. Larger human studies and parallel mechanistic studies in animals will help identify the role of specific genes.

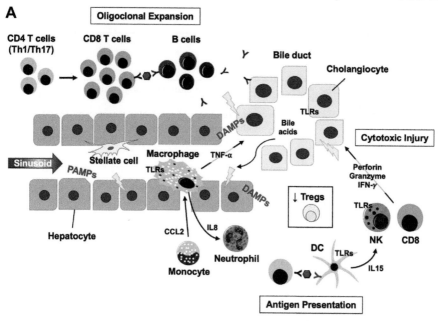

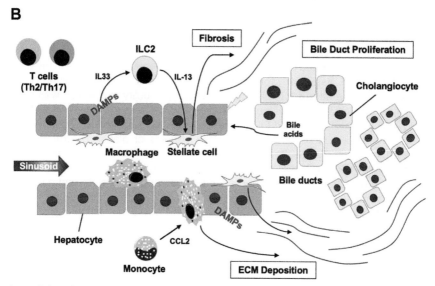

Fig. 2. (*A*) Early immune mechanism of BA is characterized by activation of innate immunity via PAMPs and DAMPs with subsequent stimulation of the adaptive immune response. (*B*). Later stages of BA exhibit a Th2/Th17 phenotype with IL-33/IL-13-driven bile duct proliferation and fibrosis. CCL2, C-C motif chemokine ligand 2; DC, dendritic cell; ECM, extracellular matrix; IFN, interferon; NK, natural killer cell.

THERAPEUTIC OPTIONS

Surgical intervention with KPE at the time of diagnosis remains the primary treatment strategy for BA. Due to our inability to prevent ongoing hepatic injury, BA remains the leading indication for pediatric liver transplantation. An isolated liver transplant without prior KPE can also achieve favorable outcomes and may be considered, particularly in

Box 2	
Genes implicated in BA	
Gene	**Function**
PKD1L1, CFC1, ZIC3, ZEB2, FOXA2, HNF1B, KIF3B, TTC17[53–55]	Regulation of laterality ciliogenesis, and development
ARF6, EFEMP1[55]	Cytoskeleton and extracellular matrix modeling
ADD3[55]	Cell contact and membrane structure
GPC1, JAG1[55,56]	Hedgehog and Wnt signaling pathways
STIP1, REV1[55]	Stress response and DNA repair

BA patients with late diagnoses.[58] Medical management after KPE includes the prevention and treatment of complications such as cholangitis and optimization of nutrition and fat-soluble vitamin supplementation.[59–64] Management of portal hypertension and timing for liver transplantation parallel standard medical care as in other etiologies of end-stage liver disease and have been reviewed comprehensively by Sundaram and colleagues.[65] We highlight the previously studied and emerging medical therapies that target-specific pathways of disease pathogenesis in the following discussion.

Investigational Medical Therapies

Generalized immune modulating therapies previously tested in BA have included steroids and intravenous immunoglobulin (IVIG). Theoretic benefits of using steroids include improving biliary inflammation to promote choleresis; however, their benefit in BA remains unclear. Davenport and colleagues[66,67] studied the effect of oral prednisolone after KPE and found that while there was improvement in jaundice in the early postoperative period, particularly for infants less than 70 day old, there was no significant reduction in the need for liver transplantation. The utility of steroids was most extensively examined in the multicenter, double-blind Steroids in Biliary Atresia Randomized Trial (START; Childhood Liver Disease Research Network), in which infants received a 13-week course of either high-dose steroids or placebo starting within 72 hours after KPE.[68] The results from START showed no difference in total bilirubin at 6 months post-KPE or 2-year survival with native liver in those that received steroids. Furthermore, the treatment group experienced impaired growth and a shorter time to first serious adverse event.[68,69] While a small clinical benefit could not be excluded by the authors, the results did not establish a role for routine use of high-dose steroids after KPE.

IVIG has been associated with clinical benefits in many inflammatory and autoimmune diseases and can interfere with phagocytosis by the cells of the innate immune system, neutralize autoantibodies, and modulate the adaptive immune response.[70] In murine BA, administration of high-dose immunoglobulin resulted in decreased bilirubin, less bile duct inflammation and obstruction, and lower levels of cytokines associated with CD4+ Th1-mediated inflammation, although overall survival did not differ.[71] However, a prospective multicenter open-label human trial in the Childhood Liver Disease Research Network (Safety Study of Intravenous Immunoglobulin Post-Portoenterostomy in Infants with Biliar Atresia; PRIME) found no improvement in bilirubin levels at 90 days post-KPE or 1-year survival with native liver in participants that received IVIG after KPE compared with a placebo-arm group.[72]

More recent studies include use of immune cell subset-specific therapies in BA. A limited study examining the effect of B cell depleting agents in BA showed that one dose of rituximab was safe and well-tolerated; however, long-term clinical outcomes were not reported.[42] A possible beneficial role of hematopoietic stem cell recruitment via granulocyte-colony stimulating factor (GCSF) in liver disease has been supported by various studies in adults. Based on this experience, a clinical trial using GCSF in patients with BA is ongoing with initial phase 1 data demonstrating safety and perhaps some improvement in early biliary drainage and frequency of cholangitis.[73]

Additional therapeutic targets in BA include interrupting ongoing hepatic injury induced through oxidative injury and bile acid toxicity. N-acetylcysteine (NAC) is an antioxidant that has been shown to improve hepatic injury and fibrosis, reduce biliary obstruction, and increase survival in murine BA.[36] A single-center, open-label, phase 2 trial is currently investigating whether NAC given after KPE may improve bile flow in humans.[74] Ursodiol has the various proposed mechanisms to reduce cholestatic liver injury and is standard supportive medical therapy after KPE. Newer agents that inhibit the ileal apical sodium-dependent bile acid transporter to interrupt enterohepatic bile acid recirculation include maralixibat and odevixibat, both with ongoing clinical trials in BA.[75] Lastly, farnesoid X receptor agonists control metabolic homeostasis and inhibit bile acid synthesis and may be considered as future therapeutic options for pediatric cholestatic liver disease.[75]

PREDICTING PROGNOSIS IN BILIARY ATRESIA

Prognosis in BA remains difficult to predict due to disease heterogeneity and the contribution of multiple clinical variables. Ongoing work to strengthen screening practices and develop targeted therapies for modifiable clinical factors is needed to further improve patient outcomes.

Patient Variables

A defining clinical variable associated with the duration of transplant-free survival is the age at which KPE is performed. KPE performed before 30 to 60 days of life improves outcomes; however, late KPE can still achieve biliary drainage.[2,76] Center expertise, patient anatomy, and BA subtype can also impact patient outcomes.[77] BA characterized by atresia of the hepatic duct and porta hepatis (Ohi type II and III) and syndromic BA have been associated with lower rates of transplant-free survival.[27] Growth failure after KPE is another well-established risk factor for death or transplant and highlights the critical importance of accurate anthropometric measurements to institute early nutritional support.[61] More recently, cardiomyopathy has been identified as a prevalent comorbidity in infants with BA and is associated with higher risk for serious adverse event and peri-transplant death.[78] In a study population of children with cirrhosis in BA of which 71% of children were less than 1 year of age, the presence of ascites, a lower serum sodium, higher bilirubin, and increased pediatric end-stage liver disease score were associated with higher mortality.[79] A summary of key clinical variables and their impact on prognosis is illustrated in **Fig. 3**.

Biochemical Markers

One of the most widely studied factors in the prognosis of BA is the bilirubin level after KPE.[80] Total bilirubin less than 2 mg/dL by 3 months post-KPE is associated with greater transplant-free survival at 2 years of age (86%) compared with bilirubin $\geq$ 2 mg/dL (20%). In addition, infants with a total bilirubin $\geq$ 2 mg/dL have a higher likelihood of developing complications of liver disease including ascites, hypoalbuminemia, or coagulopathy. Elevated GGT levels and the aspartate aminotransferase-to-platelet ratio index (APRI) after KPE have been associated with a lower rate of survival with native liver.[15,81] Other studied but not yet widely established markers for poor prognosis after KPE in BA include positive CMV serology, high IL-8, reduced number

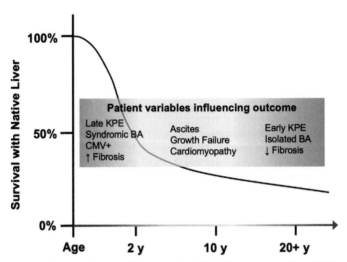

Fig. 3. Cumulative data on the overall prognosis of BA demonstrate about 50% of patients require liver transplantation by 2 years of age.

of Tregs, low IL12 B levels, increased serum hyaluronic acid, and elevated MMP-7 levels.[81–84]

Hepatic Phenotype

The extent of hepatic fibrosis at diagnosis of BA has also been associated with worse prognosis. Russo and colleagues[25] identified that a higher stage of fibrosis as well as the findings of ductal plate configuration, and moderate to severe bile duct injury on diagnostic needle liver biopsies correlated with a higher risk of transplantation. Noninvasive modalities to measure fibrosis such as APRI or liver stiffness by transient elastography have also demonstrated prognostic utility.[81] Furthermore, transcriptional profiling of the liver in BA demonstrated that a fibrotic gene signature is associated with poor outcome, whereas a more inflammatory gene signature and increased gene expression for pathways of glutathione metabolism have been associated with higher rates of transplant-free survival.[36,57] Different hepatic immune phenotypes have also been associated with patient outcomes. For example, high amounts of macrophages and IL-17+ immune cells in the portal tracts of infants with BA have been associated with worse outcome, demonstrating the clinical relevance of different immune phenotypes.[46,85] While specific transcriptional or immune signatures have not been established in clinical use, further research may better define their prognostic role in BA.

PATIENT OUTCOMES

Overall, about half of patients with BA require a liver transplant by 2 years of age, and most are transplanted by early adulthood (see **Fig. 3**).[86,87] Rates of graft and patient survival in BA after liver transplantation are excellent with a recent report from Society of Pediatric Liver Transplantation (SPLIT) of graft and patient survival at 90% and 97%, respectively.[88] At 10 years posttransplant in the SPLIT registry, more than 80% of patients had normal liver and kidney function, 89% had height z-scores greater than the third percentile, and 94% had weight z-scores for age greater than the 3rd percentile.[89]

In addition, there is growing recognition of the need to improve outcomes in patients that survive with their native liver beyond the age of 2 years. Patients surviving without transplant continue to experience complications of chronic liver disease including clinical manifestations of cirrhosis, portal hypertension, cholangitis, and pruritus. Prognostic models have recently been developed to risk stratify poor outcomes in patients with their native liver after the age of 2 years.[90] Cumulative incidence of liver transplant or death was 23.7% and predicted by increased total bilirubin, low albumin, decreased platelet count, and a history of either cholangitis or ascites.[90]

Children with BA are also at risk for impairments in neurodevelopmental outcomes and decreased quality of life. Multiple studies have shown variable levels of impairment in motor and/or language skills in infants with BA at diagnosis up to the time of transplant as well as school-age children with or without transplant.[91–93] Importantly, a 2013 cross-sectional study from the Childhood Liver Disease Research Network found that BA patients had poorer health-related quality of life compared with healthy children across all domains.[94] Similar findings have been validated by other groups and highlight the need for ongoing multidisciplinary support for this vulnerable patient population.

SUMMARY

BA remains the leading cause of neonatal obstructive jaundice and is the most common indication for pediatric liver transplantation. While outcomes after liver transplantation for BA are excellent, there remains an unmet need to develop medical therapies to prolong transplant-free survival and reduce the incidence of adverse events in patients surviving with their native liver. Significant research is needed to establish new therapies for BA that account for the multifactorial nature of disease progression and heterogeneity of immune phenotypes.

CLINICS CARE POINTS

- New diagnostic biomarkers may facilitate earlier diagnosis to improve outcomes after KPE.
- Variable contribution of immune, genetic, and environmental factors accounts for disease heterogeneity in BA and may influence response to medical therapies.
- Risk stratification of outcomes for BA patients before and after transplant is critical to reduce occurrence of serious adverse events, prolong survival with native liver, and improve neurodevelopmental outcomes.

FINANCIAL SUPPORT

S.A. Taylor is supported by funding from NIH NIDDK (1K08DK121937).

DISCLOSURE

The authors report no conflict of interest.

REFERENCES

1. The NS, Honein MA, Caton AR, et al. Risk factors for isolated biliary atresia, national birth defects prevention study, 1997-2002. Am J Med Genet A 2007; 143A(19):2274–84.
2. Schreiber RA, Barker CC, Roberts EA, et al. Biliary atresia: the Canadian experience. J Pediatr 2007;151(6):659–65, 665 e651.

3. Lin YC, Chang MH, Liao SF, et al. Decreasing rate of biliary atresia in Taiwan: a survey, 2004-2009. Pediatrics 2011;128(3):e530–6.

4. Hopkins PC, Yazigi N, Nylund CM. Incidence of biliary atresia and timing of hepatoportoenterostomy in the United States. J Pediatr 2017;187:253–7.

5. Chiu CY, Chen PH, Chan CF, et al. Taiwan infant stool color card study G. Biliary atresia in preterm infants in taiwan: a nationwide survey. J Pediatr 2013;163(1): 100–103 e101.

6. van Wessel DBE, Boere T, Hulzebos CV, et al. Preterm infants with biliary atresia: a nationwide cohort analysis from The Netherlands. J Pediatr Gastroenterol Nutr 2017;65(4):370–4.

7. Durkin N, Deheragoda M, Davenport M. Prematurity and biliary atresia: a 30-year observational study. Pediatr Surg Int 2017;33(12):1355–61.

8. Schwarz KB, Haber BH, Rosenthal P, et al. Extrahepatic anomalies in infants with biliary atresia: results of a large prospective North American multicenter study. Hepatology 2013;58(5):1724–31.

9. Fawaz R, Baumann U, Ekong U, et al. Guideline for the evaluation of cholestatic jaundice in infants: joint recommendations of the north american society for pediatric gastroenterology, hepatology, and nutrition and the european society for pediatric gastroenterology, hepatology, and nutrition. J Pediatr Gastroenterol Nutr 2017;64(1):154–68.

10. Harpavat S, Garcia-Prats JA, Anaya C, et al. Diagnostic yield of newborn screening for biliary atresia using direct or conjugated bilirubin measurements. JAMA 2020;323(12):1141–50.

11. Rendon-Macias ME, Villasis-Keever MA, Castaneda-Mucino G, et al. Improvement in accuracy of gamma-glutamyl transferase for differential diagnosis of biliary atresia by correlation with age. Turk J Pediatr 2008;50(3):253–9.

12. Tang KS, Huang LT, Huang YH, et al. Gamma-glutamyl transferase in the diagnosis of biliary atresia. Acta Paediatr Taiwan 2007;48(4):196–200.

13. Chen X, Dong R, Shen Z, et al. Value of gamma-glutamyl transpeptidase for diagnosis of biliary atresia by correlation with age. J Pediatr Gastroenterol Nutr 2016; 63(3):370–3.

14. Lertudomphonwanit C, Mourya R, Fei L, et al. Large-scale proteomics identifies MMP-7 as a sentinel of epithelial injury and of biliary atresia. Sci Transl Med 2017;9(417):eaan8462.

15. He L, Ip DKM, Tam G, et al. Biomarkers for the diagnosis and post-Kasai portoenterostomy prognosis of biliary atresia: a systematic review and meta-analysis. Sci Rep 2021;11(1):11692.

16. Urushihara N, Iwagaki H, Yagi T, et al. Elevation of serum interleukin-18 levels and activation of Kupffer cells in biliary atresia. J Pediatr Surg 2000;35(3):446–9.

17. Bessho K, Mourya R, Shivakumar P, et al. Gene expression signature for biliary atresia and a role for interleukin-8 in pathogenesis of experimental disease. Hepatology 2014;60(1):211–23.

18. Muraji T, Harada T, Miki K, et al. Urinary sulfated bile acid concentrations in infants with biliary atresia and breast-feeding jaundice. Pediatr Int 2003;45(3):281–3.

19. Fukuoka T, Bessho K, Tachibana M, et al. Total bile acid concentration in duodenal fluid is a useful preoperative screening marker to rule out biliary atresia. J Pediatr Gastroenterol Nutr 2018;67(3):383–7.

20. Zahm AM, Hand NJ, Boateng LA, et al. Circulating microRNA is a biomarker of biliary atresia. J Pediatr Gastroenterol Nutr 2012;55(4):366–9.

21. Peng X, Yang L, Liu H, et al. Identification of circulating MicroRNAs in biliary atresia by next-generation sequencing. J Pediatr Gastroenterol Nutr 2016; 63(5):518–23.
22. Zhao D, Zhou K, Chen Y, et al. Development and validation of bile acid profile-based scoring system for identification of biliary atresia: a prospective study. BMC Pediatr 2020;20(1):255.
23. Wang L, Yang Y, Chen Y, et al. Early differential diagnosis methods of biliary atresia: a meta-analysis. Pediatr Surg Int 2018;34(4):363–80.
24. Okazaki T, Ochi T, Nakamura H, et al. Needle liver biopsy has potential for delaying Kasai portoenterostomy and Is obsolete for diagnosing biliary atresia in the laparoscopic era. J Pediatr Surg 2019;54(12):2570–3.
25. Russo P, Magee JC, Anders RA, et al. Key histopathologic features of liver biopsies that distinguish biliary atresia from other causes of infantile cholestasis and their correlation with outcome: a multicenter study. Am J Surg Pathol 2016; 40(12):1601–15.
26. Lee JY, Sullivan K, El Demellawy D, et al. The value of preoperative liver biopsy in the diagnosis of extrahepatic biliary atresia: a systematic review and meta-analysis. J Pediatr Surg 2016;51(5):753–61.
27. Superina R, Magee JC, Brandt ML, et al. The anatomic pattern of biliary atresia identified at time of Kasai hepatoportoenterostomy and early postoperative clearance of jaundice are significant predictors of transplant-free survival. Ann Surg 2011;254(4):577–85.
28. Mysore KR, Shneider BL, Harpavat S. Biliary atresia as a disease starting in utero: implications for treatment, diagnosis, and pathogenesis. J Pediatr Gastroenterol Nutr 2019;69(4):396–403.
29. Harpavat S, Finegold MJ, Karpen SJ. Patients with biliary atresia have elevated direct/conjugated bilirubin levels shortly after birth. Pediatrics 2011;128(6): e1428–33.
30. Riepenhoff-Talty M, Schaekel K, Clark HF, et al. Group A rotaviruses produce extrahepatic biliary obstruction in orally inoculated newborn mice. Pediatr Res 1993;33(4 Pt 1):394–9.
31. Saito T, Terui K, Mitsunaga T, et al. Evidence for viral infection as a causative factor of human biliary atresia. J Pediatr Surg 2015;50(8):1398–404.
32. Jain V, Alexander EC, Burford C, et al. Gut microbiome: a potential modifiable risk factor in biliary atresia. J Pediatr Gastroenterol Nutr 2021;72(2):184–93.
33. Harper P, Plant JW, Unger DB. Congenital biliary atresia and jaundice in lambs and calves. Aust Vet J 1990;67(1):18–22.
34. Waisbourd-Zinman O, Koh H, Tsai S, et al. The toxin biliatresone causes mouse extrahepatic cholangiocyte damage and fibrosis through decreased glutathione and SOX17. Hepatology 2016;64(3):880–93.
35. Yang Y, Wang J, Zhan Y, et al. The synthetic toxin biliatresone causes biliary atresia in mice. Lab Invest 2020;100(11):1425–35.
36. Luo Z, Shivakumar P, Mourya R, et al. Gene expression signatures associated with survival times of pediatric patients with biliary atresia identify potential therapeutic agents. Gastroenterology 2019;157(4):1138–1152 e1114.
37. Kilgore A, Mack CL. Update on investigations pertaining to the pathogenesis of biliary atresia. Pediatr Surg Int 2017;33(12):1233–41.
38. Ortiz-Perez A, Donnelly B, Temple H, et al. Innate immunity and pathogenesis of biliary atresia. Front Immunol 2020;11:329.
39. Saito T, Hishiki T, Terui K, et al. Toll-like receptor mRNA expression in liver tissue from patients with biliary atresia. J Pediatr Gastroenterol Nutr 2011;53(6):620–6.

40. Mack CL, Falta MT, Sullivan AK, et al. Oligoclonal expansions of CD4+ and CD8+ T-cells in the target organ of patients with biliary atresia. Gastroenterology 2007;133(1):278–87.

41. Taylor SA, Malladi P, Pan X, et al. Oligoclonal immunoglobulin repertoire in biliary remnants of biliary atresia. Sci Rep 2019;9(1):4508.

42. Wang J, Xu Y, Chen Z, et al. Liver immune profiling reveals pathogenesis and therapeutics for biliary atresia. Cell 2020;183(7):1867–1883 e1826.

43. Lu BR, Brindley SM, Tucker RM, et al. alpha-enolase autoantibodies cross-reactive to viral proteins in a mouse model of biliary atresia. Gastroenterology 2010;139(5):1753–61.

44. Pang SY, Dai YM, Zhang RZ, et al. Autoimmune liver disease-related autoantibodies in patients with biliary atresia. World J Gastroenterol 2018;24(3):387–96.

45. Luo Y, Brigham D, Bednarek J, et al. Unique cholangiocyte-targeted igm autoantibodies correlate with poor outcome in biliary atresia. Hepatology 2021;73(5):1855–67.

46. Lages CS, Simmons J, Maddox A, et al. The dendritic cell-T helper 17-macrophage axis controls cholangiocyte injury and disease progression in murine and human biliary atresia. Hepatology 2017;65(1):174–88.

47. Li J, Bessho K, Shivakumar P, et al. Th2 signals induce epithelial injury in mice and are compatible with the biliary atresia phenotype. J Clin Invest 2011; 121(11):4244–56.

48. Tucker RM, Feldman AG, Fenner EK, et al. Regulatory T cells inhibit Th1 cell-mediated bile duct injury in murine biliary atresia. J Hepatol 2013;59(4):790–6.

49. Bednarek J, Traxinger B, Brigham D, et al. Cytokine-producing B cells promote immune-mediated bile duct injury in murine biliary atresia. Hepatology 2018; 68(5):1890–904.

50. Li J, Razumilava N, Gores GJ, et al. Biliary repair and carcinogenesis are mediated by IL-33-dependent cholangiocyte proliferation. J Clin Invest 2014;124(7): 3241–51.

51. Taylor SA, Chen SY, Gadhvi G, et al. Transcriptional profiling of pediatric cholestatic livers identifies three distinct macrophage populations. PLoS One 2021; 16(1):e0244743.

52. Mack CL, Anderson KM, Aubrey MT, et al. Lack of HLA predominance and HLA shared epitopes in biliary Atresia. Springerplus 2013;2(1):42.

53. Berauer JP, Mezina AI, Okou DT, et al. Identification of polycystic kidney disease 1 like 1 Gene variants in children with biliary atresia splenic malformation syndrome. Hepatology 2019;70(3):899–910.

54. Lam WY, Tang CS, So MT, et al. Identification of a wide spectrum of ciliary gene mutations in nonsyndromic biliary atresia patients implicates ciliary dysfunction as a novel disease mechanism. EBioMedicine 2021;71:103530.

55. Rajagopalan R, Tsai EA, Grochowski CM, et al. Exome sequencing in individuals with isolated biliary atresia. Sci Rep 2020;10(1):2709.

56. Kohsaka T, Yuan ZR, Guo SX, et al. The significance of human jagged 1 mutations detected in severe cases of extrahepatic biliary atresia. Hepatology 2002;36(4 Pt 1): 904–12.

57. Moyer K, Kaimal V, Pacheco C, et al. Staging of biliary atresia at diagnosis by molecular profiling of the liver. Genome Med 2010;2(5):33.

58. LeeVan E, Matsuoka L, Cao S, et al. Biliary-enteric drainage vs primary liver transplant as initial treatment for children with biliary atresia. JAMA Surg 2019;154(1): 26–32.

59. Baek SH, Kang JM, Ihn K, et al. The epidemiology and etiology of cholangitis after kasai portoenterostomy in patients with biliary atresia. J Pediatr Gastroenterol Nutr 2020;70(2):171–7.
60. Decharun K, Leys CM, West KW, et al. Prophylactic antibiotics for prevention of cholangitis in patients with biliary atresia status post-kasai portoenterostomy: a systematic review. Clin Pediatr (Phila) 2016;55(1):66–72.
61. DeRusso PA, Ye W, Shepherd R, et al. Growth failure and outcomes in infants with biliary atresia: a report from the Biliary Atresia Research Consortium. Hepatology 2007;46(5):1632–8.
62. Mouzaki M, Bronsky J, Gupte G, et al. Nutrition support of children with chronic liver diseases: a joint position paper of the north american society for pediatric gastroenterology, hepatology, and nutrition and the european society for pediatric gastroenterology, hepatology, and nutrition. J Pediatr Gastroenterol Nutr 2019; 69(4):498–511.
63. Sullivan JS, Sundaram SS, Pan Z, et al. Parenteral nutrition supplementation in biliary atresia patients listed for liver transplantation. Liver Transpl 2012;18(1): 120–8.
64. Wendel D, Mortensen M, Harmeson A, et al. Resolving malnutrition with parenteral nutrition before liver transplant in biliary atresia. J Pediatr Gastroenterol Nutr 2018;66(2):212–7.
65. Sundaram SS, Mack CL, Feldman AG, et al. Biliary atresia: indications and timing of liver transplantation and optimization of pretransplant care. Liver Transpl 2017; 23(1):96–109.
66. Davenport M, Stringer MD, Tizzard SA, et al. Randomized, double-blind, placebo-controlled trial of corticosteroids after Kasai portoenterostomy for biliary atresia. Hepatology 2007;46(6):1821–7.
67. Davenport M, Parsons C, Tizzard S, et al. Steroids in biliary atresia: single surgeon, single centre, prospective study. J Hepatol 2013;59(5):1054–8.
68. Bezerra JA, Spino C, Magee JC, et al. Use of corticosteroids after hepatoportoenterostomy for bile drainage in infants with biliary atresia: the START randomized clinical trial. JAMA 2014;311(17):1750–9.
69. Alonso EM, Ye W, Hawthorne K, et al. Impact of steroid therapy on early growth in infants with biliary atresia: the multicenter steroids in biliary atresia randomized trial. J Pediatr 2018;202:179–185 e174.
70. Schwab I, Nimmerjahn F. Intravenous immunoglobulin therapy: how does IgG modulate the immune system? Nat Rev Immunol 2013;13(3):176–89.
71. Fenner EK, Boguniewicz J, Tucker RM, et al. High-dose IgG therapy mitigates bile duct-targeted inflammation and obstruction in a mouse model of biliary atresia. Pediatr Res 2014;76(1):72–80.
72. Mack CL, Spino C, Alonso EM, et al. A phase I/IIa trial of intravenous immunoglobulin following portoenterostomy in biliary atresia. J Pediatr Gastroenterol Nutr 2019;68(4):495–501.
73. Holterman A, Nguyen HPA, Nadler E, et al. Granulocyte-colony stimulating factor GCSF mobilizes hematopoietic stem cells in Kasai patients with biliary atresia in a phase 1 study and improves short term outcome. J Pediatr Surg 2021;56(7):1179–85.
74. Tessier MEM, Shneider BL, Brandt ML, et al. A phase 2 trial of N-Acetylcysteine in Biliary atresia after Kasai portoenterostomy. Contemp Clin Trials Commun 2019; 15:100370.
75. Burns J, Davenport M. Adjuvant treatments for biliary atresia. Transl Pediatr 2020; 9(3):253–65.

76. Serinet MO, Wildhaber BE, Broue P, et al. Impact of age at Kasai operation on its results in late childhood and adolescence: a rational basis for biliary atresia screening. Pediatrics 2009;123(5):1280–6.
77. Kelly DA, Davenport M. Current management of biliary atresia. Arch Dis Child 2007;92(12):1132–5.
78. Gorgis NM, Kennedy C, Lam F, et al. Clinical consequences of cardiomyopathy in children with biliary atresia requiring liver transplantation. Hepatology 2019;69(3): 1206–18.
79. Guedes RR, Kieling CO, Dos Santos JL, et al. Severity of ascites is associated with increased mortality in patients with cirrhosis secondary to biliary atresia. Dig Dis Sci 2020;65(11):3369–77.
80. Shneider BL, Magee JC, Karpen SJ, et al. Total serum bilirubin within 3 months of hepatoportoenterostomy predicts short-term outcomes in biliary atresia. J Pediatr 2016;170:211–7.e1-2.
81. Hukkinen M, Pihlajoki M, Pakarinen MP. Predicting native liver injury and survival in biliary atresia. Semin Pediatr Surg 2020;29(4):150943.
82. Kim S, Moore J, Alonso E, et al. Correlation of immune markers with outcomes in biliary atresia following intravenous immunoglobulin therapy. Hepatol Commun 2019;3(5):685–96.
83. Lopez RN, Ooi CY, Krishnan U. Early and peri-operative prognostic indicators in infants undergoing hepatic portoenterostomy for biliary atresia: a review. Curr Gastroenterol Rep 2017;19(4):16.
84. Wu JF, Jeng YM, Chen HL, et al. Quantification of serum matrix metallopeptide 7 levels may assist in the diagnosis and predict the outcome for patients with biliary atresia. J Pediatr 2019;208:30–37 e31.
85. Kobayashi H, Puri P, O'Briain DS, et al. Hepatic overexpression of MHC class II antigens and macrophage-associated antigens (CD68) in patients with biliary atresia of poor prognosis. J Pediatr Surg 1997;32(4):590–3.
86. Shneider BL, Brown MB, Haber B, et al. A multicenter study of the outcome of biliary atresia in the United States, 1997 to 2000. J Pediatr 2006;148(4):467–74.
87. Fanna M, Masson G, Capito C, et al. Management of biliary atresia in France 1986 to 2015: long-term results. J Pediatr Gastroenterol Nutr 2019;69(4):416–24.
88. Taylor SA, Venkat V, Arnon R, et al. Improved outcomes for liver transplantation in patients with biliary atresia since pediatric end-stage liver disease implementation: analysis of the society of pediatric liver transplantation registry. J Pediatr 2020;219:89–97.
89. Ng VL, Alonso EM, Bucuvalas JC, et al. Health status of children alive 10 years after pediatric liver transplantation performed in the US and Canada: report of the studies of pediatric liver transplantation experience. J Pediatr 2012;160(5): 820–826 e823.
90. Venkat V, Ng VL, Magee JC, et al. Modeling outcomes in children with biliary atresia with native liver after 2 years of age. Hepatol Commun 2020;4(12):1824–34.
91. Rodijk LH, Bos AF, Verkade HJ, et al. Early motor repertoire in infants with biliary atresia: a nationwide prospective cohort study. J Pediatr Gastroenterol Nutr 2021;72(4):592–6.
92. Ng VL, Sorensen LG, Alonso EM, et al. Neurodevelopmental outcome of young children with biliary atresia and native liver: results from the ChiLDReN Study. J Pediatr 2018;196:139–147 e133.
93. Rodijk LH, den Heijer AE, Hulscher JBF, et al. Long-term neurodevelopmental outcomes in children with biliary atresia. J Pediatr 2020;217:118–124 e113.
94. Sundaram SS, Alonso EM, Haber B, et al. Health related quality of life in patients with biliary atresia surviving with their native liver. J Pediatr 2013;163(4): 1052–1057 e1052.

Alagille Syndrome

Current Understanding of Pathogenesis, and Challenges in Diagnosis and Management

Mohammed D. Ayoub, MD, FRCPC[a,b],
Binita M. Kamath, MBBChir, MRCP, MTR[a,*]

KEYWORDS

- Alagille syndrome • Liver transplant • JAG1 • NOTCH2 • IBAT inhibitor

KEY POINTS

- Alagille syndrome (ALGS) is a cholestatic liver disease with variable expressivity. With advances in genetic testing, a liver biopsy is no longer required for diagnosis. Histopathologic findings also do not predict the natural history of liver disease.
- Distinguishing ALGS from biliary atresia (BA) in infants with high gamma-glutamyl transferase-cholestasis remains critical and is achievable in most cases with early use of next-generation sequencing.
- Treatment of ALGS remains supportive. However, ileal bile acid transport inhibitors are promising therapeutic agents for pruritus.

INTRODUCTION

Alagille syndrome (ALGS) is the most common inherited cholestatic liver disease encountered by pediatric hepatologists. Unlike most other causes of cholestasis, the involvement of multiorgan systems in ALGS, albeit with variable severity, makes it particularly challenging to manage. Our understanding of ALGS pathobiology, presentation, and management has greatly grown since the early reports by Daniel Alagille in 1969.[1] Establishing the diagnosis initially required a liver biopsy showing intrahepatic bile duct paucity, in addition to the involvement of 3 out of 5 organ systems: chronic cholestasis, cardiac disease, skeletal anomalies, ocular abnormalities, and characteristic facial features. Descriptive studies have since recognized renal and vascular involvement in these patients,[2,3] identifying these as disease-defining features, and resulting in the expansion of the Alagille clinical criteria.[4]

[a] Division of Gastroenterology, Hepatology, and Nutrition, The Hospital for Sick Children, University of Toronto, 555 University Avenue, Toronto, Ontario M5G 1X8, Canada; [b] Department of Pediatrics, Rabigh Branch, King Abdulaziz University, PO Box 80205, Jeddah 21589, Saudi Arabia
* Corresponding author. Division of Gastroenterology, Hepatology and Nutrition, The Hospital for Sick Children, 555 University Avenue, Toronto, Ontario M5G 1X8 Canada.
E-mail address: binita.kamath@sickkids.ca

Clin Liver Dis 26 (2022) 355–370
https://doi.org/10.1016/j.cld.2022.03.002
1089-3261/22/© 2022 Elsevier Inc. All rights reserved.

ALGS is inherited in an autosomal dominant manner with variable penetrance. The incidence of ALGS was traditionally thought to be 1 in 70,000 live births, based on the identification of patients with neonatal cholestasis and before the discovery of JAG-GED1 (*JAG1*) mutations as disease-causing.[5] In 2003, Kamath and colleagues evaluated mutation-positive relatives of ALGS probands and found that 47% did not meet classic clinical criteria, thus suggesting the true frequency of ALGS to be 1 in 30,000.[6]

In this article, we provide an overview of ALGS, with a specific focus on clinically relevant approaches to diagnostic testing, advances and challenges in management, and disease outcomes in the modern era.

Clinical Features of Alagille Syndrome

A broad range of clinical manifestations is associated with ALGS. The pattern and the degree of organ involvement may be different among patients, including those sharing the same mutation.[7,8] In the absence of a genetic diagnosis, or a family history of ALGS in a first-degree relative, a clinical diagnosis can be made from clinical findings in 3 out of 7 organ systems (listed below).[9]

Hepatic features

The pattern of hepatic involvement in ALGS is diverse; however, neonatal cholestasis with high gamma-glutamyl transferase (GGT) remains the most common presentation, affecting 80% to 100% of patients.[8,10–13] In a large descriptive ALGS cohort study by Subramaniam and colleagues (n = 117), where the most patients were less than 1 year of age, scleral icterus and hepatomegaly were present in approximately 90%, and 70%, respectively.[8] In contrast, splenomegaly is quite rare in early childhood but may manifest in more than two-thirds of patients with advancing age, secondary to progressive hepatic fibrosis, and portal hypertension.[13] Synthetic liver function is maintained earlier on in the disease course. Therefore, coagulopathy at a young age is usually secondary to fat-soluble-vitamin deficiency (FSVD) rather than liver dysfunction, which is easily corrected with vitamin K supplementation.[14]

Clinically, complications secondary to chronic cholestasis are the most troublesome in early childhood, resulting in FSVD, poor growth, fractures, and pruritus. Pruritus is among the worst of any cholestatic liver disease in childhood and is the most serious and debilitating symptom. It is typically present after 4 months of age and can occur even in the absence of jaundice (anicteric cholestasis).[9] It has significant impact on quality of life, causing severe sleep disruption and skin excoriations, most commonly found on the feet, trunk, and in the ears.[4] Xanthomas may also develop secondary to hypercholesterolemia as a consequence of cholestasis. These correspond to a serum cholesterol level of 500 mg/dL or higher and are typically yellowish painless plaques found on extremities and inguinal creases, which can be painful, and may interfere with motor development.[9,15] They resolve with improvement of cholestasis and disappear following liver transplantation (LT).[4]

Until recently, the outcome of liver disease due to ALGS was viewed as relatively favorable, with only 21% to 33% of patients requiring LT due to severe cholestasis.[13,16] However, these studies included heterogenous cohorts of ALGS patients. A recent prospective multicenter North American study from tertiary level centers examined the outcome of 293 patients with ALGS, all of whom had a history of cholestasis.[17] Surprisingly, only 24.5% of subjects survived with their native liver at 18.5 years. Long-term follow-up of these patients into the second decade revealed a significant improvement in total bilirubin and cholestasis in survivors and an increased frequency of variceal bleeding, ascites, and thrombocytopenia. This study highlighted the historically underappreciated burden of liver disease that takes place in later childhood, and thus recognizing a second "wave" of liver disease in ALGS secondary to portal hypertension and advanced liver fibrosis in this age group.[17] The recent formation of an international multicentered collaborative ALGS consortium, The Global ALagille Alliance (GALA), has permitted analysis of "real-world" outcomes in ALGS. Transplant-free survival at 10 and 18 years among 1154 ALGS patients with cholestasis from 25 countries were found to be 57% and 41%, respectively.[18] GALA has built a robust foundation for future clinical studies on ALGS.

Cardiac features

Cardiac involvement is one the most penetrant features in ALGS, affecting 94% of patients.[19] Similar to liver involvement, the degree and severity of cardiac anomalies vary widely. Peripheral pulmonary artery stenosis and/or hypoplasia (PPS) is the most commonly detected anomaly, with a frequency of 76%.[19] Fortunately, complex intracardiac anomalies are less common. In a large descriptive study of 200 *JAG1*-positive ALGS patients, 12% had Tetralogy of Fallot (TOF), and 7% had valvular/supravalvular aortic stenosis.[19]

Most early deaths in ALGS are due to severe cardiac anomalies. Interestingly, the TOF phenotype in ALGS is more severe than TOF in the general population, where 40% are associated with pulmonary atresia (PA) in ALGS compared with 20% in the latter.[20] Death rates reach as high as one-third of ALGS patients with TOF and up to 75% in patients with TOF/PA.[13] Collectively, survival rates are poor, with less than half of patients with severe intracardiac lesions surviving to 6 years of age.[13]

Facial features

Patients with ALGS harbor distinct facial characteristics that differentiate them from cholestasis due to other conditions and are correctly identified as ALGS facies by geneticists in almost 80% of cases.[21] An inverted triangular face is classically described, shaped by a prominent forehead, deep set eyes with hypertelorism, and a pointed chin. Features are subtle in infancy but become more obvious with age.

Ocular features

Many ocular abnormalities have been described in ALGS. The most common finding is posterior embryotoxon seen in 55% to 95% of patients and is generally of no visual consequence.[11,22] Posterior embryotoxon is detected by slit-lamp examination and can be seen in 22% of the general population and up to 70% in patients with 22q11 syndrome.[23,24] Thus, although not specific to ALGS, it is a useful diagnostic tool. Other ocular anomalies described in ALGS include peripheral chorioretinal changes[25] and optic nerve drusen. The latter is identified by ocular ultrasonography in 80% to 95% of ALGS patients compared with none in other cholestatic conditions and only 2.5% in the general population.[26,27]

Skeletal features

Vertebral anomalies have been well described in ALGS. Butterfly vertebrae, caused by failure of fusion of the anterior arches, have been found in 30% to 90% of patients.[8,10] Similar to posterior embryotoxon, they are of no consequence, and are found in other cholestatic liver diseases and genetic syndromes.[28,29] A range of other skeletal anomalies have also been reported such as radio-ulnar synostosis and rib abnormalities.

Pathologic fractures are common in ALGS. In a report by Bales and colleagues, approximately one-third of ALGS patients without a preceding significant traumatic event, experienced a fracture at a mean age of 5, with a predilection for lower extremities in 70% of cases.[30] The cause of such bone fragility is multifactorial, arising likely from chronic cholestasis and vitamin D deficiency. A multicenter study identified lower

Z-scores of bone mineral density and content in children with ALGS compared with other causes of cholestasis.[31] This correlated negatively with serum bile acids and total bilirubin in children with previous fractures, even after adjusting for weight and height. A more recent study by Kindler and colleagues revealed deficits in cortical bone size and trabecular bone architecture in 10 patients with ALGS compared with healthy controls.[32] These intrinsic bone defects may be secondary to disrupted Notch signaling.[33]

Renal features

Renal disease has been described in the early reports of patients with ALGS.[10] It has since been recognized as a disease-defining feature with an estimated prevalence of 40%, resulting in expansion of ALGS clinical criteria.[2,9] Both structural and functional abnormalities have been reported. In a large cohort study,[2] renal dysplasia was most common abnormality identified, affecting 59%, followed by renal tubular acidosis (RTA; 10%), and urinary obstruction with vesicoureteric reflux (8%). Systemic hypertension may occur secondary to renovascular disease in 2% to 8%.[34] Chronic kidney disease in ALGS progressing to renal transplantation is relatively rare. The significance of kidney involvement in the peri-LT and post-LT setting will be discussed further below.

Vascular features

Intracranial and systemic vascular abnormalities have both been documented in ALGS. Intracranial bleeding is a well-recognized complication occurring in 15% of patients, of which half are fatal (from small series).[12,13] Clinical presentation, locations, and severity of bleeding vary widely among patients, ranging from silent infarcts to catastrophic unprovoked bleeding events. Emerick and colleagues, reported that even 50% of asymptomatic patients can have detectable lesions.[35] Hence, it has been recommended that children undergo routine screening with brain magnetic resonance imaging (MRI) and angiography (MRA) at 8 years of age (when general anesthesia is not required), and before major surgeries.[36] Lesions that have been described include internal carotid artery stenosis, middle cerebral and basilar artery aneurysms, moyamoya disease, as well as established bleeding in the subdural, epidural, or subarachnoid space.[3,13,35] Patients harboring CNS vascular malformations are at heightened risk of ischemic and hemorrhagic stroke.

The Genetics of Alagille Syndrome

ALGS is caused by heterozygous mutations in either *JAG1* or *NOTCH2*. *JAG1* mutations account for 94% of reported cases, whereas *NOTCH2* variants are found in 2% to 4%.[37,38] ALGS is inherited in an autosomal dominant manner and 60% of mutations are *de novo*. Since the identification of JAG1 in 1997, more than 700 *JAG1* pathogenic variants have been identified.[38–40] These mutations encode for the extracellular domain of *JAG1*, an area that is crucial for *NOTCH2* binding and initiation of the Notch signaling pathway. Protein-truncating mutations are the most common, affecting 75% of *JAG1* mutations.[38] *NOTCH2* was described as a second disease gene 9 years later when *JAG1* mutation-negative patients were screened for *NOTCH2*.[41] Only a handful of patients with NOTCH-2 associated ALGS have been described to date.

Mechanistically, the genetic pathobiological basis of ALGS is a subject of some debate. However, the finding of different pathogenic mutations causing identical ALGS clinical phenotypes suggests that haploinsufficiency, rather than a dominant negative mechanism as the primary disease mechanism.[38,42]

The Notch Signaling Pathway

This is an evolutionary, highly conserved signaling pathway that is critical for cell–cell communication during embryogenesis.[43,44] The binding of ligands (JAG1 and 2, Delta-like 1, 3, and 4) and 4 Notch receptors, activates an intracellular cascade leading to transcription of downstream genes and cell fate determination.[45] Numerous studies have confirmed the expression of *JAG1* in organs affected in ALGS, and in particular, Notch signaling is crucial in the development of intrahepatic bile ducts.[46]

Diagnostic Testing

Diagnostic testing in ALGS fall under 1 of 2 categories; investigations to evaluate organ involvement (ie, for the purpose of fulfilling clinical diagnostic criteria), and genetic testing for molecular confirmation of ALGS (**Table 1**). The shift in recent years has been to adopt a "sequence early" approach, where genetic testing is prioritized early when evaluating cholestatic infants. This approach is useful in the common scenario of neonatal cholestasis where BA and ALGS can have overlapping clinical features.

Clinical Investigations

ALGS liver disease typically manifests as elevated markers of cholestasis (serum bile acids, bilirubin, cholesterol, and GGT). These markers typically exceed those of hepatocellular injury. Having a normal GGT, however, does not rule out ALGS.[8] Markers of cholestasis, if elevated, may improve in childhood with improvement of pruritus, jaundice, and xanthomas.[17] Biochemical parameters have been evaluated to predict outcome. Mouzaki and colleagues identified that serum bilirubin of 3.8 mg/dL or higher measured between 12 and 24 months in 144 children with ALGS, is associated with poor hepatic outcome later in life (LT or biliary diversion).[47]

Liver ultrasonography may show a hypoplastic gallbladder, which has been reported in 28% of patients.[8] Additionally, hepatic regenerative nodules, which can look similar to hepatocellular carcinoma are present in 30%. They are distinguishable by normal tumor markers (alpha-fetoprotein) and having an isoechoic texture to surrounding liver without vascular invasion on imaging studies.[48,49] Hepatobiliary scintigraphy is usually performed early in the disease course to help differentiate ALGS from BA but it may add to the diagnostic confusion. Approximately 60% of ALGS patients have been reported to have nonexcretion of isotope into the bowel after 24 hours.[13]

To evaluate for extrahepatic features, all patients with suspected ALGS should undergo slit-lamp examination, echocardiography, spinal X-ray, and renal ultrasonography. Brain imaging with MRI/MRA may be considered in the presence of neurologic symptoms.

Liver histopathology

A liver biopsy is no longer required for the diagnosis of ALGS but is often performed to help differentiate ALGS from BA. The classic finding in ALGS is bile duct paucity, and it is necessary to have no less than 6 to 10 portal tracts in the liver biopsy specimen to confirm this finding. The normal ratio of interlobular ducts to portal tracts is 0.9 to 1.8 and bile duct paucity is present if this ratio is less than 0.9 in full-term infants.[50]

Bile duct paucity has been reported in 75% to 90% of patients with ALGS.[7,8,10–12] However, it is found less commonly in infants younger than 6 months of age (60%) compared with almost 95% in those older than 6 months of age.[13] True causes for this progression are unknown but is thought to be secondary to continued postnatal ductal destruction and/or differential maturation of portal tracts.[9,13] There are other less commonly reported histologic changes seen with ALGS such as giant cell

Table 1
Summary of diagnostic testing in Alagille syndrome

Test Category	Test	Findings/Comments
Biochemical markers of cholestasis	Serum GGT, bile acids, conjugated bilirubin	Markedly elevated GGT compared with other causes of cholestasis, although not specific to ALGS
Imaging studies	Hepatic scintigraphy	May show nonexcretion of isotope in up to 60% of ALGS cases
	Operative cholangiogram	Nonopacification of intrahepatic ducts in 74%[13] Nonopacification/hypoplasia of proximal extrahepatic ducts in 37%[13]
Liver histopathology	Immunohistochemistry	Bile duct paucity: increased frequency in ALGS with advancing age Not pathognomonic for ALGS (see Table 2)
Genetic testing	JAG1 and NOTCH2 NGS	Presence of pathogenic variants is diagnostic for ALGS

hepatitis and ductular proliferation. These findings can lead to further diagnostic uncertainty, as they are typical of BA.

Genetic testing

Molecular testing reveals an ALGS disease-causing mutation in 95% of cases.[38] If testing is carried out in a stepwise approach, Sanger sequencing of the *JAG1* gene will identify 85% of pathogenic variants. If equivocal, then large deletion/duplication analyses (chromosomal microarray, multiplex ligation-dependent probe amplification, fluorescence in-situ hybridization) are performed, which will identify an additional 9% of pathogenic variants.[38,51] *NOTCH2* gene sequencing identifies 2.5% additional mutations. Because no large deletions of *NOTCH2* have been reported in the ALGS literature, large deletion/duplication analysis is not carried out. In clinical practice, testing for both genes is performed simultaneously, by using commercially available comprehensive cholestasis next generation sequencing panels (NGS).[52] As reported by Karpen and colleagues, they carry a diagnostic yield of 12% for all diagnoses and results are available within a median of 3 weeks. Use of these panels is more cost-effective than following a stepwise approach and avoids delays in ALGS diagnosis.

Although only less than 40 patients worldwide have been reported with the *NOTCH2* mutation,[18] facial characteristics and skeletal anomalies seem to be less common in *NOTCH2* than in *JAG1* mutations; 20% vs 97% and 10% vs 65%, respectively.[53,54]

Challenging Scenarios in Alagille Syndrome

The absence of genotype–phenotype correlations

Despite the broad clinical phenotype of ALGS and large number of mutations identified to date, there have been no genotype–phenotype correlations identified.[38] This suggests the presence of genetic modifiers or epigenetic factors that may explain the phenotypic variability. A few reports have even shown different clinical presentations in monozygotic twins sharing the same mutation.[55] Therefore, it is not possible to predict disease course and natural history based on genotype. This is particularly relevant during genetic counseling and in the context of prenatal genetic diagnosis of ALGS.

The diagnostic value of histopathology in Alagille syndrome

It is important to note that bile duct paucity is not synonymous with or pathognomonic for ALGS. It has been reported in other cholestatic, infectious/immune disorders, and drug-induced liver injury (**Table 2**).[4,56] In addition, healthy preterm neonates (<38 weeks) and small for gestational age infants may have physiologic bile duct paucity, which is due to immature bile ducts that continue to develop postnatally.[57,58]

The histologic overlap of ALGS and BA, however, remains the most important area of diagnostic uncertainty. Bile duct paucity has been reported in up to 10% of BA patients, typically as a late finding.[59] In addition, common features of BA such as ductular proliferation and giant cell hepatitis have been observed in infants with ALGS.[7,12,13] This is the situation where a "sequence early" approach is crucial.

The noncommunicating cholangiogram

Operative cholangiograms are considered the gold standard for assessment of the intrahepatic and extrahepatic biliary tree and to diagnose BA. However, in ALGS, the biliary tree can be hypoplastic and cholangiograms may show noncommunication with the small bowel. Early studies have demonstrated this with approximately 40% patients having abnormally small proximal extrahepatic ducts (hepatic duct to hilum), and a similar rate of complete nonopacification proximally has been observed.[13] More commonly, the intrahepatic ducts are not visualized in almost 75% of ALGS patients. This can be thought of as a BA phenotype occurring in ALGS (which is genetically defined), rather than the coexistence of 2 different diseases as has been reported in the literature.[60] In these difficult time-sensitive situations, KPE is sometimes performed in ALGS, and it is clear that KPE adversely affects disease course in ALGS.[61,62] As reported by Kaye and colleagues, ALGS patients who underwent a KPE had higher rates of LT (47% vs 14%) and mortality (32% vs 3%) compared with age-matched ALGS controls, suggesting that the procedure itself changes the natural history.

Management of Alagille Syndrome

Treatment strategies in ALGS aim at managing cholestasis and its associated complications, such as nutritional support, FSVD, and pruritus.

Nutritional management

Children with ALGS have normal energy expenditure. However, they require at least 125% of the recommended daily allowance and may need more for catch up growth. This is typically secondary to decreased intake, fat malabsorption, and cardiac disease.[63–65] Medium chain triglyceride-rich foods are encouraged for ease of absorption (as micellar formation is not required), as well as other calorie dense foods. In children not being able to meet their caloric demands, tube feeding (nasogastric or via gastrostomy) is often required, especially in the context of end-stage liver disease.

Supplementation with fat-soluble vitamins is crucial. To aid with adherence and cost, cholestasis-specific formulations are available in the North American market (eg, DEKAs). However, individual vitamin supplementation is preferred if generic multivitamins is the only available option.

Management of pruritus

Pharmacologic treatments. Treatment of pruritus requires a stepwise approach (**Table 3**). Antihistamines are typically not effective but can be considered in mild cases and to augment sleep. Ursodeoxycholic acid promotes bile excretion rendering it more hydrophilic.[66] Due to its attractive safety profile, it is typically used as a first-line agent. Next, cholestyramine, a bile salt-binding agent may be considered. It

Table 2
Causes of nonsyndromic bile duct paucity

Disease Category	Cause
Genetic	Trisomy 21 William syndrome Peroxisomal disorders
Metabolic	α-1 antitrypsin deficiency Cystic fibrosis Hypothyroidism
Infectious	Congenital rubella Congenital syphilis Congenital cytomegalovirus
Inflammatory/immune-mediated	Graft-versus-host disease (late finding) Chronic graft rejection Hemophagocytic lymphohistiocytosis Sclerosing cholangitis
Other	Biliary atresia (late finding) Drug-induced liver injury

decreases bile acid pool size by binding bile salts in the ileum. However, poor palatability and interference with absorption of other drugs (specifically fat-soluble vitamins) limits its use.[66] Rifampin is often used instead of cholestyramine. It has been reported to improve pruritus in 50% of ALGS patients (n = 39).[66] Through enzymatic induction of 6(α)-hydroxylase of bile acids in the liver, it increases bile acid metabolism, making them less pruritogenic and facilitates their excretion by the kidneys. Opioid antagonists, such as naltrexone, are sometimes added to the regimen if pruritus persists and may provide some additional benefit. It has been shown to be effective in approximately 40% of patients in small studies (n = 14).[66] Opioid withdrawal symptoms that may occur in one-third of patients limit its use in clinical practice.[66] Finally, sertraline, a selective serotonin reuptake inhibitor (SSRI), has been used in refractory cases. Its mechanism of action is poorly understood. Limited pediatric studies support its use as adjunctive therapy intractable pruritus.[67]

Surgical interventions. In patients with drug-refractory pruritus, biliary diversion procedures that interrupt the EHC and decrease bile pool size are considered. Partial external biliary diversion, where a jejunal conduit is used to drain the gallbladder externally, is the most commonly performed procedure. In a large multicentered North American study examining biliary diversion procedures among cholestatic infants, biliary diversion in 20 ALGS patients resulted in decreased serum cholesterol, resolution of xanthomas, and a significant drop in patient-reported pruritus.[68]

It should be noted that due to the biliary hypoplasia in ALGS, less bile acids reach the small intestine in some patients. Therefore, these procedures are generally less effective in ALGS than in other cholestatic liver diseases such as progressive familial intrahepatic cholestasis. These procedures therefore may not alleviate pruritus or prevent the progression of liver disease in some ALGS patients.[4,69]

Advancements in pruritus management. Ileal bile acid transport (IBAT) inhibitors are exciting novel treatments for pruritus in ALGS. Similar to surgical diversion, the concept of IBAT inhibitors is to promote intestinal wasting of pruritogenic bile acid through inhibition of bile acid uptake by enterocytes and "chemically" disrupting the enterohepatic circulation (EHC).[70,71] Maralixibat (MRX) and Odevixibat are 2 drugs

Table 3
Pharmacologic therapy for cholestasis in Alagille syndrome

Medication Class	Medication	Dose	Adverse Effects
Choleretics	Ursodeoxycholic acid	10–20 mg/kg/d divided in 2 doses	Diarrhea, abdominal pain, vomiting
Bile salt-binding agents	Cholestyramine	240 mg/kg/d divided in 3 doses	Poor palatability, worsening FSVD, abdominal pain, constipation
Hepatic bile acid 6 (α)-hydroxylation	Rifampin	10 mg/kg/d divided in 2 doses	Hepatitis, idiosyncratic hypersensitivity reaction, red discoloration of urine
Opioid antagonist	Naltrexone	0.25–0.5 mg/kg once daily	Limited data, opioid withdrawal symptoms (nausea, irritability, diarrhea)
SSRI	Sertraline	Starting dose 1 mg/kg once daily, escalated to target dose 4 mg/kg once daily	Limited data, drug eruption, GI upset, agitation
IBAT inhibitors	MRX Odevixibat	Starting dose 380 µg/kg/d once daily; up to 760 µg/kg/d divided in 2 doses in phase II extension studies	Abdominal pain, diarrhea, hepatitis, staphylococcal hand infection

within this class that are under study, although more data currently exist with MRX in subjects with ALGS.

MRX has been evaluated in 2 phase II trials. The ITCH trial was a double-blinded placebo-controlled multicentered study that examined the efficacy of 3 different MRX dosages (up to 280 µg/kg/d) in 37 children with ALGS during 13 weeks.[72] Although the study failed to meet its prespecified primary endpoint, there was a statistically significant 1-point reduction in pruritus scores in all MRX-treated patients than placebo. Similarly, the ICONIC study evaluated 31 ALGS patients in a randomized placebo-controlled multicentered study but used a 4-week randomized drug withdrawal period, where patients were randomized to MRX vs placebo. This was followed by an open label extension period up to 204 weeks.[73] Expectedly, all MRX-treated patients had reduced serum bile acids and pruritus scores. However, during the randomized drug withdrawal period, both parameters returned to baseline in the placebo group but remained persistently low in the MRX group. Long-term follow-up data revealed a significant improvement in growth, xanthomas, fatigue, and quality of life, along with sustained low serum bile acids and itch scores. The adoption of higher doses of MRX (380 µg/kg/d up to 48 weeks and 760 µg/kg/d in the extension period) and the implementation of a randomized withdrawal window in the ICONIC trial, likely contributed to the positive changes seen in this study because this limited a positive placebo-response in the setting of patient-reported outcomes.

These preliminary studies show that IBAT inhibitors are well tolerated with comparable adverse events (AEs) to placebo. Reported AEs included vomiting, diarrhea, and hepatitis, with no worsening in fat-soluble vitamin levels. The results of these studies show that IBAT inhibitors are promising novel agents in the toolkit available to clinicians to treat cholestatic pruritus. MRX (Livmarli) was recently approved by the FDA for the treatment of cholestatic pruritus in patients with ALGS who are aged 1 year or older.

Liver transplantation

The main indications for LT in ALGS fall under 2 categories: (1) patients with severe cholestasis and/or associated complications (growth failure, FSVD, and intractable pruritus) and (2) patients with cirrhosis and complications secondary to portal hypertension (ascites and variceal bleeding).

In children with cholestasis from tertiary referral centers, LT is required in up to 75% of patients by the age of 18.[17] Outcomes post-LT is similar to most other indications of pediatric LT.[74] Arnon and colleagues analyzed the largest ALGS cohort to date with 461 children over a 21-year period.[75] One-year and 5-year patient survival were 83% and 78%, and 1-year and 5-year graft survival were 75% and 62%, respectively. Higher rates of mortality were recognized in the first 30 days post-LT, particularly when compared with the outcome of LT for patients with BA. Identified risk factors for early death in ALGS recipients included higher pre-LT serum creatinine level, longer cold ischemia time of more than 12 hours, and prior LT. A similar clustering of deaths was also reported by the SPLIT group, which may be explained by early vascular complications.[76]

Liver Transplant Special Considerations and Challenges

Living-related donor selection

Caution should be taken when considering living-related liver transplantation in ALGS. Because 40% of JAG1 mutations in a child are inherited the likelihood of one of the parents being affected is not trivial. Therefore, genetic screening is recommended for potential living-related donors. This is of particular importance because related donors may be asymptomatic or without overt clinical findings despite carrying an ALGS causing mutation.[77]

Implications of Renal Involvement in Liver Transplantation

Due to intrinsic renal abnormalities in ALGS, preexisting renal insufficiency may not recover post-LT. In a large North American study by Kamath and colleagues, 91 ALGS patients were age-matched with 236 BA patients.[76] Pre-LT glomerular filtration rate of less than 90 mL/min/1.73 m^2 was found in 18% of ALGS subjects and 5% of BA. Renal disease in fact worsened 1-year post-LT in ALGS patients (22%) compared with their BA counterparts (8%). This strongly suggests the adoption of renal-sparing immunosuppression protocol in ALGS patients and highlights the vulnerability of the intrinsically abnormal kidneys to calcineurin inhibitors in these children.

Complex cardiac disease in the face of liver transplant candidacy

The predominance of right-sided intracardiac anomalies and right ventricular outflow tract obstruction (RVOTO) secondary to PPS can lead to elevated right ventricular (RV) pressure, resulting in RV hypertrophy, volume overload, and eventually RV failure. When assessing such ALGS patients for LT candidacy, attention should be turned to the functional capacity and compliance of the RV because the rapidly fluctuating hemodynamic changes associated with transplant surgery, particularly associated with clamping the inferior vena cava can lead to marked increase in preload. To simulate these conditions before LT surgery, cardiac catherization and a dynamic stress exercise (DSE) with dobutamine have been suggested to inform decision-making.[78] DSE mimics the increased cardiac output associated with graft reperfusion intraoperatively. Cardiac reserve is considered sufficient if cardiac output reaches more than

40% with DSE. In other situations where complete surgical repair for severe cardiac disease is not feasible, balloon valvuloplasty and stenting in cases of PPS and RVOTO can be considered to mitigate the adverse outcome associated with hemodynamic instability post-LT.[19,76]

The risk and benefits of LT and/or corrective cardiac surgery should always be considered. Multidisciplinary approach in consultation with expert cardiology and cardiovascular surgery should always be sought for optimal management strategies of cardiac anomalies pre-LT. Few reports exist for successful combined heart–liver transplantation in ALGS.[79]

Surgical considerations for vasculopathy and bleeding risk

Vascular anomalies can extend beyond the CNS in ALGS. Anomalies have been well described involving the subclavian, celiac trunk (48%), renal, and superior mesenteric veins (8%).[80,81] These may require surgical modifications during LT surgery. In a retrospective study by Kohaut and colleagues, almost 65% of children with ALGS (n = 35/55) required aortic conduit reconstruction during surgery.[81] Most importantly, these patients had a significantly lower rate of hepatic artery thrombosis, compared with patients in which a standard arterial anastomosis was performed (6% vs 35%). It is therefore imperative, that children with ALGS considered for LT listing, should undergo detailed abdominal vascular imaging (eg, triphasic computed tomography scan) to help aid in surgical planning, in addition to screening brain MRI/MRA (if not previously done). If vascular anomalies are detected, consultation with the respective multidisciplinary teams should be sought before listing.

Patients with ALGS are at special risk for bleeding even in the absence of vascular anomalies, with spontaneous intracranial bleeding being the most common. Interestingly, as reported by Lykaavieris and colleagues, spontaneous systemic bleeding events occurred in 22% of ALGS patients who had no evidence of coagulopathy or a low platelet count.[82] The mechanism for excessive bleeding is unclear but may be due to hemostatic dysfunction secondary to abnormal JAG1 signaling.

Concluding Remarks

ALGS is a complex heterogenous disease, creating numerous challenges to clinicians in diagnosis and management, especially in the setting of LT. IBAT inhibitors offer a major therapeutic advancement in the treatment of cholestatic pruritis in ALGS. It remains to be seen if altering the bile salt pool with these agents also improves liver disease natural history in ALGS. The lack of genotype–phenotype correlations has steered the focus of studies toward genetic modifiers in ALGS, and it is likely that organ-specific modifiers will be identified. This will deepen our understanding of the variable expressivity of this disease and may pave the way toward precision medicine management in ALGS. International collective efforts, such as GALA, will serve as platform for future clinical studies to help overcome the challenges of a rare and variable disease and expand our understanding of ALGS natural history.

CLINICS CARE POINTS

- A diagnosis of ALGS should be considered in all cholestatic infants, especially if the GGT is high.

- A "sequence early" approach is cost-effective and can avoid unnecessary procedures such as Kasai portoenterostomy.
- A multidisciplinary approach is crucial in the management of patients with ALGS in the peri-transplant setting.

DISCLOSURE

B.M. Kamath is a Consultant for Mirum, Albireo, Audentes and Third Rock Ventures. The author receives unrestricted educational grant funding from Mirum and Albireo. The funders had no role in the design of the study; in the collection, analyses, or interpretation of data; in the writing of the article, or in the decision to publish the results. M.D. Ayoub has nothing to disclose.

REFERENCES

1. Alagille D, Habib E, Thomassin N. L'atresie des voies biliaires intrahepatiques avec voies biliaires extrahepatiques permeables chez l'enfant. J Par Pediatr 1969;301:301–18.
2. Kamath BM, Podkameni G, Hutchinson AL, et al. Renal anomalies in Alagille syndrome: a disease-defining feature. Am J Med Genet A 2012;158A(1):85–9.
3. Kamath BM, Spinner NB, Emerick KM, et al. Vascular anomalies in Alagille syndrome: a significant cause of morbidity and mortality. Circulation 2004;109(11): 1354–8.
4. Kriegermeier A, Wehrman A, Kamath BM, et al. Liver disease in alagille syndrome. In: Alagille syndrome. Cham, Switzerland: Springer; 2018. p. 49–65.
5. Danks D, Campbell P, Jack I, et al. Studies of the aetiology of neonatal hepatitis and biliary atresia. Arch Dis Child 1977;52(5):360–7.
6. Kamath B, Bason L, Piccoli D, et al. Consequences of JAG1 mutations. J Med Genet 2003;40(12):891–5.
7. Quiros-Tejeira RE, Ament ME, Heyman MB, et al. Variable morbidity in Alagille syndrome: a review of 43 cases. J Pediatr Gastroenterol Nutr 1999;29(4):431–7.
8. Subramaniam P, Knisely A, Portmann B, et al. Diagnosis of alagille syndrome—25 years of experience at King's college hospital. J Pediatr Gastroenterol Nutr 2011; 52(1):84–9.
9. Kamath BM, Piccoli DA. Alagille syndrome. In: Diseases of the liver in children. New York: Springer; 2014. p. 227–46.
10. Alagille D, Estrada A, Hadchouel M, et al. Syndromic paucity of interlobular bile ducts (Alagille syndrome or arteriohepatic dysplasia): review of 80 cases. J Pediatr 1987;110(2):195–200.
11. Deprettere A, Portmann B, Mowat AP. Syndromic paucity of the intrahepatic bile ducts: diagnostic difficulty; severe morbidity throughout early childhood. J Pediatr Gastroenterol Nutr 1987;6(6):865–71.
12. Hoffenberg EJ, Narkewicz MR, Sondheimer JM, et al. Outcome of syndromic paucity of interlobular bile ducts (Alagille syndrome) with onset of cholestasis in infancy. J Pediatr 1995;127(2):220–4.
13. Emerick KM, Rand EB, Goldmuntz E, et al. Features of Alagille syndrome in 92 patients: frequency and relation to prognosis. Hepatology 1999;29(3):822–9.
14. Ayoub MD, Kamath BM. Alagille syndrome: diagnostic challenges and advances in management. Diagnostics 2020;10(11):907.

15. Garcia MA, Margarita R, Mirta C, et al. Alagille syndrome: cutaneous manifestations in 38 children. Pediatr Dermatol 2005;22(1):11–4.
16. Lykavieris P, Hadchouel M, Chardot C, et al. Outcome of liver disease in children with Alagille syndrome: a study of 163 patients. Gut 2001;49(3):431–5.
17. Kamath BM, Ye W, Goodrich NP, et al. Outcomes of childhood cholestasis in Alagille syndrome: results of a multicenter observational study. Hepatol Commun 2020;4(3):387–98.
18. Vandriel SM, Liting L, She H, et al. Clinical features and natural history of 1154 Alagille syndrome patients: results from the international multicenter GALA study group. J Hepatol 2020;73:S554–5.
19. McElhinney DB, Krantz ID, Bason L, et al. Analysis of cardiovascular phenotype and genotype-phenotype correlation in individuals with a JAG1 mutation and/or Alagille syndrome. Circulation 2002;106(20):2567–74.
20. Ferencz C. Genetic and environmental risk factors of major cardiovascular malformations: the Baltimore-Washington infant study 1981-1989. Perspect Pediatr Cardiol 1997;5:346–7.
21. Kamath BM, Loomes KM, Oakey RJ, et al. Facial features in Alagille syndrome: specific or cholestasis facies? Am J Med Genet 2002;112(2):163–70.
22. Hingorani M, Nischal KK, Davies A, et al. Ocular abnormalities in Alagille syndrome. Ophthalmology 1999;106(2):330–7.
23. Rennie CA, Chowdhury S, Khan J, et al. The prevalence and associated features of posterior embryotoxon in the general ophthalmic clinic. Eye (Lond) 2005;19(4):396–9.
24. McDonald-McGinn D, Kirschner R, Goldmuntz E, et al. The Philadelphia story: the 22q11. 2 deletion: report on 250 patients. Genet Couns (Geneva, Switzerland) 1999;10(1):11.
25. da Palma MM, Igelman AD, Ku C, et al. Characterization of the spectrum of ophthalmic changes in patients with alagille syndrome. Invest Ophthalmol Vis Sci 2021;62(7):27.
26. Nischal KK, Hingorani M, Bentley CR, et al. Ocular ultrasound in Alagille syndrome. Ophthalmology 1997;104(1):79–85.
27. Chang MY, Pineles SL. Optic disk drusen in children. Surv Ophthalmol 2016;61(6):745–58.
28. Delgado A, Mokri B, Miller GM. Butterfly vertebra. J Neuroimaging 1996;6(1):56–8.
29. Sandal G, Aslan N, Duman L, et al. VACTERL association with a rare vertebral anomaly (butterfly vertebra) in a case of monochorionic twin. Genet Couns 2014;25(2):231–5.
30. Bales CB, Kamath BM, Munoz PS, et al. Pathologic lower extremity fractures in children with Alagille syndrome. J Pediatr Gastroenterol Nutr 2010;51(1):66–70.
31. Loomes KM, Spino C, Goodrich NP, et al. Bone density in children with chronic liver disease correlates with growth and cholestasis. Hepatology 2019;69(1):245–57.
32. Kindler JM, Mitchell EL, Piccoli DA, et al. Bone geometry and microarchitecture deficits in children with Alagille syndrome. Bone 2020;141:115576.
33. Youngstrom D, Dishowitz M, Bales C, et al. Jagged1 expression by osteoblast-lineage cells regulates trabecular bone mass and periosteal expansion in mice. Bone 2016;91:64–74.
34. Romero R. The renal sequelae of Alagille syndrome as a product of altered notch signaling during kidney development. In: Alagille syndrome. Cham, Switzerland: Springer; 2018. p. 103–20.

35. Emerick KM, Krantz ID, Kamath BM, et al. Intracranial vascular abnormalities in patients with Alagille syndrome. J Pediatr Gastroenterol Nutr 2005;41(1):99–107.

36. Vandriel SM, Ichord RN, Kamath BM. Vascular manifestations in alagille syndrome. In: Alagille syndrome. Cham, Switzerland: Springer; 2018. p. 91–102.

37. Li L, Krantz ID, Deng Y, et al. Alagille syndrome is caused by mutations in human Jagged1, which encodes a ligand for Notch1. Nat Genet 1997;16(3):243–51.

38. Gilbert MA, Bauer RC, Rajagopalan R, et al. Alagille syndrome mutation update: comprehensive overview of JAG1 and NOTCH2 mutation frequencies and insight into missense variant classification. Hum Mutat 2019;40(12):2197–220.

39. Micaglio E, Andronache AA, Carrera P, et al. Novel JAG1 deletion variant in patient with atypical Alagille syndrome. Int J Mol Sci 2019;20(24):6247.

40. Chen Y, Liu X, Chen S, et al. Targeted sequencing and RNA assay reveal a noncanonical JAG1 splicing variant causing Alagille Syndrome. Front Genet 2019;10: 1363.

41. McDaniell R, Warthen DM, Sanchez-Lara PA, et al. NOTCH2 mutations cause Alagille syndrome, a heterogeneous disorder of the notch signaling pathway. Am J Hum Genet 2006;79(1):169–73.

42. Oda T, Elkahloun AG, Pike BL, et al. Mutations in the human Jagged1 gene are responsible for Alagille syndrome. Nat Genet 1997;16(3):235–42.

43. Chiba S. Concise review: notch signaling in stem cell systems. Stem cells 2006; 24(11):2437–47.

44. Huppert SS, Campbell KM. Bile duct development and the notch signaling pathway. In: Alagille syndrome. Cham, Switzerland: Springer; 2018. p. 11–31.

45. Gridley T. Notch signaling in vascular development and physiology. Development 2007;134(15):2709–18.

46. Crosnier C, Attie-Bitach T, Encha-Razavi F, et al. JAGGED1 gene expression during human embryogenesis elucidates the wide phenotypic spectrum of Alagille syndrome. Hepatology 2000;32(3):574–81.

47. Mouzaki M, Bass LM, Sokol RJ, et al. Early life predictive markers of liver disease outcome in an International, Multicentre Cohort of children with Alagille syndrome. Liver Int 2016;36(5):755–60.

48. Andrews AR, Putra J. Central hepatic regenerative nodules in Alagille syndrome: a clinicopathological review. Fetal Pediatr Pathol 2019;40(1):1–11.

49. Alhammad A, Kamath BM, Chami R, et al. Solitary hepatic nodule adjacent to the right portal vein: a common finding of Alagille syndrome? J Pediatr Gastroenterol Nutr 2016;62(2):226–32.

50. Alagille D, Odievre M, Gautier M, et al. Hepatic ductular hypoplasia associated with characteristic facies, vertebral malformations, retarded physical, mental, and sexual development, and cardiac murmur. J Pediatr 1975;86(1):63–71.

51. Gilbert MA, Spinner NB. Genetics of alagille syndrome. In: Alagille syndrome. Cham, Switzerland: Springer; 2018. p. 33–48.

52. Karpen SJ, Kamath BM, Alexander JJ, et al. Use of a comprehensive 66-gene cholestasis sequencing panel in 2171 cholestatic infants, children, and young adults. J Pediatr Gastroenterol Nutr 2021;72(5):654–60.

53. Saleh M, Kamath BM, Chitayat D. Alagille syndrome: clinical perspectives. Appl Clin Genet 2016;9:75.

54. Kamath BM, Bauer RC, Loomes KM, et al. NOTCH2 mutations in Alagille syndrome. J Med Genet 2012;49(2):138–44.

55. Izumi K, Hayashi D, Grochowski CM, et al. Discordant clinical phenotype in monozygotic twins with Alagille syndrome: possible influence of non-genetic factors. Am J Med Genet A 2016;170(2):471–5.

56. Russo P, Ruchelli ED, Piccoli DA. Pathology of pediatric gastrointestinal and liver disease. Berlin, Heidelberg: Springer; 2014.

57. Kahn E, Markowitz J, Aiges H, et al. Human ontogeny of the bile duct to portal space ratio. Hepatology 1989;10(1):21–3.

58. Sergi C, Bahitham W, Al-Bahrani R. Bile duct paucity in infancy. Liver biopsy in modern medicine rijeka. Croatia: InTech; 2011. p. 295–304.

59. Russo P, Magee JC, Anders RA, et al. Key histopathological features of liver biopsies that distinguish biliary atresia from other causes of infantile cholestasis and their correlation with outcome: a multicenter study. Am J Surg Pathol 2016; 40(12):1601.

60. Lin H, Zoll B, Russo P, et al. A challenging case of focal extrahepatic duct obstruction/hypoplasia in Alagille syndrome. J Pediatr Gastroenterol Nutr 2017; 64(1):e18–22.

61. Kaye AJ, Rand EB, Munoz PS, et al. Effect of Kasai procedure on hepatic outcome in Alagille syndrome. J Pediatr Gastroenterol Nutr 2010;51(3):319–21.

62. Fujishiro J, Suzuki K, Watanabe M, et al. Outcomes of Alagille syndrome following the Kasai operation: a systematic review and meta-analysis. Pediatr Surg Int 2018;34(10):1073–7.

63. Rovner AJ, Schall JI, Jawad AF, et al. Rethinking growth failure in Alagille syndrome: the role of dietary intake and steatorrhea. J Pediatr Gastroenterol Nutr 2002;35(4):495–502.

64. Feranchak AP, Sokol R. Medical and nutritional management of cholestasis in infants and children. Liver Dis Child 2007;3:190–231.

65. Wasserman D, Zemel BS, Mulberg AE, et al. Growth, nutritional status, body composition, and energy expenditure in prepubertal children with Alagille syndrome. J Pediatr 1999;134(2):172–7.

66. Kronsten V, Fitzpatrick E, Baker A. Management of cholestatic pruritus in paediatric patients with alagille syndrome: the King's College Hospital experience. J Pediatr Gastroenterol Nutr 2013;57(2):149–54.

67. Thebaut A, Habes D, Gottrand F, et al. Sertraline as an additional treatment for cholestatic pruritus in children. J Pediatr Gastroenterol Nutr 2017;64(3):431–5.

68. Wang KS, Tiao G, Bass LM, et al. Analysis of surgical interruption of the enterohepatic circulation as a treatment for pediatric cholestasis. Hepatology 2017; 65(5):1645–54.

69. Sheflin-Findling S, Arnon R, Lee S, et al. Partial internal biliary diversion for Alagille syndrome: case report and review of the literature. J Pediatr Surg 2012; 47(7):1453–6.

70. Karpen SJ, Kelly D, Mack C, et al. Ileal bile acid transporter inhibition as an anticholestatic therapeutic target in biliary atresia and other cholestatic disorders. Hepatol Int 2020;14(5):677–89.

71. Trauner M, Fuchs CD, Halilbasic E, et al. New therapeutic concepts in bile acid transport and signaling for management of cholestasis. Hepatology 2017;65(4): 1393–404.

72. Shneider BL, Spino C, Kamath BM, et al. Placebo-controlled randomized trial of an intestinal bile salt transport inhibitor for pruritus in alagille syndrome. Hepatol Commun 2018;2(10):1184–98.

73. Gonzales E, Sturm E, Stormon M, et al. PS-193-Phase 2 open-label study with a placebo-controlled drug withdrawal period of the apical sodium-dependent bile acid transporter inhibitor maralixibat in children with Alagille Syndrome: 48-week interim efficacy analysis. J Hepatol Suppl 2019;70:e119.

74. Hori T, Egawa H, Takada Y, et al. Long-term outcomes after living-donor liver transplantation for Alagille syndrome: a single center 20-year experience in Japan. Am J Transplant 2010;10(8):1951–2.
75. Arnon R, Annunziato R, Miloh T, et al. Orthotopic liver transplantation for children with Alagille syndrome. Pediatr Transpl 2010;14(5):622–8.
76. Kamath BM, Yin W, Miller H, et al. Outcomes of liver transplantation for patients with Alagille syndrome: the studies of pediatric liver transplantation experience. Liver Transpl 2012;18(8):940–8.
77. Gurkan A, Emre S, Fishbein TM, et al. Unsuspected bile duct paucity in donors for living-related liver transplantation: two case reports. Transplantation 1999; 67(3):416–8.
78. Razavi RS, Baker A, Qureshi SA, et al. Hemodynamic response to continuous infusion of dobutamine in Alagille's syndrome. Transplantation 2001;72(5):823–8.
79. Gandhi SK, Reyes J, Webber SA, et al. Case report of combined pediatric heart-lung-liver transplantation. Transplantation 2002;73(12):1968–9.
80. Bérard E, Sarles J, Triolo V, et al. Renovascular hypertension and vascular anomalies in Alagille syndrome. Pediatr Nephrol 1998;12(2):121–4.
81. Kohaut J, Pommier R, Guerin F, et al. Abdominal arterial anomalies in children with Alagille syndrome: surgical aspects and outcomes of liver transplantation. J Pediatr Gastroenterol Nutr 2017;64(6):888–91.
82. Lykavieris P, Crosnier C, Trichet C, et al. Bleeding tendency in children with Alagille syndrome. Pediatrics 2003;111(1):167–70.

Overview of Progressive Familial Intrahepatic Cholestasis

Sara Hassan, MD[a], Paula Hertel, MD[b],*

KEYWORDS

- PFIC • Cholestasis • FIC1 • BSEP • MDR3 • TJP2 • MYO5B • FXR • USP53

KEY POINTS

- The progressive familial intrahepatic cholestasis disorders are a heterogeneous group of disorders that result from disruption of bile secretion and lead to cholestasis, pruritus, and/or progressive liver disease.
- Management includes supportive care, including treatment of pruritus, and addressing complications of chronic liver disease. Liver transplant may be required for end-stage liver disease, intractable pruritus, and/or hepatocellular carcinoma.
- Surgical interruption of enterohepatic circulation or novel pharmacotherapy resulting in inhibition of ileal bile acid transporters lead to increased excretion of bile acids from the gut and may improve pruritus.
- Although liver transplantation remains the definitive therapy for medically refractory disease, it does not alleviate extrahepatic manifestations associated with familial intrahepatic cholestasis 1 (FIC1) or tight junction protein 2 disease and carries a risk of disease in the transplanted organ in certain patients with FIC1, bile salt export pump, or farnesoid X receptor disease.

INTRODUCTION

Progressive familial intrahepatic cholestasis (PFIC) is a label applied to a heterogenous group of monogenic disorders that cause impaired intrahepatic bile flow or cholestasis.[1–4] These cholestasis syndromes result from defects in canalicular bile acid trafficking and/or secretion, and comprise a broad clinical spectrum ranging from a nonprogressive, intermittent cholestatic jaundice (benign recurrent intrahepatic cholestasis, or "BRIC"), to chronic liver disease (PFIC).[5,6] Their heterogeneity and rarity have made study of these disorders challenging but collaborative, multicenter

[a] Department of Pediatrics, Division of Gastroenterology, Hepatology and Nutrition, Mayo Clinic, 200 First Street Southwest, Rochester, MN 55905, USA; [b] Department of Pediatrics, Division of Gastroenterology, Hepatology and Nutrition, Baylor College of Medicine, Texas Children's Hospital, 6621 Fannin Street, Houston, TX 77030, USA
* Corresponding author.
E-mail address: phertel@bcm.edu
Twitter: @SaraHassanMD (S.H.)

Clin Liver Dis 26 (2022) 371–390
https://doi.org/10.1016/j.cld.2022.03.003
1089-3261/22/© 2022 Elsevier Inc. All rights reserved.

studies such as the Natural Course and Prognosis of PFIC and Effect of Biliary Diversion (NAPPED) and the Childhood Liver Disease Research Network consortia have enabled study of larger cohorts. The PFIC disorders are autosomal recessive but individuals with heterozygous mutations in these genes may present with transient neonatal cholestasis, intrahepatic cholestasis of pregnancy (ICP), drug-induced liver injury, cholelithiasis/choledocholithiasis, predisposition to parenteral nutrition associated liver disease, or milder forms of chronic multidrug resistance 3 (MDR3) liver disease.[7–12] Homozygous nonsense or frameshift mutations or large deletions, resulting in a nonfunctional protein, may be more likely to result in severe disease than mutations that only partially affect function but clear genotype–phenotype relationships are not always present.[13–15] Pruritus remains one of the most significant clinical manifestations of these disorders, and may severely affect sleep, school performance, and overall quality of life. Severe, refractory pruritus may be an indication for liver transplant. End-stage liver disease and/or liver cancer also necessitate liver transplant. With advances in molecular genetics, additional PFIC disorders have been identified in recent years, further highlighting the burden of genetic causes of intrahepatic cholestasis.[2,5,6] The purpose of this review is to provide a comprehensive outline of genetic causes, clinical manifestations, and management strategies for the evolving class of monogenic intrahepatic cholestasis disorders referred to as PFIC.

DISCUSSION
Bile Flow and Metabolism

Bile, an alkaline fluid, is a robust detergent that is produced by hepatocytes and contains bilirubin, bile acids, cholesterol, and other lipids.[5,16] It is typically transported via the biliary tree and stored in the gallbladder, where it is released into the small intestine to aid in lipid digestion and fat-soluble vitamin absorption.[17] Additionally, it removes toxins from the liver and facilitates their excretion into the gut.[18] Once excreted, some bile acids are reabsorbed in the ileum and transported back to the liver via enterohepatic circulation by the apical sodium-dependent bile transporter (ASBT).[2,3,5]

Bile acid trafficking is a complex physiologic process that depends on intricate machinery to ensure smooth transport out of the hepatocyte. The bile salt export pump (BSEP) is essential in transporting bile salts formed by hepatocytes across the canalicular membrane, the stability of which rests on an adequate enclosure and dispersal of the phosphatidylcholine molecule regulated by MDR3 and familial intrahepatic cholestasis 1 (FIC1) proteins, respectively.[3,5,19] BSEP expression itself is controlled by farnesoid X receptor (FXR), and its localization on the canalicular membrane depends on myosin 5B (MYO5B).[2] The integrity of hepatocytes is partially determined by tight junctions (whose integrity depends on tight junction protein 2 [TJP2]) that protect hepatocytes from the detergent properties of bile and, likely, ubiquitin-specific protease 53 (USP53), which has been shown to colocalize and interact with TJP2 in mice.[20] Genetic defects in any of these proteins may lead to intrahepatic cholestasis.

Epidemiology and Prevalence

Incidence of the PFIC disorders is difficult to precisely determine due to relative infrequency and heterogeneity of this class of disorders, and lack of genetic data to confirm diagnosis in many older studies. As cited in a recent systematic review, the local population prevalence of PFIC was between 9% and 12.9% of children admitted to hospital with cholestasis, liver failure, or splenomegaly based on 3 studies.[21] The first 3 identified PFIC disorders, FIC1 disease, BSEP disease, and MDR3 disease are the most common, with BSEP disease being the most common out of these 3 diseases.[7,22] For patients with severe FIC1 or BSEP deficiency, survival with native liver (SNL) beyond childhood is not expected in most cases, with only 50% surviving with their native liver up to 10 years and nearly none to 20 years of age in one study.[23] Patients with milder forms of disease can be expected to survive with their native liver well into adulthood.

Pruritus in Progressive Familial Intrahepatic Cholestasis Disorders

Pruritus is a hallmark symptom of the PFIC disorders, and it can be severely debilitating.[22] It is treated with medications and/or nontransplant surgery (surgical interruption of enterohepatic circulation; sEHC) to interrupt enterohepatic circulation of bile acids. In the most severe and refractory cases, it can be an indication for liver transplant. The pathophysiology of pruritus in cholestatic liver disease is not well understood. It is thought that circulating bile acids play a role but serum bile acid levels do not always correlate with pruritus symptoms. There is a more direct correlation between itching and circulating levels of lysophosphatidic acid (LPA), a neuronal activator, and levels of autotaxin, the enzyme responsible for the formation of LPA.[24] The ItchRO scale was recently developed as a tool to objectively assess pruritus, and it has proven useful in assessing response to treatment.[25]

Medications for Pruritus

Table 1 summarizes medications commonly used to manage pruritus in PFIC disorders. Ursodeoxycholic acid, or ursodiol, is a synthetic hydrophilic bile acid used in many cholestatic liver disorders used to alleviate pruritus and improve bile flow. It renders bile more hydrophilic (less toxic to cell membranes) and promotes bile flow by stimulating cholangiocyte bicarbonate secretion and upregulating BSEP and MRP2.[26] It can prevent biliary stone formation (BSEP and MDR3 disease) and, in some cases, it may slow or reverse the progression of disease.[27] Rifampicin (rifampin) may exert antipruritic effects via its enhancement of hepatic cytochrome P450 activity and increased 6-a hydroxylation and 2-a glucuronidation of bile acids and/or by its effects on intestinal flora and secondary bile acids.[28] Other therapies for pruritus include bile acid-binding resins (including cholestyramine), antihistamines (hydroxyzine, diphenhydramine), naltrexone, and sertraline. Therapy using molecular chaperones such as 4-phenylbutyrate, which may rescue protein function associated with missense BSEP and FIC1 mutations in vitro, has promise but caution and further study are warranted after the first participant (with FIC1 deficiency) enrolled in a 4-phenylbutyrate trial developed severe, acute, reversible liver injury after withdrawal of rifampin, which had been prescribed concomitantly. It was hypothesized that discontinuation of the rifampin, a strong inducer of CYP3A4, resulted in phenylacetate toxicity.[29] Ileal apical sodium-dependent intestinal bile acid transporters inhibitors (iBAT inhibitors) are a newer class of antipruritus medications that work by reducing bile reabsorption, which occurs primarily in the ileum, back into enterohepatic circulation. Odevixibat is the first FDA-approved (July 2021) medical therapy for pruritus in patients 3 months of age and older with all types of PFIC.[30] In trials, once-daily administration was shown to reduce serum bile acids and improve pruritus and associated sleep disturbance in children with cholestasis. It may also improve hepatic fibrosis, although the mechanism remains unclear. Drug is primarily confined to the intestinal lumen and is generally well tolerated, with diarrhea, fat-soluble vitamin deficiency, and transient increases in aminotransferases being the most common side effects. No serious adverse events were reported in trials before FDA approval.[30] There are several other iBAT inhibitors currently in development.[22]

Table 1
Pharmacotherapy for alleviating pruritus

Drug Name	Mechanism of Action	Comments
Ursodeoxycholic acid (ursodiol)	Choleretic	Promotes bile flow May improve hepatic fibrosis in some case
Hydroxyzine	Antihistamine	May cause drowsiness
Cholestyramine Colesevelam Colestipol	Bile-acid binding resin/ sequestrant	Gastrointestinal side effects include nausea, vomiting, bloating and constipation May be unpalatable Administer at least 1 h after and 4 h before other medications
Rifampicin, Rifampin	Antibiotic, potent agonist of pregnane-X-receptor, which promotes detoxification	Association with development of hepatotoxicity 10%–15% Contraindicated in patients with advanced liver disease
Naltrexone, Naloxone	Opioid antagonist	Can be associated with opioid withdrawal-like symptoms Variable rates of elevated liver enzymes in some cases. Use of opioid antagonists may complicate control of acute or postoperative pain unless dosong held at least 72 h
Sertraline	Selective serotonin reuptake inhibitor	Mechanism of action in treatment of pruritus is unclear
Odevixibat	Intestinal bile acid transport inhibitor	Diarrhea or other GI discomfort is most common side effect. May cause elevated liver enzymes. Limited efficacy in patients with BSEP deficiency with complete absence of BSEP protein

Nontransplant Surgery for Pruritus

Surgical interventions ("sEHC" hereafter) are available when medical management has been maximized but incompletely effective and include partial biliary diversion (PEBD) and ileal bypass.[22,31] PEBD can decrease serum bile acids by disrupting the enterohepatic circulation via surgical placement of an external biliary conduit.[32,33] Complications may include diarrhea, profuse stoma output with dehydration and/or electrolyte abnormalities, and surgical complications necessitating revisions.[34,35] A trial of nasobiliary drainage, using a nasogastric feeding tube, may be attempted in surgical candidates to assess response before committing to surgery.[36] PEBD should be avoided in patients with cirrhosis because a beneficial response may be less likely, and varices can develop at the stoma site and cause bleeding if portal hypertension is present. Partial internal biliary diversion is a more recently developed surgical procedure that consists of creating an internal conduit between the gallbladder and the colon and bypassing the terminal ileum, the site of bile acid reabsorption, thereby effectively disrupting the enterohepatic circulation but without necessitating creation of an external ostomy.[35,37] Choleretic diarrhea may result from bile flow directly into the colon, for which bile acid sequestrants may be helpful in management. There is also a theoretic long-term cancer risk associated with bile flowing directly into the colon, which should be considered after internal diversion.[38] Both types of sEHC surgeries may lead to improved laboratory and growth parameters, improved hepatic fibrosis, and better control of pruritus.[15,32,35,39] Ileal exclusion is performed to decrease bile acid reabsorption by surgically bypassing 15% to 20% of the distal ileum, where most bile acid reabsorption occurs. It is favored in patients with gallbladder anomalies or, particularly before the development of internal biliary diversion, in those who wished to avoid or to close an existing PEBD stoma. It can, however, lead to significant diarrhea and malabsorption, and its effectiveness in controlling pruritus is often transient.[40]

Specific Progressive Familial Intrahepatic Cholestasis Syndromes

Here forth, specific PFIC syndromes, listed based on affected protein and gene, are discussed. **Table 2** summarizes several genetic variants that may cause intrahepatic cholestasis and cites associated clinical manifestations of each disorder.

Familial intrahepatic cholestasis 1 (Byler) disease: ATPase phospholipid transporting 8B1 gene (OMIM 211600, 243300)

Originally identified in the family of Jacob Byler in Western Pennsylvania in late 1960s, FIC1 deficiency, also commonly known as "Byler" disease, represents the first recognized type of progressive intrahepatic familial cholestasis. It is also termed PFIC 1.[16]

Familial intrahepatic cholestasis 1 disease genetics and pathophysiology. Mutations in the *ATPase phospholipid transporting 8B1 gene (ATP8B1)* gene on chromosome 8 cause FIC 1 disease, also called PFIC 1 or "Byler" disease. The protein FIC1 is expressed on hepatocytes and contributes to the stability of the canalicular membrane. It is a member of the ATP-dependent membrane transporters; specifically, ATP8B1—a phospholipid flippase, which translocates phospholipids inward on the cell membrane.[6] Both flippases and floppases, the latter of which translocate phospholipids outward on the cell membrane, maintain a balanced distribution of lipids in the cell membrane. It is hypothesized that mutations in FIC1 result in impaired bile flow due to membrane instability and resultant inability to effectively traffic bile acids, which accumulate intracellularly and become cytotoxic. In addition to its hepatic expression, FIC1 is also expressed in the ear, pancreas, small intestine, and bladder, which is relevant to its role in extrahepatic disease and in complications that may develop following liver transplant [12]. A mild disease phenotype is commonly associated with at least one mutation that affects protein function only moderately, including common missense mutation I661 T, which is the most common mutation associated with a BRIC phenotype.[36] Genotype alone does not, however, tend to reliably predict disease course or response to sEHC in FIC1 disease in general.[15,32,39]

Familial intrahepatic cholestasis 1 disease clinical manifestations, laboratory findings, and histology. Patients with PFIC 1 usually present with cholestasis during the first few months of life.[41] Intense pruritus, hepatosplenomegaly, and portal hypertension

Table 2

Summary of genetic causes, clinical characteristics, and histologic features of progressive familial intrahepatic cholestasis Disorders

Disorder	Gene	Clinical Manifestations	Laboratory Findings	Cancer Risk	Response to sEHC	Histology
FIC1 disease (PFIC 1,Byler disease)	ATP8B1	Severe pruritus Extrahepatic manifestations(diarrhea, pancreatitis, sensorineural hearing loss) Diarrhea and/or hepatic steatosis with progressive fibrosis posttransplant DILI, low-GGT ICP, contraceptive-induced cholestasis	Normal GGt	Not reported	Yes	Bland cholestasis Coarse and granular intracanalicular bile (EM)
BSEP disease (PFIC 2)	ABCB11	Sever pruritus Risk of recurrence following OLT due to anti-BSEP antibodies Cholelithiasis ILI, low-GGT ICP, contraceptive cholestasis	Normal GGT AST and ALT may be more elevated than in other PFIC disorders	HCC Cholangiocarcinoma Pancreatic adeno-carcinoma	Yes (more likely if "mild" mutation such as E297 G or D482 G)	Giant cell hepatitis Amorphous bile (EM)
MDR3 disease (PFIC 3)	ABCB4	Moderate-to-severe pruritus Progressive biliary disease with generally later onset than other PFIC disorders Cholelithiasis (LPAC) DILI, high-GGT ICP, contraceptive-induced cholestasis	Elevated GGT	Cholangiocarcinoma	No	Changes in cholangiocytes Bile duct proliferation

TJP2 disease (PFIC 4)	TJP2	Cholestatic liver disease with characteristics overlapping with FIC1 and BSEP disease Sensorineural hearing loss Low-GGT ICP Cholelithiasis per one report	Normal GGT	HCC	Not reported	Bland cholestasis
FXR disease (PFIC 5)	NR1H4	Early infantile onset with rapid progression to liver failure (coagulopathy with low factor 5 levels and vitamin K refractoriness) Hepatic steatosis posttransplant Biliary stones ICP	Normal GGT	Not reported	Not reported	Giant cell transformation Bile duct proliferation
MYO5B disease (PFIC 6)	MYO5B	Many present as isolated cholestatic liver disease or in patients with MVID May present or worsen following intestinal transplant for MVID Neurologic involvement in a few cases Biliary stones per one report	Normal GGT	Not reported	Yes (very limited data)	Giant cell hepatitis Canalicular and hepatocellular cholestasis
USP53 (PFIC 7)	USP53	Self-limited cholestasis, or episodic BRIC-like course in many Some with excellent response to rifampin Cholelithiasis Sensorineural hearing loss	Normal GGT	Not reported	Not reported	Mild ductular reaction Periportal fibrosis Mild lobular inflammation

Abbreviations: AFP, alpha fetoprotein; BSEP, bile salt export pump; FIC1, Familial Intrahepatic Cholestasis 1; FXR, Farnesoid X Receptor; GGT, gamma glutamyl transferase; HCC, hepatocellular carcinoma; ICP, intrahepatic cholestasis of pregnancy; LPAC, low-phospholipid associated cholelithiasis; MDR3; Multidrug Resistance 3, MYO5B; myosin 5B, PI; pancreatic insufficiency, TJP2; Tight Junction Protein 2, USP53; ubiquitin-specific protease 53.

may develop. Extrahepatic manifestations can include diarrhea, pancreatitis, exocrine pancreatic insufficiency, elevated sweat chloride, pneumonia, and/or sensorineural hearing loss.[23] Growth failure with stunting is more predominant in FIC1 disease than in BSEP or MDR3 disease.[7] Laboratory findings are remarkable for elevated conjugated bilirubin and serum bile acids at presentation, and mildly to moderately elevated aminotransferases in the setting of normal gamma-glutamyl transferase (GGT) levels. Liver biopsy typically reveals bland canalicular cholestasis, and granular "Byler" bile may be noted on electron microscopy.[5,42] Hepatic manifestations may progress to chronic end-stage liver disease requiring transplantation; Van Wessel and colleagues, in the NAPPED consortium, observed that fewer than half of FIC1 patients survived to adulthood with native liver.[41] However, prognosis seems difficult to determine in individuals with this disorder; neither *ATP8B1* mutation nor serum bile acid level at presentation predicted prognosis in FIC1 patients in the NAPPED study. Similarly, responses to sEHC, although generally more favorable in FIC1 disease than in BSEP disease, have been reported as variable among FIC1 disease recipients, even in patients with identical genotype.[15,32,39] Patients with milder phenotypes of FIC1 disease can develop recurrent episodes of cholestasis without progressive liver disease. This is typically referred to as benign recurrent intrahepatic cholestasis or "BRIC" (type 1).[16] Some patients presenting with a BRIC phenotype, however, may evolve to a more persistent and progressive PFIC phenotype.[23] Low-GGT ICP is another manifestation of FIC1 disease. Liver cancer has not been reported in children with isolated FIC1 disease.

Familial intrahepatic cholestasis 1 disease management. Supportive therapies are the cornerstone for managing FIC1 disease.[22] These include medical management of pruritus and, if ineffective, nontransplant surgery (see dedicated discussion on this topic above). Biliary diversion (sEHC) generally has higher success rates in FIC1 disease than in BSEP disease, and it should be strongly considered in lieu of liver transplant in appropriate candidates who do not have cirrhosis, given the potentially severe complications that can develop posttransplant in patients with FIC1 disease (discussed below). Following sEHC, some patients with FIC1 disease have shown a dramatic reduction in serum bile acids and complete resolution of pruritus; many have followed a course of relapsing/remitting cholestasis and pruritus resembling BRIC.[32,35,39] Addressing nutritional deficiencies (screening for fat-soluble vitamin deficiencies and prescribing replacement when required, prescribing medium chain triglyceride (MCT) oil or MCT-enriched formulas), assessing bone mineral density, screening for extrahepatic manifestations of disease, and managing sequelae of portal hypertension and end-stage liver disease are imperative. Liver transplantation is often reserved for patients who develop cirrhosis and end-stage liver disease.[2,5,22] It is important to note that extrahepatic manifestations of FIC1 disease do not improve after transplantation, and diarrhea and/or hepatic steatosis can become significant complications in many patients posttransplant. Diarrhea is likely due to bile acid diarrhea secondary to normalized bile flow into the FIC1-deficient intestine from the healthy transplanted liver and has been shown to improve with bile acid binding resins such as cholestyramine, or with PEBD.[16,43] FGF19 analogs have also been proposed as a putative therapy; this requires further investigation. Additionally, hepatic steatosis may develop in the allograft and may be associated with progressive fibrosis, and, in some cases, cirrhosis, which may necessitate retransplantation.[39,43,44] The precise mechanisms for this are unclear but, as in the case with diarrhea posttransplant, are likely related to restoration of normal bile flow from the transplanted liver into the FIC1-deficient gut and disordered enterohepatic circulation. As is the case for FIC1 disease postliver transplant diarrhea, sEHC has shown promise in reversing posttransplant hepatic steatosis in FIC1 disease and should be considered. Preventive internal diversion at the time of transplant was successfully performed in one case, although efficacy of this procedure in preventing allograft steatosis requires further study.[44,45]

Bile salt export pump disease: ATP binding cassette subfamily B member11 (OMIM 601847, 605479)

Bile salt export pump disease genetics and pathophysiology. Mutations in the *ATP binding cassette subfamily B member11 (ABCB11)* gene on chromosome 2 result in BSEP disease, also termed PFIC 2. This leads to impaired bile salt transport into the canaliculus and translates into hepatocellular injury and pruritus.[7] A clear relationship between gene mutation severity and disease severity has been demonstrated in BSEP disease, unlike in FIC1 disease.[14] Mutations that result in only partial loss of BSEP function, with p.D482 G and p.E297 G being notable examples, are generally associated with less severe disease (including BRIC, which is characterized by nonprogressive, episodic cholestasis), good response to ursodiol, longer SNL, and more consistent improvement in SNL following sEHC.[14,39] Variants A590 T and R1050 C have also been reported in association with a BRIC phenotype. Conversely, individuals with at least one severe mutation leading to a predicted nonfunctional protein (often frameshift, protein-truncating mutations or large deletions) tend to have shorter SNL, more frequent hepatocellular carcinoma (HCC), and less favorable response to sEHC. Mild or heterozygous mutations may result in other manifestations of this disease including transient neonatal cholestasis.[12,46] Some variants, including the relatively common V444 A, may be associated with drug-induced hepatic cholestasis or with low-GGT ICP.[8,47,48]

Bile salt export pump disease clinical manifestations, laboratory findings, and histology. Patients with BSEP disease typically present during infancy and frequently have progressive chronic liver disease, including pruritus, jaundice, fat-soluble vitamin deficiencies, portal hypertension, and cirrhosis.[31,41] Serum bile acids are elevated but GGT is normal. Giant cell hepatitis is a notable finding on liver biopsy, as well as canalicular cholestasis with amorphous (rather than coarse and granular) bile, and absence of BSEP protein. AST and ALT are more elevated than observed in FIC1 disease, and early progression to advanced liver disease and liver transplantation are reported more frequently than in FIC1 or MDR3 disease.[7,23] Initial presentation with severe bleeding due to vitamin K deficiency, in the absence of other significant stigmata of liver disease, has been reported.[49] Because BSEP protein is expressed exclusively in the liver, deficiency does not present with extrahepatic manifestations, as observed in FIC1 disease.[2,5,16] Patients with BSEP disease are at particular risk for HCC, even in the absence of cirrhosis, and HCC may develop even in very young patients[50] [6]. Cholangiocarcinoma and pancreatic adenocarcinoma have also been reported.[51,52]

Bile salt export pump disease management. Supportive care for BSEP disease is similar to what is recommended for other PFIC disorders, with emphasis on pruritus management, nutrition optimization, fat-soluble vitamin supplementation, and expectant management of complications associated with cirrhosis and portal hypertension.[5,53] Ursodiol is a mainstay of therapy and may have a particularly significant beneficial effect in those with less severe mutations. Screening for hepatic malignancies with tumor markers (including alpha-fetoprotein [AFP]) and abdominal imaging is critical for children with BSEP disease and has been recommended beginning at around 12 months of age.[16] Response to sEHC in BSEP disease depends on degree of BSEP activity retention, with worse outcomes in patients with absent protein but more consistently good outcomes in those with D482 G and/or E297 G or other less severe mutations. Although liver transplantation is generally curative, especially given that BSEP is expressed exclusively in the liver and that there are no extrahepatic manifestations of BSEP disease, up to 10% of PFIC2 patients develop recurrent liver disease with evidence of anti-BSEP antibodies after liver transplant. This phenomenon has been termed autoimmune BSEP disease, and it has been effectively managed with B-cell depleting antibody therapy (rituximab), IVIG, plasmapheresis, steroids, and/or use of mycophenolate as part of the posttransplant immunosuppression regimen.[54–56]

Multidrug resistance 3 disease: ATP binding cassette subfamily B member 4 (OMIM 602347)

Tight Junction protein 2 disease genetics and pathophysiology. Mutations in the *ATP binding cassette subfamily B member 4 (ABCB4)* gene, on chromosome 7, cause MDR3 disease, also known as PFIC 3. *ABCB4* encodes phospholipid transporter MDR3, which is located on the canalicular membrane of hepatocytes and is critical for bile acid transport.[6,16,41] Mutations in *ABCB4* can lead to defective MDR3 and impaired neutralization of free bile acids, resulting in so-called toxic, low-phospholipid bile with resultant biliary injury.

Multidrug resistance 3 disease clinical manifestations, laboratory findings, and histology. MDR3 deficiency causes low phospholipid-associated cholestasis and/or cholelithiasis (both also sometimes referred to as low phospholipid-associated cholelithiasis [LPAC]). It may manifest with pruritus and jaundice but progressive hepatic fibrosis with portal hypertension is a more salient feature of this disorder compared with FIC1 and BSEP disease.[7] Age of onset is later than observed in FIC1 and BSEP disease, with clinical findings usually first notable in childhood or adolescence rather than during infancy. Unlike in FIC1 and BSEP disease, GGT is elevated in MDR3 deficiency. Hepatic aminotransferases and serum bile acids are commonly elevated, and bilirubin is sometimes elevated. Liver biopsy may demonstrate bile duct proliferation, intraductal stone formation, and giant cell hepatitis.[16] Cholestasis leads to impaired copper excretion in bile and may lead to hepatic copper accumulation, and patients with MDR3 disease may present with hepatic copper overload and clinical features overlapping with Wilson disease.[57–59] *ABCB4* variants may be associated with LPAC, drug-induced liver injury, transient neonatal cholestasis, increased susceptibility to parenteral nutrition-associated cholestasis, and high-GGT ICP, and these disorders may be responsive to ursodiol.[4,8,11,36,47,60,61]

Multidrug resistance 3 disease management. Management focuses on supportive care including pruritus management[41] and ursodiol, which may not only help to alleviate pruritus but also to reduce hepatic fibrosis in some cases; it has even been reported to reverse cirrhosis this disorder.[27] Surgical diversion (sEHC) does not improve liver disease in this disorder, and transplantation remains the only therapy in medically refractory cases with end-stage liver disease or cancer. Screening for cholangiocarcinoma is warranted, as this has been reported.[60]

Tight junction protein 2 disease: tight junction protein 2 (OMIM 615878)

Multidrug resistance 3 disease genetics and pathophysiology. First described in 2014, mutations and loss of function in the *TJP2* gene on chromosome 9 lead to deficiency of TJP2 protein, a cytoplasmic component of the hepatocyte cellular junctions, that prevents leaking of bile between the cells and into the liver parenchyma.[6]

Complete TJP2 deficiency results in severe and progressive liver disease, although other mutations present with milder liver disease or hypercholanemia with fat-soluble vitamin deficiencies.[62,63] There may also be variable disease penetrance, as evidenced in one large family with consanguineous parents, in whom some homozygous adult offspring had developed cirrhosis, whereas others had elevated liver enzymes but no cirrhosis.[64]

Tight junction protein 2 disease clinical manifestations, laboratory findings, and histology. Patients with severe TJP2 deficiency most commonly present during early infancy with low-GGT cholestasis with elevated serum bile acids, pruritus, and progressive liver disease.[62,65] Liver biopsy demonstrates nonspecific findings including intracellular cholestasis. Other variations of TJP2 disease may present as cirrhosis with portal hypertension or as mild liver disease in young adulthood,[64] and heterozygous or homozygous TJP2 mutations in women may result in low-GGT ICP.[8] Cholelithiasis has been reported, as well.[62] Extrahepatic manifestations may include respiratory disease, hearing loss, and/or neurologic symptoms.[66] HCC has been reported in young patients with severe liver disease.[65,67]

Tight junction protein 2 disease management. As for other PFIC disorders, supportive care, including management of fat-soluble vitamin deficiencies and malnutrition, pruritus, and sequelae of portal hypertension when it develops. Early screening for malignancy beginning in the first year of life is recommended, as HCC has been reported in TJP2 deficiency at a very young age.[65,67] Liver transplantation offers definitive treatment of liver disease with or without localized malignancy, although it does not resolve extrahepatic findings. Hepatic steatosis and diarrhea posttransplant have not been reported posttransplant. There have been no reports, at the time of this writing, of outcomes following sEHC in patients with TJP2 disease.

Farnesoid X receptor disease: nuclear receptor subfamily 1, group H, member 4 (OMIM 617049)

Farnesoid X receptor disease genetics and pathophysiology. FXR is a nuclear transcription factor encoded by the *nuclear receptor subfamily 1, group H, member 4 (NR1H4)* gene on chromosome 12 and responsible for regulation of bile salt metabolism. FXR disease, or PFIC 5, results in inappropriate regulation of BSEP and causes a severe variety of neonatal cholestatic liver disease.[6]

Farnesoid X receptor disease clinical manifestations, laboratory findings, and histology. Loss of FXR results in severely impaired bile flow in the neonatal period, coagulopathy refractory to vitamin K supplementation and with evidence of hepatic synthetic dysfunction, and rapid progression to end-stage liver disease.[5] Serum GGT levels are low and serum bile acid levels are elevated. Serum AFP is elevated, often markedly so.[5,68] Liver biopsy shows giant cell hepatitis and hepatocyte ballooning, bile duct proliferation, cholestasis, and absent BSEP and FXR on immunostaining.[2,68] Infants typically present with severe cholestatic liver disease before 2 months of age but onset as late as the second year of life has also been reported. Mutations in NR1H4 may also cause ICP or cholelithiasis.[16]

Farnesoid X receptor disease management. Liver transplant is the definitive therapy for this disorder.[68] Due to its typically rapidly progressive course, diagnosis may not be determined before transplant but outcomes have reportedly been good in the transplant recipients reported in the medical literature thus far. FXR does have extrahepatic expression, and hepatic steatosis has been reported in a few transplant recipients in the posttransplant period. More data are required to determine prognosis for this complication in children transplanted for FXR disease.

Myosin 5B disease, myosin 5B (MIM 251850)

Myosin 5B disease genetics and pathophysiology. MYO5B, encoded by the MYO5B gene on chromosome 18, plays an important role in cell membrane trafficking and localization of BSEP and other canalicular proteins via its interaction with rab11a.[69] With inappropriate canalicular protein localization and hepatocyte membrane polarization, adequate bile acid secretion is impaired and results in hepatotoxicity.[70] Defects in MYO5B historically have been associated with intestinal microvillous inclusion disorder (MVID), which causes severe congenital diarrhea that may necessitate parenteral nutrition and intestinal transplant. In 2013, Girard and colleagues reported a PFIC-like cholestatic liver disease in 8 children out of a cohort of 28 patients with MVID that was apparently unrelated to parenteral nutrition.[71] Subsequently, isolated cholestatic liver disease in patients with MYO5B mutations, but without apparent intestinal disease, was reported in 5 children.[70] The patients in this series had either compound heterozygous or homozygous mutations in MYO5B, all of which were previously unreported in patients with either isolated MVID or MVID with cholestasis. As such, a distinct disorder was identified. Interestingly, MYO5B's role in the development of cholestasis seems to rely solely on its interaction with active rab11a, rather than on its loss of motor function.[69] Thus, although severe (eg, biallelic nonsense or frameshift) mutations in the MYO5B gene consistently result in MVID, this genotype–phenotype relationship does not apply to MYO5B liver disease.[69]

Myosin 5B disease clinical manifestations, laboratory findings, and histology. Patients with MYO5B liver disease present with low-GGT cholestasis and elevated serum bile acids, typically in late infancy or early in the second year of life, and may have hepatomegaly, pruritus, and/or pale stools. In patients with MYO5B cholestasis and MVID, cholestasis with significant pruritus may worsen or may newly develop following intestinal transplant.[71] AFP levels have been normal in cases reported to-date. Liver biopsy demonstrates canalicular cholestasis and giant cell transformation, with abnormal MYO5B, RAB11a, MDR3, and BSEP immunostaining.[2,5,42,70] Extraintestinal manifestations reported include episodic diarrhea, which resolved after 3 years of age in one infant who had normal duodenal histology, and neurologic symptoms of unclear cause in one child with a normal vitamin E level.[70] Cholelithiasis was reported in a child with MYO5B disease in one case series, with recurrent "mild and self-limiting" diarrhea before 3 years of age, who was not diagnosed with MVID and presumably not treated with parenteral nutrition, although this was not explicitly stated.[72] Cancer has not been reported in MYO5B liver disease at the time of this writing.

Myosin 5B disease management. Management consists of supportive care targeting pruritus, fat-soluble vitamin deficiencies, controlling diarrhea, and optimizing nutrition.[70] Ursodiol and/or rifampin has improved cholestasis and pruritus but episodic cholestasis may occur despite its continuous use. In patients with both MVID and cholestatic liver disease (with onset either before or after intestinal transplant), medical therapy for pruritus has shown inconsistent effectiveness, pruritus may worsen following intestinal transplant, and hepatic fibrosis may progress.[71] As such, it has been suggested that combined intestinal/liver transplant should be considered in patients with MVID and severe cholestatic liver disease who are being considered for intestinal transplant. In small bowel transplant patients with cholestasis and pruritus posttransplant, removal of a failed bowel graft has resulted in complete or partial remission of pruritus, presumably due, at least in part, to loss of enterohepatic circulation of bile acids.[71] Nontransplant surgery such as partial external biliary drainage (PEBD) may improve cholestasis and alleviate pruritus in medically refractory cases of isolated MYO5B liver disease, as well as in patients with MVID and MYO5B cholestasis, either before or after intestinal transplant.[70,71] For patients with MVID undergoing intestinal transplant, conservation of the gallbladder should be considered so that PEBD can be considered if cholestasis worsens after transplant. Ileal exclusion has effectively alleviated pruritus in MYO5B liver disease but only transiently in at least one case in which it was reported.[71] Combined small bowel and liver transplant for MVID with advanced liver disease have been performed effectively; isolated liver transplant has not yet been reported.

Ubiquitin-specific protease 53 deficiency, ubiquitin-specific protease 53
Ubiquitin-specific protease 53 disease genetics and pathophysiology. USP53 is encoded by the *USP53* gene on chromosome 4. In mice, it has been shown to colocalize and interact with TJP2 and to contribute to tight junction function in the ear.[83] USP53 liver disease was first reported in 2019, in 3 infants from a single family from Saudi Arabia in whom a novel, homozygous truncating mutation in the *USP53* gene was detected by whole exome sequencing.[73] Subsequently, additional cases of cholestatic liver disease in children with biallelic mutations in *USP53* have been reported.[20,62,74,75]

Ubiquitin-specific protease 53 disease clinical manifestations, laboratory findings, and histology. At the time of this writing, 19 cases of USP53 liver disease have been described.[20,74–76] The disorder manifests as low GGT cholestasis, with elevated serum bile acids and modestly elevated aminotransferases. USP53 disease reportedly presents during infancy in most patients but during childhood or adolescence in some. Disease course is self-limiting or episodic in many and may respond well to rifampin.[20,76] Although fibrosis on liver biopsy and splenomegaly were reported in several affected patients in one report, no descriptions yet of complications of end-stage liver disease or significant portal hypertension have been reported for in this disorder. Cholelithiasis was reported in several patients.[20,74,75] Liver biopsy demonstrates periportal fibrosis and mild lobular activity in most, variable lobular and canalicular cholestasis, and ductular reaction. In one series, evidence of cholangiopathy was observed on liver biopsies, and its potential cause, especially in the setting of normal GGT, was discussed. The authors noted that loss of USP53 or TJP2 may cause secondary deficiency of the tight junction protein claudin 1, deficiency of which causes neonatal sclerosing cholangitis, a cholangiopathy. The latter disorder, however, is characterized by high GGT, unlike USP53 and TJP2 deficiencies, and there is no evidence of cholangiopathy in TJP2 deficiency.[74] Autoimmune cause was described as another possible mechanism but no definite evidence for this was described. Extrahepatic manifestations reported included hearing loss in several patients described in 2 of the articles, including one patient who was deaf from birth and later received a cochlear implant.[74,76] Developmental and speech delay was reported in a single patient. None of the patients cited so far have developed cancer or end-stage liver disease. One received liver transplant at 6 years of age for intractable pruritus.[74]

Ubiquitin-specific protease 53 disease management. Recommended medical management for USP53 disease should be similar to the other PFIC disorders, focused on optimizing fat-soluble vitamin levels and nutrition in the setting of cholestasis and associated malabsorption, and relieving pruritus. Ursodiol has been used in many of the patients described thus far, and rifampin has shown excellent benefit in some, including in one child who developed complete normalization of liver enzymes and bilirubin along with complete resolution of pruritus while taking rifampin.[20,74,76] Another had resolution of disease while taking ursodiol and rifampin, then experienced relapse of pruritus on cessation of these medications, and experienced resolution of pruritus again after restarting rifampin. Nontransplant management of cholestasis and pruritus using sEHC has not yet been reported in USP53 disease.

Other Intrahepatic Cholestasis Genes

Recently, mutations in the lipolysis-stimulated lipoprotein receptor (LSR) gene (encoding LSR) have been reported in 2 patients (in separate publications).[73,77] LSR is a tight junction protein whose complete absence causes liver hypoplasia and fetal death in mice. Both patients presented during the first year of life with low-GGT cholestasis with elevated serum bile acids and severe pruritus that was unresponsive to ursodiol.[73,77] Mutations were biallelic and predicted to be pathogenic in both patients, who had nonprogressive disease course at last follow-up. Both also had mild speech and cognitive delay but hearing deficits were not reported.

Four patients with infantile cholestasis and diarrhea, with biallelic mutations in the Unc-45 myosin chaperone (UNC45 A) gene, were described in 2018.[78] GGT was normal in 3 patients but elevated in the fourth as early as 7 days of age; this patient received parenteral nutrition although timing of its initiation and its potential contribution to liver disease was not discussed. Two patients with intractable pruritus had good response to PEBD. Severe congenital diarrhea necessitating parenteral nutrition was present in 3 patients; this persisted to at least 5 years of age in one and resolved in the others. Other associated findings included hearing loss, mild developmental delay, and bone fragility, without evidence of vitamin D deficiency or parathyroid dysfunction in at least one patient.

In another report, homozygous truncating mutations in the SLC51 B gene (encoding organic solute transporter beta [OSTb]) were identified in 2 siblings with high-GGT cholestasis, fat-soluble vitamin deficiencies, and chronic diarrhea (with normal intestinal histology) with infantile onset.[79] Serum bile acid levels were low. OSTb, similar to ASBT, is an intestinal bile acid transporter; its dysfunction, in these cases, presumably caused disruption of enterohepatic circulation of bile acids, with resultant bile acid and fat-soluble vitamin malabsorption, and cholestasis.

SUMMARY

PFIC represents a heterogenous group of monogenic disorders stemming from defects in bile acid transport/secretion.[3,5] The availability of rapid genetic diagnostics has yielded further understanding of defects impacting bile acid trafficking and contributing to the clinical phenotype of cholestasis and progressive liver disease,[2,6,80] and it is expected that the number of identified PFIC disorders will continue to grow. The mainstay of treatment remains supportive, including management of pruritus, malnutrition, fat-soluble vitamin deficiencies, and sequelae of end-stage liver disease, as well as cancer screening—particularly in BSEP, TJP2, and MDR3 disease. Liver transplant is a definitive treatment of end-stage liver disease, malignancy confined to the liver, and medically refractory disease. Nontransplant surgery (such as PEBD) may be successful in certain types of PFIC (MDR3 disease is a notable exception) and may be especially suited to patients with FIC1 disease, in whom many have a good response, and in whom liver transplant should be carefully considered due to the possibility of chronic diarrhea and/or hepatic steatosis with progressive fibrosis posttransplant in this disorder. iBAT inhibitors are a novel class of pharmacologic therapy that interrupt enterohepatic circulation and reduce serum bile acids and pruritus.[22] More studies are needed to determine effects on the progression of liver disease. Other prospective future treatments, such as gene therapy or hepatocyte transplantation, could potentially prove effective. These would be particularly desirable for FIC1 disease, in which liver transplant is often fraught with postoperative complications but residual cancer risk in BSEP and TJP2 diseases may render new nontransplant therapies for these disorders less attractive.[31,81,82]

CLINICS CARE POINTS

- Familial intrahepatic cholestasis 1 (FIC1), bile salt export pump (BSEP), tight junction protein 2 (TJP2), myosin 5B (MYO5B), farnesoid X receptor, and ubiquitin-specific protease 53 disease are all characterized by defects in canalicular bile transport and/or secretion with low-normal gamma-glutamyl transferase (GGT) level (usually <100 IU/L), whereas patients with multidrug resistance 3 (MDR3) disease typically have elevated GGT associated with biliary injury due to low-phospholipid bile.

- Patients with progressive familial intrahepatic cholestasis (PFIC) may develop jaundice and/or hepatic fibrosis, and pruritus is a significant disease complication. Lack of adequate intestinal bile may cause malabsorption of fat and fat-soluble vitamins with consequent malnutrition, low bone mineral density, vitamin-K responsive coagulopathy, and/or complications of vitamin A or E deficiency.

- BSEP and TJP2 disease are associated with cancer risk, and affected individuals should undergo regular cancer screening, including laboratory evaluation and imaging, from a young age.

- Biliary diversion surgery (enterohepatic circulation; PEBD, PIBD, or ileal exclusion) may alleviate symptoms and/or slow disease progression in FIC1, BSEP, and possibly MYO5B deficiency but it should not be performed in patients with cirrhosis and/or MDR3 deficiency and may be less effective in some patients with severe (no residual protein function) mutations.

- Liver transplant is recommended in the setting of end-stage liver disease, refractory pruritus, and/or cancer confined to the liver but should be approached with caution in FIC1 disease given the possibility of posttransplant diarrhea and/or hepatic steatosis, and autoimmune BSEP disease should be screened for in posttransplant BSEP-deficient patients.

- Odevixibat, an ileal apical sodium-dependent intestinal bile acid transporter inhibitor, medically impairs enterohepatic circulation and has proven promising as a new and safe therapy for pruritus in the PFIC disorders.

DISCLOSURE

The authors have nothing to disclose.

REFERENCES

1. Squires RH, Monga SP. Progressive familial intrahepatic cholestasis: is it time to transition to genetic cholestasis? J Pediatr Gastroenterol Nutr 2021;72(5):641–3.
2. Bull LN, Thompson RJ. Progressive familial intrahepatic cholestasis. Clin Liver Dis 2018;22(4):657–69.
3. Karpen SJ. Pediatric cholestasis: epidemiology, genetics, diagnosis, and current management. Clin Liver Dis (Hoboken) 2020;15(3):115–9.
4. Fawaz R, Baumann U, Ekong U, et al. Guideline for the evaluation of cholestatic jaundice in infants: joint recommendations of the north American society for

pediatric gastroenterology, hepatology, and nutrition and the european society for pediatric gastroenterology, hepatology, and nutrition. J Pediatr Gastroenterol Nutr 2017;64(1):154–68.

5. Henkel SA, Squires JH, Ayers M, et al. Expanding etiology of progressive familial intrahepatic cholestasis. World J Hepatol 2019;11(5):450–63.

6. Amirneni S, Haep N, Gad MA, et al. Molecular overview of progressive familial intrahepatic cholestasis. World J Gastroenterol 2020;26(47):7470–84.

7. Hertel PM, Bull LN, Thompson RJ, et al. Mutation analysis and disease features at presentation in a multi-center cohort of children with monogenic cholestasis. J Pediatr Gastroenterol Nutr 2021;73(2):169–77.

8. Dixon PH, Sambrotta M, Chambers J, et al. An expanded role for heterozygous mutations of ABCB4, ABCB11, ATP8B1, ABCC2 and TJP2 in intrahepatic cholestasis of pregnancy. Sci Rep 2017;7(1):11823.

9. Waisbourd-Zinman O, Surrey LF, Schwartz AE, et al. A rare BSEP mutation associated with a mild form of progressive familial intrahepatic cholestasis type 2. Ann Hepatol 2017;16(3):465–8.

10. Jacquemin E, Malan V, Rio M, et al. Heterozygous FIC1 deficiency: a new genetic predisposition to transient neonatal cholestasis. J Pediatr Gastroenterol Nutr 2010;50(4):447–9.

11. Sticova E, Jirsa M. ABCB4 disease: many faces of one gene deficiency. Ann Hepatol 2020;19(2):126–33.

12. Liu LY, Wang XH, Lu Y, et al. Association of variants of ABCB11 with transient neonatal cholestasis. Pediatr Int 2013;55(2):138–44.

13. Klomp LW, Vargas JC, van Mil SW, et al. Characterization of mutations in ATP8B1 associated with hereditary cholestasis. Hepatology 2004;40(1):27–38.

14. van Wessel DBE, Thompson RJ, Gonzales E, et al. Genotype correlates with the natural history of severe bile salt export pump deficiency. J Hepatol 2020;73(1): 84–93.

15. van Wessel DBE, Thompson RJ, Gonzales E, et al. Impact of genotype, serum bile acids, and surgical biliary diversion on native liver survival in FIC1 deficiency. Hepatology 2021;74(2):892–906.

16. Sticova E, Jirsa M, Pawlowska J. New Insights in genetic cholestasis: from molecular mechanisms to clinical implications. Can J Gastroenterol Hepatol 2018;2018: 2313675.

17. Dawson PA, Karpen SJ. Intestinal transport and metabolism of bile acids. J Lipid Res 2015;56(6):1085–99.

18. Linton KJ. Lipid flopping in the liver. Biochem Soc Trans 2015;43(5):1003–10.

19. Sticova E, Jirsa M, Pawłowska J. New insights in genetic cholestasis: from molecular mechanisms to clinical implications. Can J Gastroenterol Hepatol 2018;2313675. https://doi.org/10.1155/2018/2313675.

20. Bull LN, Ellmers R, Foskett P, et al. Cholestasis due to USP53 deficiency. J Pediatr Gastroenterol Nutr 2021;72(5):667–73.

21. Jones-Hughes T, Campbell J, Crathorne L. Epidemiology and burden of progressive familial intrahepatic cholestasis: a systematic review. Orphanet J Rare Dis 2021;16(1):255.

22. Baker A, Kerkar N, Todorova L, et al. Systematic review of progressive familial intrahepatic cholestasis. Clin Res Hepatol Gastroenterol 2019;43(1):20–36.

23. Pawlikowska L, Strautnieks S, Jankowska I, et al. Differences in presentation and progression between severe FIC1 and BSEP deficiencies. J Hepatol 2010;53(1): 170–8.

24. Levy C. Management of pruritus in patients with cholestatic liver disease. Gastroenterol Hepatol (N Y) 2011;7(9):615–7.
25. Kamath BM, Abetz-Webb L, Kennedy C, et al. Development of a novel tool to assess the impact of itching in pediatric cholestasis. Patient 2018;11(1):69–82.
26. Paumgartner G, Beuers U. Ursodeoxycholic acid in cholestatic liver disease: mechanisms of action and therapeutic use revisited. Hepatology 2002;36(3): 525–31.
27. Frider B, Castillo A, Gordo-Gilart R, et al. Reversal of advanced fibrosis after long-term ursodeoxycholic acid therapy in a patient with residual expression of MDR3. Ann Hepatol 2015;14(5):745–51.
28. Khurana S, Singh P. Rifampin is safe for treatment of pruritus due to chronic cholestasis: a meta-analysis of prospective randomized-controlled trials. Liver Int 2006;26(8):943–8.
29. Shneider BL, Morris A, Vockley J. Possible phenylacetate hepatotoxicity during 4-phenylbutyrate therapy of byler disease. J Pediatr Gastroenterol Nutr 2016;62(3): 424–8.
30. Baumann U, Sturm E, Lacaille F, et al. Effects of odevixibat on pruritus and bile acids in children with cholestatic liver disease: phase 2 study. Clin Res Hepatol Gastroenterol 2021;45(5):101751.
31. van der Woerd WL, Houwen RH, van de Graaf SF. Current and future therapies for inherited cholestatic liver diseases. World J Gastroenterol 2017;23(5):763–75.
32. Squires JE, Celik N, Morris A, et al. Clinical variability after partial external biliary diversion in familial intrahepatic cholestasis 1 deficiency. J Pediatr Gastroenterol Nutr 2017;64(3):425–30.
33. Davis AR, Rosenthal P, Newman TB. Nontransplant surgical interventions in progressive familial intrahepatic cholestasis. J Pediatr Surg 2009;44(4):821–7.
34. Gunaydin M, Tander B, Demirel D, et al. Different techniques for biliary diversion in progressive familial intrahepatic cholestasis. J Pediatr Surg 2016;51(3):386–9.
35. Wang KS, Tiao G, Bass LM, et al. Analysis of surgical interruption of the enterohepatic circulation as a treatment for pediatric cholestasis. Hepatology 2017; 65(5):1645–54.
36. Alissa FT, Jaffe R, Shneider BL. Update on progressive familial intrahepatic cholestasis. J Pediatr Gastroenterol Nutr 2008;46(3):241–52.
37. Foroutan HR, Bahador A, Ghanim SM, et al. Effects of partial internal biliary diversion on long-term outcomes in patients with progressive familial intrahepatic cholestasis: experience in 44 patients. Pediatr Surg Int 2020;36(5):603–10.
38. Ajouz H, Mukherji D, Shamseddine A. Secondary bile acids: an underrecognized cause of colon cancer. World J Surg Oncol 2014;12:164.
39. Bull LN, Pawlikowska L, Strautnieks S, et al. Outcomes of surgical management of familial intrahepatic cholestasis 1 and bile salt export protein deficiencies. Hepatol Commun 2018;2(5):515–28.
40. Hollands CM, Rivera-Pedrogo FJ, Gonzalez-Vallina R, et al. Ileal exclusion for Byler's disease: an alternative surgical approach with promising early results for pruritus. J Pediatr Surg 1998;33(2):220–4.
41. Srivastava A. Progressive familial intrahepatic cholestasis. J Clin Exp Hepatol 2014;4(1):25–36.
42. Squires JE, McKiernan P. Molecular mechanisms in pediatric cholestasis. Gastroenterol Clin North Am 2018;47(4):921–37.
43. Knisely AS, Houwen RHJ. Liver Steatosis and diarrhea after liver transplantation for progressive familial intrahepatic cholestasis type 1: can biliary diversion solve these problems? J Pediatr Gastroenterol Nutr 2021;72(3):341–2.

44. Alrabadi LS, Morotti RA, Valentino PL, et al. Biliary drainage as treatment for allograft steatosis following liver transplantation for PFIC-1 disease: a single-center experience. Pediatr Transplant 2018;22(4):e13184.

45. Mali VP, Fukuda A, Shigeta T, et al. Total internal biliary diversion during liver transplantation for type 1 progressive familial intrahepatic cholestasis: a novel approach. Pediatr Transplant 2016;20(7):981–6.

46. Li LT, Li ZD, Yang Y, et al. ABCB11 deficiency presenting as transient neonatal cholestasis: correlation with genotypes and BSEP expression. Liver Int 2020; 40(11):2788–96.

47. Nayagam JS, Williamson C, Joshi D, et al. Review article: liver disease in adults with variants in the cholestasis-related genes ABCB11, ABCB4 and ATP8B1. Aliment Pharmacol Ther 2020;52(11–12):1628–39.

48. Meier Y, Zodan T, Lang C, et al. Increased susceptibility for intrahepatic cholestasis of pregnancy and contraceptive-induced cholestasis in carriers of the 1331T>C polymorphism in the bile salt export pump. World J Gastroenterol 2008;14(1):38–45.

49. Tibesar E, Karwowski C, Hertel P, et al. Two cases of progressive familial intrahepatic cholestasis type 2 presenting with severe coagulopathy without jaundice. Case Rep Pediatr 2014;2014:185923.

50. Knisely AS, Strautnieks SS, Meier Y, et al. Hepatocellular carcinoma in ten children under five years of age with bile salt export pump deficiency. Hepatology 2006;44(2):478–86.

51. Bass LM, Patil D, Rao MS, et al. Pancreatic adenocarcinoma in type 2 progressive familial intrahepatic cholestasis. BMC Gastroenterol 2010;10:30.

52. Scheimann AO, Strautnieks SS, Knisely AS, et al. Mutations in bile salt export pump (ABCB11) in two children with progressive familial intrahepatic cholestasis and cholangiocarcinoma. J Pediatr 2007;150(5):556–9.

53. Bergasa NV. The pruritus of cholestasis: from bile acids to opiate agonists: relevant after all these years. Med Hypotheses 2018;110:86–9.

54. Stindt J, Kluge S, Droge C, et al. Bile salt export pump-reactive antibodies form a polyclonal, multi-inhibitory response in antibody-induced bile salt export pump deficiency. Hepatology 2016;63(2):524–37.

55. Kubitz R, Droge C, Kluge S, et al. Autoimmune BSEP disease: disease recurrence after liver transplantation for progressive familial intrahepatic cholestasis. Clin Rev Allergy Immunol 2015;48(2–3):273–84.

56. Kubitz R, Droge C, Kluge S, et al. High affinity anti-BSEP antibodies after liver transplantation for PFIC-2 - successful treatment with immunoadsorption and B-cell depletion. Pediatr Transplant 2016;20(7):987–93.

57. Shneider BL. ABCB4 disease presenting with cirrhosis and copper overload-potential confusion with Wilson disease. J Clin Exp Hepatol 2011;1(2):115–7.

58. Ramraj R, Finegold MJ, Karpen SJ. Progressive familial intrahepatic cholestasis type 3: overlapping presentation with Wilson disease. Clin Pediatr (Phila) 2012; 51(7):689–91.

59. Boga S, Jain D, Schilsky ML. Presentation of progressive familial intrahepatic cholestasis type 3 mimicking Wilson disease: molecular genetic diagnosis and response to treatment. Pediatr Gastroenterol Hepatol Nutr 2015;18(3):202–8.

60. Stattermayer AF, Halilbasic E, Wrba F, et al. Variants in ABCB4 (MDR3) across the spectrum of cholestatic liver diseases in adults. J Hepatol 2020;73(3):651–63.

61. Lang C, Meier Y, Stieger B, et al. Mutations and polymorphisms in the bile salt export pump and the multidrug resistance protein 3 associated with drug-induced liver injury. Pharmacogenet Genomics 2007;17(1):47–60.

62. Zhang J, Liu LL, Gong JY, et al. TJP2 hepatobiliary disorders: novel variants and clinical diversity. Hum Mutat 2020;41(2):502–11.

63. Carlton VE, Harris BZ, Puffenberger EG, et al. Complex inheritance of familial hypercholanemia with associated mutations in TJP2 and BAAT. Nat Genet 2003; 34(1):91–6.

64. Wei CS, Becher N, Friis JB, et al. New tight junction protein 2 variant causing progressive familial intrahepatic cholestasis type 4 in adults: a case report. World J Gastroenterol 2020;26(5):550–61.

65. Zhou S, Hertel PM, Finegold MJ, et al. Hepatocellular carcinoma associated with tight-junction protein 2 deficiency. Hepatology 2015;62(6):1914–6.

66. Sambrotta M, Strautnieks S, Papouli E, et al. Mutations in TJP2 cause progressive cholestatic liver disease. Nat Genet 2014;46(4):326–8.

67. Tang J, Tan M, Deng Y, et al. Two novel pathogenic variants of TJP2 gene and the underlying molecular mechanisms in progressive familial intrahepatic cholestasis type 4 patients. Front Cell Dev Biol 2021;9:661599.

68. Gomez-Ospina N, Potter CJ, Xiao R, et al. Mutations in the nuclear bile acid receptor FXR cause progressive familial intrahepatic cholestasis. Nat Commun 2016;7:10713.

69. Overeem AW, Li Q, Qiu YL, et al. A Molecular mechanism underlying genotype-specific intrahepatic cholestasis resulting from MYO5B mutations. Hepatology 2020;72(1):213–29.

70. Gonzales E, Taylor SA, Davit-Spraul A, et al. MYO5B mutations cause cholestasis with normal serum gamma-glutamyl transferase activity in children without microvillous inclusion disease. Hepatology 2017;65(1):164–73.

71. Girard M, Lacaille F, Verkarre V, et al. MYO5B and bile salt export pump contribute to cholestatic liver disorder in microvillous inclusion disease. Hepatology 2014;60(1):301–10.

72. Wang L, Qiu YL, Xu HM, et al. MYO5B-associated diseases: novel liver-related variants and genotype-phenotype correlation. Liver Int 2021;42(2):402–11.

73. Maddirevula S, Alhebbi H, Alqahtani A, et al. Identification of novel loci for pediatric cholestatic liver disease defined by KIF12, PPM1F, USP53, LSR, and WDR83OS pathogenic variants. Genet Med 2019;21(5):1164–72.

74. Alhebbi H, Peer-Zada AA, Al-Hussaini AA, et al. New paradigms of USP53 disease: normal GGT cholestasis, BRIC, cholangiopathy, and responsiveness to rifampicin. J Hum Genet 2021;66(2):151–9.

75. Porta G, Rigo PSM, Porta A, et al. Progressive familial intrahepatic cholestasis associated with USP53 gene mutation in a brazilian child. J Pediatr Gastroenterol Nutr 2021;72(5):674–6.

76. Zhang J, Yang Y, Gong JY, et al. Low-GGT intrahepatic cholestasis associated with biallelic USP53 variants: clinical, histological and ultrastructural characterization. Liver Int 2020;40(5):1142–50.

77. Uehara T, Yamada M, Umetsu S, et al. Biallelic mutations in the LSR gene cause a novel type of infantile intrahepatic cholestasis. J Pediatr 2020;221:251–4.

78. Esteve C, Francescatto L, Tan PL, et al. Loss-of-function mutations in UNC45A cause a syndrome associating cholestasis, diarrhea, impaired hearing, and bone fragility. Am J Hum Genet 2018;102(3):364–74.

79. Sultan M, Rao A, Elpeleg O, et al. Organic solute transporter-beta (SLC51B) deficiency in two brothers with congenital diarrhea and features of cholestasis. Hepatology 2018;68(2):590–8.

80. Feldman AG, Sokol RJ. Neonatal cholestasis: emerging molecular diagnostics and potential novel therapeutics. Nat Rev Gastroenterol Hepatol 2019;16(6): 346–60.

81. Aronson SJ, Bakker RS, Shi X, et al. Liver-directed gene therapy results in long-term correction of progressive familial intrahepatic cholestasis type 3 in mice. J Hepatol 2019;71(1):153–62.

82. Bosma PJ, Wits M, Oude-Elferink RP. Gene therapy for progressive familial intra-hepatic cholestasis: current progress and future prospects. Int J Mol Sci 2020; 1:22.

83. Bull LN, Ellmers R, Foskett P, et al. Cholestasis due to USP53 deficiency. J Pediatr Gastroenterol Nutr 2021;72(5):667–73.

Alpha-1 Antitrypsin Deficiency Liver Disease

Anandini Suri, MD*, Dhiren Patel, MD, Jeffrey H. Teckman, MD

KEYWORDS

- Autophagy • Proteolysis • ERAD • Protein polymer • siRNA

KEY POINTS

- Homozygous ZZ alpha-1 antitrypsin (AAT) deficiency is a common genetic metabolic liver disease primarily affecting adults but also a minority of children. The clinical manifestations are highly variable, with many patients remaining healthy or exhibiting only mild biochemical abnormalities.
- The genetic modifiers of protein processing are thought to be associated with severe disease.
- There is no specific treatment for AAT-associated liver disease, but there are treatment options involving supportive measures and liver transplant.
- New technologies aimed at stimulating proteolysis via autophagy, small molecule chaperones, gene therapy, RNA technologies, gene repair, or cell transplantation may hold promise for the treatment of this disease.

INTRODUCTION

Alpha-1 antitrypsin (AAT) is an abundant serum protein, secreted in large amounts daily, second only to albumin. It acts as a serine protease inhibitor (PI) and neutrophil PI, with a wide range of anti-proteolytic and anti-inflammatory actions. It is also an acute phase reactant. The liver is the primary site of synthesis of AAT protein.[1] Liver disease in adults and children with AAT deficiency (AATD) is associated with an excessive deposition of abnormally folded protein in the liver (gain of function). In contrast, lung disease, which occurs in adulthood, characterized by emphysema, is the manifestation of low serum levels of the protein, causing uninhibited protease activity in the lung (loss of function).

AATD is caused by a point mutation in the SERPINA gene. The WHO nomenclature for the alleles of this gene is based on the electrophoretic protein variants (phenotypes) and is designated as PI*.[2] The wild type allele is called the PIM allele. This codes

Division of Pediatric Gastroenterology, Hepatology and Nutrition, Department of Pediatrics, Saint Louis University School of Medicine, SSM Health Cardinal Glennon Children's Hospital, 1465 S Grand Boulevard, St. Louis, MO 63104, USA
* Corresponding author.
E-mail address: anandini.suri@gmail.com

Clin Liver Dis 26 (2022) 391–402
https://doi.org/10.1016/j.cld.2022.03.004
1089-3261/22/© 2022 Elsevier Inc. All rights reserved.

for the M protein (wild type), which successfully binds with chaperones after biosynthesis, and attains properly folded structure. It is then secreted from the liver.

PI*Z allele is associated with most of the liver disease. The AAT mutant Z protein is appropriately transcribed and translated. The Z mutation affects the conformation of the protein at the hinge region of the reactive site and impedes proper folding. Only 15% of the Z protein is secreted successfully. The remaining 85% of the molecules never reach a secretion competent conformation and are retained in the hepatocyte (**Fig. 1**). The liver injury in AATD is caused by the accumulation of Z protein polymers [globules or periodic acid-Schiff (PAS)-Digestion resistant inclusions in hepatocytes], which initiates a cascade of liver cell death, apoptosis, compensatory proliferation, and fibrosis, which predisposing to cancerous changes. However, not all patients with PIZZ phenotype develop cirrhosis and liver disease. Genetic and environmental modifiers play an important role in the disease progression.[3]

Molecular and Cellular Pathophysiology of AAT ZZ Liver Disease

Perlmutter and colleagues showed the reduced intracellular clearance of mutant Z protein correlated to life-threatening liver disease, which gave strong support to the hypothesis that an accumulation of mutant Z protein in the liver was the key trigger of liver injury.[4] The accumulation hypothesis was also dramatically illustrated in various studies of mice transgenic for the human mutant Z gene. These mice retain their endogenous anti-protease genes but develop liver injury very similar to ZZ humans which seems to be caused by hepatic accumulation of mutant Z protein.[5] The discovery by Teckman and Perlmutter that autophagy was an important route of intracellular degradation for the mutant Z protein polymers, when combined with these other concepts, has led to multiple new therapeutic approaches.[6] The documentation by Teckman and Perlmutter of the hepatocellular apoptosis and compensatory proliferation in the liver revealed how mutant Z protein accumulation was likely linked to cirrhosis and hepatocellular carcinoma (HCC).[7,8]

Most of the retained mutant Z protein molecules are eventually directed to intracellular proteolysis pathways to reduce the intracellular mutant Z protein burden and reduce injury (**Fig. 2**).[6] These include ubiquitin dependent and ubiquitin independent proteasomal pathways as well as other mechanisms sometimes referred to as "ER-

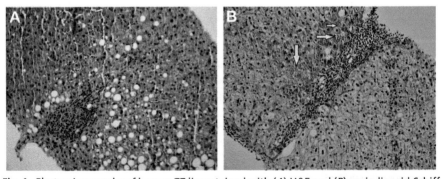

Fig. 1. Photomicrographs of human ZZ liver stained with (*A*) H&E and (*B*) periodic acid-Schiff followed by diastase digestion (PASd). PASd stains accumulations of glycoproteins red which can be easily identified on a neutral background. Normal liver is typically free of large, stainable glycoprotein masses. The globules (some highlighted by *arrows*) are variable in size and are not seen in all hepatocytes for unknown reasons.

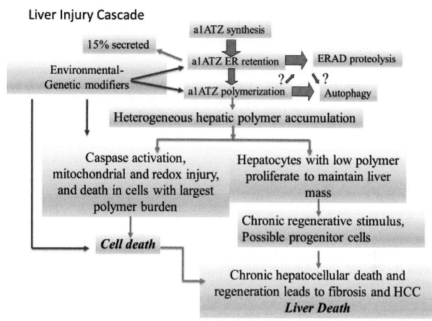

Fig. 2. Injury cascade of AAT mutant Z protein in liver. The AAT mutant Z protein is synthesized, but then 85% of the molecules are retained in the ER of hepatocytes rather than secreted. Quality control processes direct most of the mutant Z protein molecules to intracellular proteolysis (ERAD). However, some of the mutant Z protein molecules escape proteolysis and may attain a polymerized conformation forming inclusions in the ER. Autophagy is activated to degrade mutant Z polymer, but for reasons that are still unclear, some cells remain engorged with the large amount of mutant Z polymerized protein. In the population of cells with the largest polymer accumulations, hepatocellular death results from an uninhibited apoptotic cascade, redox injury, and possibly other mechanisms. Compensatory hepatocellular regeneration is stimulated to preserve functional liver mass. The chronic cycle of liver cell death and regenerations leads to fibrosis, HCC, and end organ injury. Given the variable nature of clinical liver injury between individuals with this same genotype, there are likely to be important genetic modifiers affecting the rate and magnitude of these processes.

associated degradation" (ERAD).[9] It is thought that the proteasomal pathways as a part of ERAD are the primary route for degradation for AAT mutant Z, newly synthesized, monomeric molecules, in the non-polymerized conformation. Studies in human fibroblast cell lines established from ZZ homozygous patients show that patients susceptible to liver disease have less efficient ERAD of AAT mutant Z protein than ZZ patients without liver disease.[10,11] Studies of the enzyme ManIBI also suggest that it may have a critical role in directing AAT mutant Z molecules to the proteasome for degradation.[12]

Autophagy is a highly conserved degradation system in which specialized vacuoles degrade abnormal proteins and larger structures such as senescent organelles. Studies show that the accumulation of the polymerized AAT mutant Z protein within cells induces an autophagic response and autophagy is an important route for the degradation of AAT mutant Z polymers.[6] In experimental systems, the liver injury can be reduced by the increased autophagic degradation of mutant Z polymer protein.[13–15]

In humans, some hepatocytes have more accumulation of Z protein, and others have less. Death occurs in cells with high accumulation.[8,16,17] These processes cause a low, but higher than normal, baseline rate of hepatocyte death in the ZZ liver tissue compared with normal liver. The cells with low polymer accumulation then proliferate to maintain the functional liver mass. Over time, the continued stress, death, and repair lead to liver fibrosis, cirrhosis, HCC, and chronic organ injury. Environmental and genetic modifiers of protein secretion, degradation, apoptosis, or regeneration would then by hypothesized to influence the progression of liver disease in an individual patient.[8]

Clinical Presentation

Liver disease associated with AATD is highly variable, ranging from mild self-limiting cholestasis in infancy to chronic hepatitis, cirrhosis, HCC, or the rare occurrence of fulminant hepatic failure.[18–20] The risk of life-threatening liver disease in children is about 3% to 5%.[16,21] In the neonatal period, the typical presentation is the "neonatal hepatitis syndrome," which includes cholestatic jaundice, pruritus, poor feeding, poor weight gain, hepatomegaly, and splenomegaly.[21,22] There are rare reports of severe vitamin K-deficient coagulopathic hemorrhage as the presenting feature of AATD in infants(van Hasselt, 2009 #257).

In toddlers and older children, ZZ AATD may present as asymptomatic chronic hepatitis [isolated alanine transaminase (ALT) and AST elevation], failure to thrive, possibly with poor feeding, or isolated portal hypertension, hepatomegaly, or splenomegaly. The occurrence of various liver-related abnormalities ranged from 15% to 50% in a Swedish cohort, although many were mild enough to likely escape medical attention without newborn screening.[21] Occasionally, children with previously unrecognized chronic liver disease and cirrhosis present with ascites, gastrointestinal bleeding due to portal hypertension, or hepatic failure. There has also been a common observation that some children with severe liver disease in the first few months or years of life may enter a "honeymoon period" with few signs or symptoms and normal growth, before entering a period of renewed progressive injury and decompensation as teenagers. There is recent evidence that portal hypertension may affect growth in children with AATD.[19,23–26]

AATD also causes emphysematous lung disease. Children do not develop emphysema, although they may be more prone to develop asthma. Children with AATD and pulmonary symptoms are evaluated in childhood, but most are seen by pulmonologists at age 18 years and followed by them regularly thereafter.

Natural History in Children

The best, prospective, unbiased data on the natural history of AATD are the study by Sveger and colleagues who screened 200,000 newborns in Sweden in the 1970s and identified 127 PIZZ.[20] Majority remained asymptomatic through childhood. Life-threatening liver disease occurred in about 3% to 5% of ZZ children in the first few months or years of life.[27] However, there is concern that the outcomes reported might not be fully representative of a less homogenous genetic population, such as North America, which may carry a different array of modifier genes.[28] Neonatal hepatitis seems to be the strongest factor associated with severe childhood liver disease as it was seen in the French DEFI alpha cohort.[29] Analysis of the Childhood Liver Disease Research Network (ChiLDReN) database cohort of 269 subjects showed that[30] neonatal cholestasis was only weakly associated with portal hypertension in children, with many severe subjects in later childhood without neonatal cholestasis.[23]

Adulthood and AAT-Associated Liver Disease

The exact burden of liver disease in adulthood is not well understood, as the condition seems to be underdiagnosed and commonly mistaken for NASH or alcoholic liver disease which have similar presentations but are much more common. The pathogenesis and natural history of liver disease are independent of lung disease. Liver biopsy findings in adults may include lobular inflammation, variable hepatocellular necrosis, fibrosis, cirrhosis, steatosis, and PAS-positive, diastase-resistant globules in some, but not all, hepatocytes, although rare patients may lack globules.[19]

Long-term data from the Swedish AATD cohort showed that after the childhood deaths, death compared with the population in general was the same up to middle age (43–45 years).[31] Further follow-up in the same cohort showed that age greater than 50 years, male sex, obesity, and diabetes seem to be factors which are associated with liver cirrhosis in PIZZ individuals. Seven percent had liver cirrhosis, and 2% had HCC. Data from a US study by Clark and colleagues also showed that high BMI and metabolic syndrome were associated with worse liver disease in PIZZ (Clark, 2018 #230). When data from PIZZ individuals from across Sweden outside of the birth cohort was examined, the mean age of onset of liver disease was 61 years.[32] However, AATD is still an underrecognized cause of liver disease in adults. A single-center retrospective review of 1400 pathology reports from explant livers for patients greater than 18 years of age was done by Shah and colleagues showed that 7.9% (117/1473) had PAS + globules suggestive of AATD. Only 36/117 (30.8%) had established this diagnosis before transplant.[33]

Heterozygotes and Liver Disease

Over 100 mutations in the AAT gene have been described based on the proteins isolated by gel electrophoresis which include F, S, Mmalton, Mduarte, and so forth. The ability of these proteins to cause liver disease is thought to be determined by the accumulation of heteropolymers (with Z protein) in the ER. Individuals with SZ phenotype have liver disease like ZZ phenotype due to the accumulation of SZ heteropolymers in the ER. They can have higher liver enzymes, and more frequent liver fibrosis, and primary liver cancer.[10,20,34–37] Other heterozygous phenotypes do not cause liver disease. A study done by the European AAT liver disease group Strnad and colleagues showed that PI*Z heterozygous variants were more prone to cirrhosis with NAFL and alcoholic liver disease, thus suggesting that PI*Z carriage could act as a disease modifier.[38]

The incidence of liver related outcomes in carriers of PIMZ phenotype has been described to be at least 2-fold higher and independent of factors such as age, BMI, and sex.[39] Hakim and colleagues found that the Z allele is associated with cirrhosis in a dose-dependent manner. Heterozygotes had higher odds of cirrhosis than noncarriers but much lower than PIZZ homozygotes. The liver injury markers such as ALT, AST, ALP, and gamma-glutamyl transpeptidase (GGT) were also higher in the heterozygotes than the noncarriers. They also found a significant interaction between BMI and Z allele carriage.[40] All these studies illustrate the burden of liver disease that could be related to Z allele carriage. Recent studies, however, also show that Pi*Z heterozygotes are "protected" against HCC (Rabekova, 2021 #217). Although the liver disease risk to any PIMZ individual is low, counseling about an avoidance of potential triggers like alcohol and healthy eating should be considered in those who are heterozygous for PIZ mutation.

Diagnosis and Monitoring

Laboratory evaluation in infants may reveal elevated total and/or conjugated bilirubin, serum aspartate transaminase,[41] and ALT, hypoalbuminemia, or coagulopathy due to liver synthetic dysfunction. The gold standard for the diagnosis of AATD is the analysis of the "phenotype" of AAT protein in a patient's serum or the genotype analysis of genomic DNA.[42] It is common in some liver clinics to use a serum AAT level as a screening test and then perform the gold standard test if the result is outside the normal range. Isolated, single AAT level results should be interpreted with caution as AAT is an acute phase reactant and even a ZZ patient will have modest increases in serum levels during times of systemic inflammation. Although a ZZ patient would not be expected to produce a level in the normal range, this author has seen SZ patients with liver disease occasionally have AAT levels reported in the normal range during episodes of systemic inflammation (**Table 1**). Serum AAT levels also seem to be higher in the neonatal period and then rapidly decrease to the more typical expected ranges later in the first year of life, a fact which may not be reflected in the reference ranges of some laboratories. Care should also be taken not to obtain serum for a level or phenotype if the patient has recently had a plasma transfusion, as is sometimes used to treat patients with severe liver disease, as the result will reflect the status of the plasma donor and not the host patient.

Given the unpredictability of disease progression, many authorities suggest regular monitoring of all PIZZ individuals for liver disease, on at least an annual basis, by a physician familiar with liver disease and its complications.[18] Monitoring should include history and physical examination sensitive for liver disease, such as a focus on the detection of splenomegaly. Laboratory examination including white blood cell count, platelet count, AST, ALT, alkaline phosphatase, albumin, bilirubin, and international normalized ratio.[38] Some data suggest that the GGT may be an especially sensitive indicator of liver disease.

Granulocytopenia, thrombocytopenia, climbing enzymes and bilirubin, and coagulopathy often accompany progressive liver injury in children and adults. Normal blood tests do not rule out liver disease, as it is well-known that individuals with life-threatening cirrhosis and portal hypertension can sometimes have normal blood tests, such as ALT. As in many liver diseases, a baseline liver ultrasound is considered useful as an adjunct to the physical examination to confirm spleen size and other signs of hepatobiliary health. Transient elastography is a noninvasive tool to study liver stiffness, which can be a measure of liver cirrhosis. It is validated in adults and helps identify patient with higher degree of fibrosis, who could then receive a liver biopsy. In a study done by the ChiLDReNs network, they showed that for children greater than 2 years of age, the liver stiffness measurement measure by TE correlated with liver injury markers such as GGT, INR, PELD score, and platelet count. It was also a strong predictor for poor prognostic factors like portal hypertension.

Table 1	
AAT genotypes and typical corresponding serum levels[54]	
Genotype	Level μM
PIMM	20–48 μM
PIMZ	12–35 μM
PISS	15–33 μM
PISZ	8–19 μM
PIZZ	2.5–7.0 μM
Null-Null	0

Convert μM to mg/dl by 5.2 conversion factor.

The diagnosis of AATD does not require liver biopsy. Globular eosinophilic inclusions in some but not all hepatocytes are usually seen under conventional H&E stain, which represent dilated ER membranes engorged with polymerized AAT mutant Z protein (see **Fig. 1**).[43] Staining with PAS followed by digestion with diastase, a technique which stains glycoproteins red, is used to highlight the "globules" ("PAS-positive") within hepatocytes on a neutral background. The globules are not present in all hepatocytes or can be small and "dust-like" in small infants. Globules may be absent in the neonatal liver. Liver biopsy, however, can be an important tool to assess the degree of liver injury and is still regarded as the gold standard to determine the extent of hepatic fibrosis and diagnose cirrhosis.

All AATD patients regardless of the presence of lung disease are urgently cautioned to avoid cigarette smoke and other inhalation exposures. Some studies suggest that exposure to even secondhand smoke and environmental air pollutants in childhood is an important risk factor for the development of AATD-associated adult emphysema.[20,44,45] Therefore, ZZ children and their household contacts are urgently cautioned against smoking. Children with ZZ AATD generally do not develop clinically detectable emphysema, although they may be at increased risk for childhood asthma and may report various respiratory symptoms.[46,47] ZZ children are commonly referred to an adult pulmonologist at age 18 years for a baseline evaluation, unless asthma or other respiratory symptoms are present, in which case an earlier pulmonary evaluation is recommended.

Treatment

Current treatment for progressive liver injury is primarily supportive with attention to the prevention of malnutrition, rickets, coagulopathy, or managing the complications of portal hypertension such as ascites or variceal bleeding. Monitoring growth closely is important in children with silent portal hypertension and cirrhosis. Children with splenomegaly secondary to portal hypertension should be cautioned against splenic injury from contact sports, advised to abstain from alcohol, supplemented as needed with fat-soluble vitamins, surveyed for variceal bleeding, and cautioned to avoid nonsteroidal anti-inflammatory drugs (NSAIDs), as this can result in life-threatening bleeding even in well compensated individuals. Studies in animal models of AATD suggest that NSAIDs may be uniquely toxic to the ZZ liver even if cirrhosis is not present.[3] AAT is an acute phase reactant; hence, baseline constitutive high level of synthesis is increased in the presence of inflammation. In the case of AAT, the inflammation linked synthesis is released by prostaglandin inhibition.[42] Therefore, NSAIDs would be predicted to increase AAT synthesis and in the case of ZZ would increase hepatic accumulation and augment liver injury. Although never tested in humans, this process of increased ZZ liver injury associated with NSAIDs has been observed in animal model systems of AAT disease. Whereas high doses of acetaminophen might also be injurious, normal doses seem less likely to be toxic that normal doses of NSAIDs. Therefore, many authorities suggest overall NSAID avoidance in favor of moderate doses of acetaminophen for mild pain or fever in ZZ patients. There is no data regarding alcohol consumption in ZZ individuals who have no evidence of liver injury.

If progressive liver failure or uncompensated cirrhosis is present and becomes life-threatening, then liver transplantation is considered. In the United States, cadaveric organs are allocated by empirically derived severity scores for both children and adults, which are correlated with increasing risk of mortality without transplant. Early evaluation at a transplant center is recommended for patients with signs or symptoms of deterioration, although early listing and time on the list do not influence the severity scores in the United States. Many centers have reported excellent liver transplant outcomes for AATD, often better than the median benchmark outcomes for other liver diseases. Living-related liver transplants in infants (left lateral segment) and adults (split liver) are also reported as successful, including successful anecdotes when one of the donors is heterozygous, MZ for AAT.

New Therapeutic Technologies

Specific therapy for AATD is being investigated. The treatment options for AATD could be addressed to either reducing the production of the mutant protein, enhancing proper folding to enhance secretion or by increasing intracellular degradation of the retained, toxic protein by increasing autophagy, or other degradation pathways (**Fig. 3**).

ARO-AAT is a newly developed investigational siRNA therapeutic that showed reduction in the homopolymerized Z protein by 97.7% in mouse livers. On the repeat dosing, it also halted the accumulation of polymers in the liver and enhanced clearing of existing polymers. When administered in normal humans, there was a 90% reduction in serum AAT levels, which was sustained for 6 weeks on administration of single dose and 14 weeks if three doses were administered. Data from phase 2 human trials showed the significant reduction of Z protein from the liver, reduction of fibrosis, and improvement in liver injury markers. No significant side effects were reported. This drug is very promising, and further human trials are underway.[48]

Several gene repair technologies are also being investigated, including the recently developed clustered regularly interspersed short palindromic repeats method, but no human trials have yet begun, and in vitro reports are still limited.

There has been long-standing interest in chemical chaperone approaches to improve proper folding and to augment secretion of AAT mutant Z, instead of intrahepatic protein retention. Such an approach might treat the lung and the liver as well. The primary barrier to this approach is the sheer mass of AAT protein synthesized, which is up to 2 g/d in an adult. If a one-to-one binding stoichiometry is needed as part of the mechanism, then a huge mass of drug would need to be delivered to the ER of the hepatocytes.

Still, studies in cell culture have shown that several compounds promote the secretion of AAT, and one, 4-phenyl butyrate, was effective in the mouse model.[49] A pilot

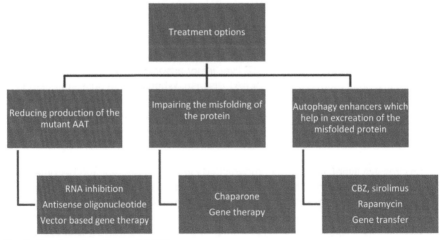

Fig. 3. Treatment options of AATD.

human trial was conducted, but no effect on secretion was detected, likely due to peak drug levels not able to reach the therapeutic range documented in the mouse.[50] Strategies designed in silico or cell-free systems for therapeutic disruption of mutant Z protein polymerization, likely an event distal to the protein retention signal, have also been examined in a number of studies.[51,52] However, many of the compounds examined have not had the predicted effect when examined in cell culture and there have been chemical hurdles to creating medicinal molecules for trials in animal models.

Autophagy is an intracellular degradation pathway known to play an importing role in trying to compensate for the accumulation of misfolded mutant Z protein in the liver. Sirolimus, carbamazepine, and the bile acid nor-UDCA, plus a genetic approach to augment expression of key autophagy regulators have all been shown to reduce mutant Z protein accumulation within cells via enhanced autophagy and to reduce liver cell injury in model systems. A human trial of low-dose carbamazepine in ZZ patients with cirrhosis was closed with no results released. Finally, several studies, including human trials, have examined strategies to synthesize WT AAT in tissues outside the liver, which might increase serum levels to protect the lung, but which would not change the risk of liver injury.[53,54] To date, these studies have only been able to generate less than 5% of the WT serum AAT level thought to be needed for therapeutic benefit.

SUMMARY

Homozygous ZZ AATD is a common genetic metabolic liver disease. The clinical manifestations are highly variable, with many patients remaining healthy or exhibiting only mild biochemical abnormalities. An accumulation of the AAT mutant Z protein within hepatocytes activates an intracellular injury cascade of apoptotic liver cell death and compensatory hepatocellular proliferation is leading to end organ injury. Genetic and environmental disease modifiers are thought to be important and are being investigated. There is no specific treatment for AAT-associated liver disease, but there are treatment options involving supportive measures and liver transplant. New technologies aimed at stimulating proteolysis via autophagy, small molecule chaperones, gene therapy, RNA technologies, gene repair, or cell transplantation may hold promise for the treatment of this disease. Many human liver studies in this disease are underway. Future research is likely to lead to studies of these new approaches, although the high degree of clinical variability will pose a challenge to the design of clinical trials.

CLINICS CARE POINTS

- Screen for alpha 1 antitrypsin deficiency in infants presenting with cholestasis.
- Monitor children with alpha 1 antitrypsin deficiency liver disease for complications like growth failure and portal hypertension, annually.
- Use of tylenol in therapeutic doses for pain control as needed is acceptable.
- NSAIDs can cause liver injury, and should be avoided.

REFERENCES

1. Teckman JH, Mangalat N. Alpha-1 antitrypsin and liver disease: mechanisms of injury and novel interventions. Expert Rev Gastroenterol Hepatol 2014;1–8.

2. JK Stoller, V Hupertz, and LS Aboussouan, Alpha-1 antitrypsin deficiency, A.H. Adam MP, Pagon RA, Editor. 2020.

3. Rudnick DA, Shikapwashya O, Blomenkamp K, et al. Indomethacin increases liver damage in a murine model of liver injury from alpha-1-antitrypsin deficiency. Hepatology 2006;44(4):976–82.

4. Wu Y, Whitman I, Molmenti E, et al. *A lag in intracellular degradation of mutant alpha 1-antitrypsin correlates with the liver disease phenotype in homozygous PiZZ alpha 1-antitrypsin deficiency.* Proc Natl Acad Sci U S A 1994;91(19): 9014–8.

5. Lomas DA, Evans DL, Finch JT, et al. The mechanism of Z alpha 1-antitrypsin accumulation in the liver. Nature 1992;357(6379):605–7.

6. Teckman JH, Perlmutter DH. Retention of mutant alpha(1)-antitrypsin Z in endoplasmic reticulum is associated with an autophagic response. Am J Physiol Gastrointest Liver Physiol 2000;279(5). G961-74.

7. Rudnick DA, Liao Y, An JK, et al. Analyses of hepatocellular proliferation in a mouse model of alpha-1-antitrypsin deficiency. Hepatology 2004;39(4):1048–55.

8. Lindblad D, Blomenkamp K, Teckman J. Alpha-1-antitrypsin mutant Z protein content in individual hepatocytes correlates with cell death in a mouse model. Hepatology 2007;46(4):1228–35.

9. Sifers RN. *Medicine.* Clearing conformational disease. Science 2010;329(5988): 154–5.

10. Teckman JH, Perlmutter DH. The endoplasmic reticulum degradation pathway for mutant secretory proteins alpha1-antitrypsin Z and S is distinct from that for an unassembled membrane protein. J Biol Chem 1996;271(22):13215–20.

11. Perlmutter DH. *Alpha-1-antitrypsin deficiency: importance of proteasomal and autophagic degradative pathways in disposal of liver disease-associated protein aggregates.* Annu Rev Med 2011;62:333–45.

12. Sifers RN. Intracellular processing of alpha1-antitrypsin. Proc Am Thorac Soc 2010;7(6):376–80.

13. Pastore N, Blomenkamp K, Annunziata F, et al. Gene transfer of master autophagy regulator TFEB results in clearance of toxic protein and correction of hepatic disease in alpha-1-anti-trypsin deficiency. EMBO Mol Med 2013;5(3): 397–412.

14. Kaushal S, Annamali M, Blomenkamp K, et al. Rapamycin reduces intrahepatic alpha-1-antitrypsin mutant Z protein polymers and liver injury in a mouse model. Exp Biol Med (Maywood) 2010;235(6):700–9.

15. Hidvegi T, Ewing M, Hale P, et al. An autophagy-enhancing drug promotes degradation of mutant alpha1-antitrypsin Z and reduces hepatic fibrosis. Science 2010; 329(5988):229–32.

16. Teckman JH, Mangalat N. *Alpha-1 antitrypsin and liver disease: mechanisms of injury and novel interventions.* Expert Rev Gastroenterol Hepatol 2015;9(2): 261–8.

17. Marcus NY, Blomenkamp K, Ahmad M, et al. Oxidative stress contributes to liver damage in a murine model of alpha-1-antitrypsin deficiency. Exp Biol Med (Maywood) 2012;237(10):1163–72.

18. Nelson DR, Teckman J, Di Bisceglie AM, et al. Diagnosis and management of patients with a(1)-antitrypsin (A1AT) deficiency. Clin Gastroenterol Hepatol 2011.

19. Perlmutter DH. Alpha-1-antitrypsin deficiency: diagnosis and treatment. Clin Liver Dis 2004;8(4):839–59, viii-ix.

20. American Thoracic Society/European respiratory Society statement: Standards for the Diagnosis and Management of Individuals with alpha-1 antitrypsin deficiency. Am J Respir Crit Care Med 2003;168(7):818–900.

21. Sveger T. Liver disease in alpha1-antitrypsin deficiency detected by screening of 200,000 infants. N Engl J Med 1976;294(24):1316–21.

22. Sveger T. Alpha 1-antitrypsin deficiency in early childhood. Pediatrics 1978; 62(1):22–5.

23. Teckman J, Rosenthal P, Hawthorne K, et al. Longitudinal outcomes in young patients with alpha-1-antitrypsin deficiency with native liver reveal that neonatal cholestasis is a poor predictor of Future portal hypertension. J Pediatr 2020; 227:81–86 e4.

24. Sveger T. The natural history of liver disease in alpha 1-antitrypsin deficient children. Acta Paediatr Scand 1988;77(6):847–51.

25. Mowat AP. Alpha 1-antitrypsin deficiency (PiZZ): features of liver involvement in childhood. Acta Paediatr Suppl 1994;393:13–7.

26. Pittschieler K, Massi G. Alpha 1 antitrypsin deficiency in two population groups in north Italy. Padiatr Padol 1988;23(4):307–11.

27. Sveger T, Eriksson S. The liver in adolescents with alpha 1-antitrypsin deficiency. Hepatology 1995;22(2):514–7.

28. Cruz PE, Mueller C, Cossette TL, et al. In vivo post-transcriptional gene silencing of alpha-1 antitrypsin by adeno-associated virus vectors expressing siRNA. Lab Invest 2007;87(9):893–902.

29. Ruiz M, Lacaille F, Berthiller J, et al. Liver disease related to alpha1-antitrypsin deficiency in French children: the DEFI-ALPHA cohort. Liver Int 2019;39(6): 1136–46.

30. Teckman JH, Rosenthal P, Abel R, et al. Baseline analysis of a young alpha-1-antitrypsin deficiency liver disease cohort reveals frequent portal hypertension. J Pediatr Gastroenterol Nutr 2015;61(1):94–101.

31. Mostafavi B, Piitulainen E, Tanash HA. Survival in the Swedish cohort with alpha-1-antitrypsin deficiency, up to the age of 43-45 years. Int J Chron Obstruct Pulmon Dis 2019;14:525–30.

32. Tanash HA, Piitulainen E. Liver disease in adults with severe alpha-1-antitrypsin deficiency. J Gastroenterol 2019;54(6):541–8.

33. Shah RS, Alsuleiman B, Bena J, et al. Alpha-1 antitrypsin deficiency is under-recognized in individuals with cirrhosis undergoing liver transplantation. Eur J Gastroenterol Hepatol 2020.

34. Lomas DA, Elliott PR, Sidhar SK, et al. Alpha 1-Antitrypsin Mmalton (Phe52-deleted) forms loop-sheet polymers in vivo. Evidence for the C sheet mechanism of polymerization. J Biol Chem 1995;270(28):16864–70.

35. Lomas DA, Finch JT, Seyama K, et al. Alpha 1-antitrypsin Siiyama (Ser53->Phe). Further evidence for intracellular loop-sheet polymerization. J Biol Chem 1993; 268(21):15333–5.

36. Mahadeva R, Chang WS, Dafforn TR, et al. Heteropolymerization of S, I, and Z alpha1-antitrypsin and liver cirrhosis. J Clin Invest 1999;103(7):999–1006.

37. Fromme M, Schneider CV, Pereira V, et al. Hepatobiliary phenotypes of adults with alpha-1 antitrypsin deficiency. Gut 2021.

38. Strnad P, Buch S, Hamesch K, et al. Heterozygous carriage of the alpha1-antitrypsin Pi*Z variant increases the risk to develop liver cirrhosis. Gut 2019; 68(6):1099–107.

39. Luukkonen PK, Salomaa V, Aberg F. The Pi *MZ Allele in alpha-1 antitrypsin increases liver-related Outcomes in a population-based study. Gastroenterology 2021;160(5):1874–5.

40. Hakim A, Moll M, Qiao D, et al. Heterozygosity of the alpha 1-antitrypsin Pi*Z allele and risk of liver disease. Hepatol Commun 2021;5(8):1348–61.

41. Schneider CV, Hamesch K, Gross A, et al. Liver phenotypes of European adults heterozygous or homozygous for Pi *Z variant of AAT (Pi *MZ vs Pi *ZZ genotype) and Noncarriers. Gastroenterology 2020;159(2):534–548 e11.

42. Shneider BL, Goodrich NP, Ye W, et al. Nonfasted liver stiffness correlates with liver disease Parameters and portal hypertension in Pediatric cholestatic liver disease. Hepatol Commun 2020;4(11):1694–707.

43. Piitulainen E, Sveger T. Respiratory symptoms and lung function in young adults with severe alpha(1)-antitrypsin deficiency (PiZZ). Thorax 2002;57(8):705–8.

44. Sveger T, Thelin T, McNeil TF. Young adults with alpha 1-antitrypsin deficiency identified neonatally: their health, knowledge about and adaptation to the high-risk condition. Acta Paediatr 1997;86(1):37–40.

45. Sveger T, Piitulainen E, Arborelius M Jr. Lung function in adolescents with alpha 1-antitrypsin deficiency. Acta Paediatr 1994;83(11):1170–3.

46. Eden E, Hammel J, Rouhani FN, et al. Asthma features in severe alpha1-antitrypsin deficiency: experience of the National Heart, lung, and blood Institute Registry. Chest 2003;123(3):765–71.

47. Wooddell CI, Blomenkamp K, Peterson RM, et al. Development of an RNAi therapeutic for alpha-1-antitrypsin liver disease. JCI Insight 2020;5(12).

48. Burrows JA, Willis LK, Perlmutter DH. Chemical chaperones mediate increased secretion of mutant alpha 1-antitrypsin (alpha 1-AT) Z: a potential pharmacological strategy for prevention of liver injury and emphysema in alpha 1-AT deficiency. Proc Natl Acad Sci U S A 2000;97(4):1796–801.

49. Teckman JH. Lack of effect of oral 4-phenylbutyrate on serum alpha-1-antitrypsin in patients with alpha-1-antitrypsin deficiency: a preliminary study. J Pediatr Gastroenterol Nutr 2004;39(1):34–7.

50. Mahadeva R, Dafforn TR, Carrell RW, et al. 6-mer peptide selectively anneals to a pathogenic serpin conformation and blocks polymerization. Implications for the prevention of Z alpha(1)-antitrypsin-related cirrhosis. J Biol Chem 2002;277(9): 6771–4.

51. Parfrey H, Dafforn TR, Belorgey D, et al. Inhibiting polymerization: new therapeutic strategies for Z alpha1-antitrypsin-related emphysema. Am J Respir Cell Mol Biol 2004;31(2):133–9.

52. Loring HS, Flotte TR. Current status of gene therapy for alpha-1 antitrypsin deficiency. Expert Opin Biol Ther 2015;15(3):329–36.

53. Flotte TR, Trapnell BC, Humphries M, et al. Phase 2 clinical trial of a recombinant adeno-associated viral vector expressing alpha1-antitrypsin: interim results. Hum Gene Ther 2011;22(10):1239–47.

54. American Thoracic S, European Respiratory S. American Thoracic Society/European Respiratory Society statement: standards for the diagnosis and management of individuals with alpha-1 antitrypsin deficiency. Am J Respir Crit Care Med 2003;168(7):818–900.

Hepatitis B and C in Children

A. Bailey Sperry[a], Aaron Bennett, MD[b], Jessica Wen, MD[b],*

KEYWORDS

- Viral hepatitis • Hepatitis B • Hepatitis C • Vertical transmission • Vaccine
- Interferon

KEY POINTS

- Hepatitis B and C in children most often occur via vertical transmission.
- There are 4 phases of chronic hepatitis B infection and treatment is indicated when there is persistent elevation in liver enzyme.
- Treatment for hepatitis C is indicated whenever there is chronic infection since cure can be achieved with anti-viral treatment.
- Direct-acting anti-viral is available for children age 3 and older and is well tolerated with high cure rate.

INTRODUCTION

Viral hepatitis is a significant global health burden. Hepatitis B and C specifically pose public health challenges given the development of chronic infections. Together, hepatitis B and C account for nearly 95% of deaths worldwide from viral hepatitis, surpassing human immunodeficiency virus (HIV) and tuberculosis. In 2016 the World Health Organization (WHO) recognized viral hepatitis as a pandemic, focusing on reducing transmission, increasing vaccination rates, and broadening access to treatment.

Hepatitis B and C are bloodborne infections. They are a particular risk to the pediatric population because of mother-to-child transmission and subsequent chronic disease. Engaging with the pediatric population plays a key role in reducing transmission and adult morbidity and mortality.

HEPATITIS B

Hepatitis B is a major contributor to acute and chronic liver disease worldwide. In 2019, the WHO estimated greater than 295 million people worldwide were living with chronic hepatitis B infections.[106] However, 90% were unaware of their infection

[a] Lewis Katz School of Medicine at Temple University, 3500 North Broad Street, Philadelphia, PA 19140, USA; [b] The Children's Hospital of Philadelphia, Perelman School of Medicine at the University of Pennsylvania, 3401 Civic Center Boulevard, Philadelphia, PA 19104, USA
* Corresponding author.
E-mail address: wenj@chop.edu

Clin Liver Dis 26 (2022) 403–420
https://doi.org/10.1016/j.cld.2022.03.005
1089-3261/22/© 2022 Elsevier Inc. All rights reserved.

due to lack of symptoms, inconsistent screening, passive surveillance, and underreporting.[1,2] Most of the chronic infections begin at birth or in the first few years of life, and pediatric patients have a much greater risk of developing complications from this disease.

Epidemiology

Hepatitis B has significant variation in prevalence by country and region. Hepatitis B surface antigen (HBsAg) positivity establishes a diagnosis of hepatitis B infection, with HBsAg positivity greater than or equal to 6 months defining a chronic infection.[3] Regions are considered endemic when the prevalence of HBsAg-positive persons is greater than or equal to 8%, intermediate if less than 8% and greater than or equal to 2%, and low endemicity if less than 2%.[4] Prevalence is highest in portions of east Asia and sub-Saharan Africa, with estimates that 5% to 10% of those adult populations have chronic hepatitis B virus (HBV) infection.[5] Regional and intercounty variation follows larger socioeconomic trends: vulnerable communities and low-income populations disproportionately live in endemic regions, and high-income regions tend to have low endemicity.[6] In developed countries, including the United States, most of the HBV infections are found among foreign-born persons who immigrated from high endemic regions or children born to immigrant parents.[3]

Mother-to-child transmission is responsible for nearly half of the global chronic HBV infections and is the primary mode of transmission worldwide.[7] In high endemic countries, particularly where vaccine coverage is poor, up to one-third of incident HBV infections may be acquired in early childhood due to horizontal transmission.[8,9]

Table 1
Geographic distribution of hepatitis B virus genotypes

Genotype	Subgenotype	Geographic Distribution
A	A1–A4	A1: Africa, South Asia A2: Europe, North America
B	B1–B5	B1: Japan B2: East Asia B3: Indonesia, Philippines, China
C	C1–C16	C1-C3: Southeast Asia, East Asia C4: Australian aborigines C6-C16: Indonesia
D	D1–D7	D1: Middle East D2: Europe/Africa D3: global D5: India D7: Africa
E	—	Western/Central Africa
F	F1–F4	South and Central Americas
G	—	France, Germany, United States
H	—	Mexico, Nicaragua
I	I1–I2	Southern China, Vietnam, Laos, India
J	—	Possibly originated from Borneo (Japanese man with HCC)

Adapted from Tong S, Revill P. Overview of hepatitis B viral replication and genetic variability. *J Hepatol.* 2016;64(1Suppl):S4-S16.

Natural History and Transmission

There are 10 identified genotypes of HBV (A–J) and each has a unique geographic profile (**Table 1**).[10] Genotype A is more prevalent in Europe, whereas B to F are more often seen in high endemicity regions.[11,12] In the United States, genotypes A to H have been documented, but A to C are most common.[13] However, increasing global travel and migration has affected geographic distribution.[11]

Genotype-specific characteristics may play a role in progression of infection, complication rates, and response to therapy.[14,15] For example, genotype A, most often found in North America or Africa, is associated with higher rates of antigen loss following interferon (IFN) therapy.[3,11] Genotype B, on the other hand, found mostly in East Asia, may have a slower progression to cirrhosis and a lower risk of development of hepatocellular carcinoma (HCC) when compared with genotype C, which is found mostly in Southeast Asia and the Western Pacific.[3,11]

Perinatal exposure and mother-to-child transmission account for most chronic infections, but HBV can also be passed through exposure to infectious bodily fluids (eg, blood, saliva, semen), nonsterile medical/dental procedures, or sharing unclean needles.[12] Although most adult infections in the United States are found in immigrant populations due to perinatal transmission in endemic countries, newly acquired adult infections are more often seen through horizontal transmission in vulnerable populations (ie, incarcerated persons) or those exhibiting high-risk behaviors (eg, unprotected sex with multiple partners, intravenous drug use).[3,6,8]

Testing

HBsAg positivity indicates HBV infection, but screening tools and chronic infection monitoring additionally use multiple antigen/antibody serologies (**Table 2**) as well as clinical markers to determine the stage of chronic infection and disease progression. The 2018 AALSD Guidance outlines high risk groups that should be screened for infection, including persons born in regions with greater than or equal to 2% HBsAg prevalence, those who have ever injected drugs, those requiring immunosuppressive therapy, those with greater than 1 sexual partner in the previous 6 months, those seeking treatment of a sexually transmitted infection or victims of sexual assault.[3]

Table 2	
Hepatitis B virus serologic markers	
HBsAg	Hepatitis B surface antigen: on the surface of the HBV virus, indicates HBV infection (acute or chronic); component of the HBV vaccine
HBsAb/anti-HBs	Hepatitis B surface antibody: indicates immunity from HBV infection
HBeAg	Hepatitis B e antigen: protein inside the nucleocapsid of HBV, when detected in serum indicates high infectivity, associated with high viral load
HBeAb/anti-HBe	Hepatitis e antibody: indicates decreasing levels of HBV DNA
HBcAg	Hepatitis B core antigen: protein on the nucleocapsid surface of HBV; indicates HBV replication during active infection
HBcAb/anti-HBc	Hepatitis B core antibody: indicates previous or ongoing HBV infection
HBcAb IgM/anti-HBc IgM	Hepatitis B core antibody (IgM): appears at the onset of acute hepatitis B infection (indicates recent infection vs chronic infection)

Table 3
Hepatitis B virus infection stage serologies

	HBsAg	HBsAb	HBeAg	HBeAb	HBcAb
Acute	+	−	+/−	−/+	+ (IgM)
Acute - Window	−	−	−	−	+ (IgM and/or IgG)
Chronic/immune tolerant	+	−	+	−	+ (IgG)
Chronic/Immune Active	+	−	+	−	+ (IgG)
Chronic/Inactive carrier	+	−	−	+	+ (IgG)
Cleared	−	+	−	+	+
Vaccinated	−	+	−	−	−

Recommended screening tests include HBsAg, anti-HBs, and anti-HBc of positive persons to distinguish their stage of infection (**Table 3**).

Vaccination

Hepatitis B is a vaccine-preventable disease. The vaccine, available since the 1980s, has shown that vaccination programs are incredibly effective at reducing childhood infections. Overall incidence dropped dramatically after the implementation of universal vaccination programs.[16] A report by the WHO in 2017 showed that HBsAg positivity in preschool children decreased from 4.7% pre-vaccination (1980s-early 2000s) to 1.3% in 2015.[107]

Perinatal transmission represents the biggest risk, and many vaccination protocols and screening guidance target pregnant women and newborns. In the United States, the 2018 AALSD Guidance supports screening all pregnant women for hepatitis B. If negative, and not previous vaccinated, vaccination is safe during pregnancy and may help protect the neonate via passive transfer of maternal antibodies.[3] In the United States, the Advisory Committee on Immunization Practices (ACIP) recommends all children should receive their first vaccine dose within 24 hours of birth, with second dose at 1 to 2 months and third dose between 6 and 18 months.[3,17]

If a pregnant woman is screened and found to be positive, the ACIP recommends her infant be vaccinated and receive hepatitis B immunoglobulin (HBIG) within 12 hours of delivery, in addition to postvaccination testing and regular completion of the vaccine series. If the mother was not screened during pregnancy and her HBsAg status is unknown, her infant should also be vaccinated within 12 hours of delivery.[3,17] HBIG is 75% effective at preventing infant infection, and together with vaccination, provides a 90% protection rate in HBeAg+ mothers and 98% protection in HBeAg− mothers.[18] Mothers of infants who received proper immunoprophylaxis at birth may breastfeed their children without an additional risk of transmission.[19]

For pregnant women who are infected with hepatitis B, antiviral therapy in their third trimester may be given to reduce perinatal transmission. For women who have high levels of HBV-DNA (>200,000 IU/mL) antiviral therapy is recommended through delivery or up to 4 weeks post partum.[3] Tenofovir disoproxil fumarate (TDF) has been shown to reduce mother-to-child transmission when given in the third trimester, without increases in adverse events for the exposed infants.[20–22] In addition, mothers on antiviral therapy may breastfeed their infants.[23,24]

Clinical Course

Most unvaccinated exposed adults, unlike children, clear an acute infection. The risk of chronic disease (≥6 months HBsAg+) is higher for infants and young children; up to

Table 4
Phases of chronic hepatitis B virus infection

	Immune-Tolerant	Immune-Active	Inactive Carrier	Reactivation
HBsAg	+ ≥6 mo	+ ≥6 mo	+ ≥6 mo	+ ≥6 mo
HBeAg	+	+ or −	−; HBeAb +	+ or −
HBV-DNA	High (>1 million IU/mL)	>20,000 IU/mL in HBeAg+ >2000 IU/mL in HbeAg−	<2000 IU/mL	Increased
ALT/AST	Normal or minimally elevated	Intermittent or persistent elevation	Normal (without intermittent elevations)	Increased
Biopsy	No fibrosis; minimal inflammation	Chronic hepatitis with inflammation; with or without fibrosis	Confirmed absence of significant inflammation; variable fibrosis	Inflammation or fibrosis
Treat?	No	Yes	No	Yes

90% of newborns exposed at birth will develop chronic HBV. The risk drops as children age, with 25% to 30% of children age 5 years or younger and less than 5% of older children exposed to HBV developing chronic infection.[18,28] Children who develop chronic infection, compared with adults, have much higher risk of cirrhosis and development of HCC. Twenty-five percent of infants who develop chronic HBV infection will die of chronic liver disease in adulthood.[12]

There are 4 phases of chronic hepatitis B infection: immune-tolerant, immune-active, inactive/carrier, and reactivation (**Table 4**). Chronicity is maintained due to HBV integration within the host genome and formation of covalently closed circular DNA (cccDNA) in hepatocellular nuclei.[25] Most children, particularly those infected at birth, are in the immune-tolerant phase. They are largely asymptomatic, without clinical evidence of infection or inflammation and normal liver function tests (LFTs) in the setting of HBeAg+ and measurable HBV-DNA levels. Many will stay in this phase until their early adult years, sometimes into their 30s.[26]

Patients are considered in the immune-active phase when they show clinical signs of hepatitis—elevated LFTs and evidence of liver inflammation and/or fibrosis. HBV-DNA levels are decreased from the immune-tolerant phase but still elevated. An extended duration of the immune-active phase, with extensive inflammation, is associated with development of cirrhosis and HCC.[27] Spontaneous seroconversion to anti-HBe is possible, although not common. Children are typically treated in this stage to reduce the risks of long-term sequelae, as elevated transaminases and increased viral load correspond with increased risk of progression to cirrhosis and development of HCC.[28]

After HBeAg/HBeAb seroconversion, children enter an inactive/chronic carrier state; this is typically accompanied by an improvement in clinical symptoms (falling LFTs, improved hepatic inflammation) and lowered HBV-DNA levels (<2000 IU/mL). Once children enter this stage, it is not recommended to treat but to instead monitor their condition for possible HBV reaction and disease progression. Because development of HCC is exceedingly rare in children, surveillance is limited to children with cirrhosis or a first-degree relative with HCC.[3]

Table 5
Approved therapies for chronic hepatitis B virus infection in children[32]

Therapeutic	Age	RoA	% Virological Response (vs Placebo)	Study
Interferon-α-2b	≥1 y	Subcutaneous injection 3x/weekly	26% (vs 11%)	Sokal EM 1998
Pegylated interferon-α-2b	≥3 y	Subcutaneous injection 1x/weekly	19.8% (vs 2%)	Wirth S 2018
Lamivudine	≥3 y	Oral solution or tables	23% (vs 13%)	Jonas MM 2002
Entecavir	≥2 y	Oral solution or tablets	24.2% (vs 3.3)	Jonas MM 2016
Adefovir	≥12 y	Tablets	10.6% (vs. 0)	Jonas MM 2008
Tenofovir disoproxil fumarate	≥12 y	Oral powder or tablets	21.2% (vs 0)	Murray KF 2012

HBV is considered cured when HBsAg and cccDNA are eliminated. More common is a "functional" cure, the loss of HBsAg and acquiring of anti-HBs antibodies. HBV genotype, HBV genomic mutations, level of viremia, and other risk factors, including genetic predispositions of the patient, will all contribute to a patient's overall lifetime risk of complications.[29]

Treatment

Treatment of HBV has progressed rapidly in the last decade, shifting from IFN therapy to nucleoside and nucleotide analogues (NAs) (**Table 5**). IFN-α and pegylated IFN (PEG-IFN) are immune modulators and encourage the host immune system to suppress replication, clear the virus, and induce seroconversion and loss of antigen positivity. IFN therapy is relatively cheaper and has limited duration of use, but it is a subcutaneous injection and has numerous systemic side effects.[8] IFN therapy is no longer considered a first-line treatment of all patients.

NAs, on the other hand, directly disrupt viral replication via DNA targets. Lamivudine and adefovir were the first generation, blocking HBV reverse transcriptase, but do not affect intrahepatic ccc-DNA, causing decreased HBsAg clearance.[30] The second generation of NAs, entecavir and tenofovir, are now considered the first-line agents with PEG-IFN during the immune-active phase. Entecavir is approved in children aged 2 years and older and has a low risk of drug resistance.[32] TDF is approved to treat infection in adults and children 2 years of age and older who weigh at least 10 kg.[32]

The goals of treatment of HBV are to reduce the risk of transmission and complications, including cirrhosis and HCC, and suppress HBV replication and therefore infectivity.[3] Recent guidelines support treating children only in an immune-active phase but not in an immune-tolerant phase. Treatment of children in the immune-tolerant phase has been tried, with the idea that breaking tolerance would lead to more rapid clearance of the infection. Studies were carried out with lamivudine and IFN-α, but the results were not promising.[33] A trial studying entecavir + PEG-IFN in immune-tolerant children had very few patients reaching the endpoint.[34]

Prevention/Prejudice

HBV is preventable with vaccination. Vaccination programs reduce new infections and overall global HBsAg seropositivity rates. However, to effectively eliminate HBV globally, improved treatments are necessary. Childhood chronic disease places significant social and economic burdens on infected children and their families. As children transition into adolescence and adulthood, increased education about horizontal and future vertical transmission is needed but is difficult due to the stigma surrounding chronic HBV infection.[35]

HEPATITIS C
Epidemiology

Hepatitis C has a global prevalence of 130 to 150 million infected persons, half being chronic infections. Three to five million are estimated to be individuals younger than 18 years.[5] Hepatitis C has been increasing in recent years, although variably among different regions.[36] Current screening methodologies and identification practices make exact calculations difficult, so these figures are likely underestimated. In the pediatric population, HCV is difficult to identify as many remain asymptomatic.[37]

Natural History

There are 6 major, and 2 newly identified, genotypes of HCV.[38–41] Genotypic variation in location (**Table 6**) is reported in adults and likely mirrors pediatric infections. Spread of globally present epidemic strains is thought to be due to infected blood and injection drug use before the identification of and testing for the virus.[40]

In adults, percutaneous blood exposure is the most common route of viral transmission. Transfusion-related transmission remains low in the United States after 1992 screening protocols were adopted.[42] Transmission is predominantly through needle-sharing—injection drug use and health care settings (eg, needlestick injuries).[43] In children, vertical transmission is most common.[44,45]

Vertical Transmission

Without universal screening at birth, HCV prevalence in infants is based on data in pregnant women.[105] Vertical transmission occurs in approximately 4% to 7% of infants born to HCV+ mothers and greater than or equal to 25% in HIV+/HCV+ mothers.[31,44,45] Although the rate of transmission remains roughly stable, the number of infected mothers is increasing correlated with the opioid epidemic, causing increasing perinatal infections and pediatric hepatitis.[46–50]

HCV can be transmitted during pregnancy or peripartum.[51,52] HCV-RNA found before day 3 of life indicates intrauterine transmission.[52] HCV-RNA positivity in the first month of life indicates peripartum infection. High viral load increases the risk of vertical transmission during pregnancy, and HIV coinfection has a 3- to 4-fold higher rate of HCV transmission.[53,54] However, antiretroviral therapy and low HIV viral loads during pregnancy have reduced the risk to comparable with HIV− women.[55,56]

Procedures that lead to fetal exposure of infected maternal blood may increase transmission risk, including both prolonged and premature rupture of membranes.[52] Amniocentesis, mode of delivery, and breastfeeding have not been shown to significantly increase the risk of vertical transmission. A mother's HCV+ status should not influence the decision to perform a C-section.[57,58] HCV+ mothers are encouraged to breastfeed their infants.[50,52]

Recent work has shown certain genetic factors may alter the risk of vertical HCV transmission.[59,60] HLA matching was greater in children who developed a chronic infection, whereas a maternal/fetal HLA mismatch was associated with increased viral clearance.[61,62] A single nucleotide polymorphism in the interleukin-28B gene was associated with spontaneous viral clearance in genotype 3 infection.[63,64] Evidence also shows pregnancy immune system modulations affect maternal HCV infection,

Table 6
Estimated global distribution of hepatitis C virus genotypes by global burden of disease region

Genotype	% of Global HCV Cases	GBD Region[a] Prevalence (in Descending Order) (N=Thousands)
1	46.2%	South & Southeast Asia (36,992)[b] South Asia (12,889) High Income Countries (9,954)[b] Central Asia/Eastern Europe (7,671)[b] Latin America (6,051)[b] Sub-Saharan Africa (6,050)[b] North Africa (3,808)
2	9.1%	South & Southeast Asia (10,016) Sub-Saharan Africa (1,879) High-income Countries (1,871) South Asia (1,333) Latin America (875) Central Asia/Eastern Europe (419) North Africa (115)
3	30.1%	South Asia (39,076)[b] South & Southeast Asia (7,093) Central Asia/Eastern Europe (2,951) High-income Countries (2,184) Latin America (1,129) North Africa (884) Sub-Saharan Africa (395)
4	8.3%	North Africa (9,118)[b] Sub-Saharan Africa (3,982) South Asia (1,413) High-income Countries (331) South & Southeast Asia (117) Central Asia/Eastern Europe (28) Latin America (27)
5	0.8%	Sub-Saharan Africa (1,328) South Asia (80) North Africa (47) High-income Countries (36) Latin America (5)
6	5.4%	South & Southeast Asia (9,711) South Asia (55) High-income Countries (31)
7	—	Found in Central African immigrants to Canada (Murphy DG 2015; Messina JP 2015)
8	—	Identified in India (Borgia SM 2018)

[a] Except Oceania.
[b] Most prevalent for the region.
Adapted from: Messina JP, Humphreys I, Flaxman A, et al. Global distribution and prevalence of hepatitis C virus genotypes. Hepatology. 2015;61(1):77-87.

Table 7
Monitoring pediatric patients with chronic hepatitis C infection before, during, and after treatment with direct-acting antivirals

Test	Before Treatment with DAAs	During DAA Treatment	Post-DAA Treatment
Liver function tests (AST, ALT, GGT, total and direct bilirubin)	At diagnosis, then every 6–12 mo	At 4 wk and as clinically indicated	12 wk posttreatment Every 6 mo (if cirrhotic)
CBC	At diagnosis, then every 6–12 mo	At 4 wk and as clinically indicated	If clinically indicated
Coagulation tests (PT, INR)	At diagnosis, then every 6–12 mo	If clinically indicated	If clinically indicated
HCV RNA (qPCR)	Annually	At 4 wk; can be considered at the end of treatment course	12 wk posttreatment, can be considered at 24 wk posttreatment, and 1 y posttreatment
Urine HCG (women of childbearing age)	Before initiating treatment	Every 4 wk (if sexually active)	N/A
Liver ultrasound (with or without alpha-fetoprotein)	Every 6 mo if cirrhotic, otherwise as needed	N/A	Every 6 mo if cirrhotic, until noncirrhotic

Adapted from Leung DH, Squires JE, Jhaveri R, et al. Hepatitis C in 2020: A North American Society for Pediatric Gastroenterology, Hepatology, and Nutrition Position Paper. *J Pediatr Gastroenterol Nutr.* 2020;71(3):407-417 and Ghany MG, Morgan TR, AASLD-IDSA Hepatitis C Guidance Panel. Hepatitis C Guidance 2019 Update: American Association for the Study of Liver Diseases-Infectious Diseases Society of America Recommendations for Testing, Managing, and Treating Hepatitis C Virus Infection. *Hepatology.* 2020;71(2):686-721.

allowing clearance and preventing transmission to her infant.[65] About 25% to 40% of children infected at birth will spontaneously clear their infection by age 2 years; afterward, 6% to 12% of children may spontaneously clear their infection before adulthood.[66]

Horizontal Transmission

Recently, the number of adolescents newly infected with hepatitis C is increasing. This trend correlates closely with increasing rates of intravenous drug use among teens and young adults and increasing numbers of children being hospitalized with HCV infections associated with substance use.[47,67,68]

HCV is associated with high-risk behaviors, such as drug use and high-risk sexual practices. Adults are often counseled on such risks, but these behaviors are commonly seen during adolescence. Greater discussion and counseling with younger patients regarding the risks of HCV transmission is needed, as worse outcomes for HCV infection are associated with these high-risk behaviors.[69–71]

As children living with chronic HCV grow into teenagers, they are at risk of spreading HCV to their peers through high-risk behaviors or passing the virus to a new generation. Harm reduction practices and prevention strategies that have previously focused on adults can, and should, also be directed at children and adolescents to prevent HCV transmission in this population.[72–74]

Screening

2020 updates to USPSTF and CDC Recommendations expanded screening criteria to better capture infections, including the screening of all pregnant women during each pregnancy. 2021 AAP recommendations indicate all children born to HCV+ mothers should be screened. Broader screening will increase identification of HCV infections, helping patients connect to treatment and halting future transmission.

Anti-HCV antibodies are used for screening, with subsequent testing for HCV-RNA to distinguish current from previous infections. Children aged 18 months or younger have waning maternal antibodies, so screening is typically not conducted until that age. Recommendations allow screening-exposed infants at 2 to 6 months of age for HCV-RNA if needed, with confirmatory follow-up serologic testing at 18 months.[75]

Infected children are evaluated annually for progression of their disease (**Table 7**). Intervention is rare at the age of 3 years and younger, given high rates of spontaneous clearance, the asymptomatic nature of most infections, and the lack of approved therapies. Untreated children are monitored with routine blood tests (eg, LFTs, complete blood count, and so forth) and HCV-RNA levels. Annual abdominal ultrasound is only indicated if there is a family history of early cirrhosis, HCC, or evidence of rapid disease progression.[50,105]

Clinical Course

Acute hepatitis C is very rare in pediatric patients. Only a single case of HCV-induced acute liver failure was documented in a database of 986 children.[76] Childhood morbidity from chronic HCV is uncommon; most remain asymptomatic.[77–79] Some patients may exhibit mild, nonspecific symptoms (eg, fatigue, abdominal pain).[80] Symptoms are more severe, and progression may be accelerated in children with comorbid conditions, such as HIV or HBV, childhood obesity, or cancer.[66,75,81,82] Worse outcomes are also associated with adverse social conditions, such as homelessness or incarceration.[69–71,83] Extrahepatic manifestations are very rare in children, but renal disease and thyroid involvement have been documented.[84–86]

Because progression is insidious, advanced liver disease is uncommon in the pediatric population, and newer treatments greatly reduce this risk.[87–89] Complications from chronic liver disease in children and adolescents are rare.[87,90,91] Children often experience transaminase elevations, which do not correlate with histologic severity seen on biopsy.[92] Cirrhosis develops in 1% to 2% of the population, but they rarely require transplantation.[93,94] In one study 30% developed cirrhosis, with median age of onset 33 years,[95] but cases of children younger than 5 years with decompensated cirrhosis are documented. Development of HCC in the pediatric population has been reported but is exceedingly rare.[90] This risk may be increased by comorbid conditions, including diabetes and obesity.[82]

Treatment

Treatment options for hepatitis C have expanded dramatically in the last decade. Eradication of the virus before adolescence decreases complication risks, reduces horizontal transmission among high-risk populations, and may help decrease the stigmatization of HCV infection.

Historically, the treatment of HCV was PEG-IFN + ribavirin. The PEDS-C trial assessing PEG-IFN + ribavirin was the first multicenter controlled trial for the treatment of pediatric chronic HCV infection in the United States.[96,97] The development and Food and Drug Administration approval of direct-acting antivirals (DAAs) for use in children has now largely replaced this therapeutic option.[98]

Table 8
Approved treatment regimens for chronic hepatitis C virus infection in children[32]

Drug Regimen	Age Range	Genotype	Duration of Treatment	Dosage	SVR12 (%)/Study
Sofosbuvir/ledipasvir (Harvoni)	≥3 y	GT 1, 4, 5, 6 without/with compensated cirrhosis; GT 1 with decompensated cirrhosis (+ribavirin)	12 wk Except: GT 1 treatment experienced with compensated cirrhosis: 24 wk	<17 kg: 150/33.75 mg/d 17–<35 kg: 200/45 mg/d>= 35 kg: 400/90 mg/d	97–99 Balistreri et al, 2017; Murray KF 2018; Schwarz KB 2020;
Glecaprevir/pibrentasvir (Mavyret)	≥3 y	GT 1–6 without/with compensated cirrhosis; GT 1 treatment experienced	Treatment naïve Without/ with compensated cirrhosis: 8 wk Treatment experienced: 8–16 wk (based on GT and presence of cirrhosis)	<20 kg: 150/60 mg/d 20–<30 kg: 200/80 mg/d 30–<45 kg: 250/100 mg/d ≥45 kg OR ≥12 yrs: 300/120 mg/d	100 Jonas MM 2019; Jonas MM 2020
Sofosbuvir/velpatasvir (Epclusa)	≥3 y	GT 1–6 without/with compensated cirrhosis; GT 1–6 with decompensated cirrhosis (+ribavirin)	12 wk	<17 kg: 150/37.5 mg/d 17–<30 kg: 200/50 mg/d ≥30 kg: 400/100 mg/d	92 Sokal EM 2020
Sofosbuvir + ribavirin (Sovaldi + ribavirin) Not recommended regimen	≥3 y	GT 2, 3 without/with compensated cirrhosis	GT 2: 12 wk GT 3: 24 wk	Sofosbuvir: <17 kg: 150 mg/d 17–<35 kg: 200 mg/d ≥35 kg: 400 mg	98 Wirth S 2017; Rosenthal P 2020;

DAAs are approved in the United States in children aged 3 years and older and have shown better response over historical treatments (**Table 8**) with fewer risks and side effects. They are easier to administer because of their short duration of treatment, oral formulation, and the lack of required monitoring during treatment.

There are currently 3 types of DAAs: NS5A inhibitors, NS5B polymerase inhibitors, and NS3/4A protease inhibitors.[99] Ledipasvir/sofosbuvir was the first DAA approved for use in the pediatric population. A once daily regimen for 12 weeks in children older than 12 years infected with genotypes 1, 4, 5, or 6 was the original indication, but approval has been extended to children aged 3 years and older.[100] Sofosbuvir/ribavirin was initially approved for genotypes 2 and 3, as an option for those ineligible for treatment with ledipasvir/sofosbuvir, but due to ribavirin side effects and the availability of newer pangenotypic DAAs, it is no longer recommended.[50,101,102] Glecaprevir/pibrentasvir is approved for all 6 genotypes in children aged 3 years and older and is only 8 weeks of treatment for treatment-naïve children with or without cirrhosis, but treatment is extended in treatment-experienced patients.[103] Sofosbuvir/velpatasvir is another pangenotypic regimen approved for children aged 3 years and older.[104]

SUMMARY

Hepatitis B and C remain a global health burden. Universal vaccination in early childhood will significantly decrease the incidence of chronic hepatitis B, whereas new therapeutic options for hepatitis C can greatly reduce morbidity and mortality. Addressing this pandemic cannot be achieved without intervention in the pediatric population.

Although mother-to-child transmission is the most common route for children to acquire a chronic hepatitis infection, special consideration must be given to adolescents. The increase in new infections in this group emphasizes the gap in treating existing infections, preventing peer-to-peer horizontal transmission and vertical transmission to the next generation. Public health interventions, educational programs, and counseling are needed in this age group and can reduce the stigma and prejudice surrounding children living with these chronic diseases.

CLINICS CARE POINTS

- Hepatitis B is a vaccine preventable disease most commonly acquired via vertical transmission.
- Defining stage of chronic hepatitis B infection can appropriately identify patients requiring therapy.
- Horizontal transmission rates of hepatitis C are growing in the pediatric population, mainly through adolescents, creating additional concern given inconsistent screening via anti-hepatitis C antibody.
- The options for hepatitis C therapy continue to expand, increasing accessible and affordable treatment opportunities for vulnerable populations.

DISCLOSURE

J. Wen is a consultant for Gilead Sciences and receives research support from Abbvie, Gilead Sciences, and Alexion.

REFERENCES

1. Bousali M, Papatheodoridis G, Paraskevis D, Karamitros T. Hepatitis B virus DNA integration, chronic infections and hepatocellular carcinoma. Microorganisms 2021;9(8):1787.
2. Polaris Observatory Collaborators. Global prevalence, treatment, and prevention of hepatitis B virus infection in 2016: a modelling study. Lancet Gastroenterol Hepatol 2018;3(6):383–403.
3. Terrault NA, Lok ASF, McMahon BJ, et al. Update on prevention, diagnosis, and treatment of chronic hepatitis B: AASLD 2018 hepatitis B guidance. Hepatology 2018;67(4):1560–99.
4. Nelson NP, Easterbrook PJ, McMahon BJ. Epidemiology of hepatitis B virus infection and impact of vaccination on disease. Clin Liver Dis 2016;20(4): 607–28.
5. Global health sector Strategy on viral hepatitis 2016-2021. Geneva (Switzerland): World Health Organization; 2016.
6. Tu T, Block JM, Wang S, et al. The lived experience of chronic hepatitis B: a broader view of its impacts and why we need a cure. Viruses 2020;12(5):515.
7. Shah U, Kelly D, Chang MH, et al. Management of chronic hepatitis B in children. J Pediatr Gastroenterol Nutr 2009;48(4):399–404.
8. Indolfi G, Easterbrook P, Dusheiko G, et al. Hepatitis B virus infection in children and adolescents. Lancet Gastroenterol Hepatol 2019;4(6):466–76.
9. Ling SC, Lin HS, Murray KF, et al. Chronic hepatitis is common and often untreated among children with hepatitis B infection in the United States and Canada. J Pediatr 2021;237:24–33.e12.
10. Kramvis A. Genotypes and genetic variability of hepatitis B virus. Intervirology 2014;57(3–4):141–50.
11. Tong S, Revill P. Overview of hepatitis B viral replication and genetic variability. J Hepatol 2016;64(1Suppl):S4–16.
12. Sokal EM, Nannini P. Chapter 6.1. Pediatric chronic hepatitis B and C: 30 Years of ESPGHAN clinical research and recommendations. J Pediatr Gastroenterol Nutr 2018;66Suppl1:S119–21.
13. Ghany MG, Perrillo R, Li R, et al. Characteristics of adults in the hepatitis B research network in North America reflect their country of origin and hepatitis B virus genotype. Clin Gastroenterol Hepatol 2015;13(1):183–92.
14. Lin CL, Kao JH. Natural history of acute and chronic hepatitis B: the role of HBV genotypes and mutants. Best Pract Res Clin Gastroenterol 2017;31(3):249–55.
15. Marcellin P, Ahn SH, Ma X, et al. Combination of tenofovir disoproxil fumarate and peginterferonα-2a increases loss of hepatitis B surface antigen in patients with chronic hepatitis B. Gastroenterology 2016;150(1):134–44.e10.
16. Zanella B, Bechini A, Boccalini S, et al. Hepatitis B seroprevalence in the pediatric and adolescent population of florence (Italy): An update 27 years after the Implementation of Universal Vaccination. Vaccines (Basel) 2020;8(2):156.
17. Schillie S, Vellozzi C, Reingold A, et al. Prevention of hepatitis B virus infection in the United States: recommendations of the advisory committee on immunization practices. MMWR Recomm Rep 2018;67(1):1–31.
18. Sokal EM, Paganelli M, Wirth S, et al. Management of chronic hepatitis B in childhood: ESPGHAN clinical practice guidelines. J Hepatol 2013;59(4):814–29.
19. Wang JS, Zhu QR, Wang XH. Breastfeeding does not pose any additional risk of immunoprophylaxis failure on infants of HBV carrier mothers. Int J Clin Pract 2003;57(2):100–2.

20. Pan CQ, Duan Z, Dai E, et al. Tenofovir to prevent hepatitis B transmission in mothers with high viral load. N Engl J Med 2016;374(24):2324–34.
21. Chen HL, Lee CN, Chang CH, et al. Efficacy of maternal tenofovir disoproxil fumarate in interrupting mother-to-infant transmission of hepatitis B virus. Hepatology 2015;62(2):375–86.
22. Jao J, Abrams EJ, Phillips T, et al. In utero tenofovir exposure is not associated with fetal long bone growth. Clin Infect Dis 2016;62(12):1604–9.
23. Benaboud S, Pruvost A, Coffie PA, et al. Concentrations of tenofovir and emtricitabine in breast milk of HIV-1-infected women in Abidjan, Cote d'Ivoire. Antimicrob Agents Chemother 2011;55(3):1315–7.
24. Mirochnick M, Taha T, Kreitchmann R, et al. Pharmacokinetics and safety of tenofovir in HIV-infected women during labor and their infants during the first week of life. J Acquir Immune Defic Syndr 2014;65(1):33–41.
25. Coffin CS, Schreiber RA. Hepatitis B in children-the pursuit of a hepatitis free future generation. J Pediatr 2021;237:9–11.
26. Bortolotti F, Guido M, Bartolacci S, et al. Chronic hepatitis B in children after e antigen seroclearance: final report of a 29-year longitudinal study. Hepatology 2006;43(3):556–62.
27. Paganelli M, Stephenne X, Sokal EM. Chronic hepatitis B in children and adolescents. J Hepatol 2012;57(4):885–96.
28. Lee MH, Yang HI, Liu J, et al. Prediction models of long-term cirrhosis and hepatocellular carcinoma risk in chronic hepatitis B patients: risk scores integrating host and virus profiles. Hepatology 2013;58(2):546–54.
29. Levrero M, Zucman-Rossi J. Mechanisms of HBV-induced hepatocellular carcinoma. J Hepatol 2016;64(1Suppl):S84–101.
30. Torre P, Aglitti A, Masarone M, Persico M. Viral hepatitis: Milestones, unresolved issues, and future goals. World J Gastroenterol 2021;27(28):4603–38.
31. Dunkelberg JC, Berkley EM, Thiel KW, Leslie KK. Hepatitis B and C in pregnancy: a review and recommendations for care. J Perinatol 2014;34(12):882–91.
32. Nicastro E, Norsa L, Di Giorgio A, et al. Breakthroughs and challenges in the management of pediatric viral hepatitis. World J Gastroenterol 2021;27(20):2474–94.
33. D'Antiga L, Aw M, Atkins M, et al. Combined lamivudine/interferon-alpha treatment in "immunotolerant" children perinatally infected with hepatitis B: a pilot study. J Pediatr 2006;148(2):228–33.
34. Rosenthal P, Ling SC, Belle SH, et al. Combination of Entecavir/Peginterferon Alfa-2a in Children With Hepatitis B e Antigen-Positive Immune-Tolerant Chronic Hepatitis B Virus Infection. Hepatology 2019;69(6):2326–37.
35. Valizadeh L, Zamanzadeh V, Bayani M, Zabihi A. The social stigma experience in patients with hepatitis B infection: a Qualitative study. Gastroenterol Nurs 2017;40(2):143–50.
36. El-Shabrawi MH, Kamal NM. Burden of pediatric hepatitis C. World J Gastroenterol 2013;19(44):7880–8.
37. Schmelzer J, Dugan E, Blach S, et al. Global prevalence of hepatitis C virus in children in 2018: a modelling study. Lancet Gastroenterol Hepatol 2020;5(4):374–92.
38. Pisano MB, Giadans CG, Flichman DM, et al. Viral hepatitis update: progress and perspectives. World J Gastroenterol 2021;27(26):4018–44.
39. Murphy DG, Sablon E, Chamberland J, et al. Hepatitis C virus genotype 7, a new genotype originating from central Africa. J Clin Microbiol 2015;53(3):967–72.

40. Messina JP, Humphreys I, Flaxman A, et al. Global distribution and prevalence of hepatitis C virus genotypes. Hepatology 2015;61(1):77–87.

41. Borgia SM, Hedskog C, Parhy B, et al. Identification of a Novel hepatitis C virus genotype from Punjab, India: Expanding classification of hepatitis C virus into 8 genotypes. J Infect Dis 2018;218(11):1722–9.

42. Luban NL, Colvin CA, Mohan P, Alter HJ. The epidemiology of transfusion-associated hepatitis C in a children's hospital. Transfusion 2007;47(4):615–20.

43. Jafari S, Copes R, Baharlou S, et al. Tattooing and the risk of transmission of hepatitis C: a systematic review and meta-analysis. Int J Infect Dis 2010; 14(11):e928–40.

44. Benova L, Mohamoud YA, Calvert C, Abu-Raddad LJ. Vertical transmission of hepatitis C virus: systematic review and meta-analysis. Clin Infect Dis 2014; 59(6):765–73.

45. Kanninen TT, Dieterich D, Asciutti S. HCV vertical transmission in pregnancy: new horizons in the era of DAAs. Hepatology 2015;62(6):1656–8.

46. Centers for Disease Control and Prevention (CDC). Hepatitis C virus infection among adolescents and young adults:Massachusetts, 2002-2009. MMWR Morb Mortal Wkly Rep 2011;60(17):537–41.

47. Suryaprasad AG, White JZ, Xu F, et al. Emerging epidemic of hepatitis C virus infections among young nonurban persons who inject drugs in the United States, 2006-2012. Clin Infect Dis 2014;59(10):1411–9.

48. Ly KN, Jiles RB, Teshale EH, et al. Hepatitis C virus infection among Reproductive-aged women and children in the United States, 2006 to 2014. Ann Intern Med 2017;166(11):775–82.

49. Patrick SW, Bauer AM, Warren MD, et al. Hepatitis C virus infection among women giving birth-Tennessee and United States, 2009-2014. MMWR Morb Mortal Wkly Rep 2017;66(18):470–3.

50. Leung DH, Squires JE, Jhaveri R, et al. Hepatitis C in 2020: a North American society for pediatric Gastroenterology, Hepatology, and Nutrition position paper. J Pediatr Gastroenterol Nutr 2020;71(3):407–17.

51. Mok J, Pembrey L, Tovo PA, et al. When does mother to child transmission of hepatitis C virus occur? Arch Dis Child Fetal Neonatal Ed 2005;90(2):F156–60.

52. Pott H, Theodoro M, de Alemida Vespoli J, et al. Mother-to-child transmission of hepatitis C virus. Eur J Obstet Gynecol Reprod Biol 2018;224:125–30.

53. Polis CB, Shah SN, Johnson K, Gupta A. Impact of maternal HIV coinfection on the vertical transmission of hepatitis C virus: a meta-analysis. Clin Infect Dis 2007;44(8):1123–31.

54. Tovo PA, Palomba E, Ferraris G, et al. Increased risk of maternal-infant hepatitis C virus transmission for women coinfected with human immunodeficiency virus type 1. Clin Infect Dis 1997;25(5):1121–4.

55. Checa Cabot CA, Stoszek SK, Quarleri J, et al. Mother-to-Child transmission of hepatitis C virus (HCV) among HIV/HCV-coinfected women. J Pediatr Infect Dis Soc 2013;2(2):126–35.

56. Snijdewind IJ, Smit C, Schutten M, et al. Low mother-to-child-transmission rate of Hepatitis C virus in cART treated HIV-1 infected mothers. J Clin Virol 2015; 68:11–5.

57. Hughes BL, Page CM, Kuller JA, Society for Maternal-Fetal Medicine (SMFM). Hepatitis C in pregnancy: screening, treatment, and management. Am J Obstet Gynecol 2017;217(5):B2–12.

58. Espinosa C, Jhaveri R, Barritt AS. Unique challenges of hepatitis C in infants, children, and adolescents. Clin Ther 2018;40(8):1299–307.

59. Ruiz-Extremera A, Muñoz-Gámez JA, Salmerón-Ruiz MA, et al. Genetic variation in interleukin 28B with respect to vertical transmission of hepatitis C virus and spontaneous clearance in HCV-infected children. Hepatology 2011;53(6): 1830–8.

60. Fitzmaurice K, Hurst J, Dring M, et al. Additive effects of HLA alleles and innate immune genes determine viral outcome in HCV infection. Gut 2015;64(5):813–9.

61. Bevilacqua E, Fabris A, Floreano P, et al. Genetic factors in mother-to-child transmission of HCV infection. Virology 2009;390(1):64–70.

62. Ruiz-Extremera A, Pavón-Castillero EJ, Florido M, et al. Influence of HLA class I, HLA class II and KIRs on vertical transmission and chronicity of hepatitis C virus in children. PLoS One 2017;12(2):e0172527.

63. Resti M, Jara P, Hierro L, et al. Clinical features and progression of perinatally acquired hepatitis C virus infection. J Med Virol 2003;70(3):373–7.

64. Indolfi G, Mangone G, Calvo PL, et al. Interleukin 28B rs12979860 single-nucleotide polymorphism predicts spontaneous clearance of hepatitis C virus in children. J Pediatr Gastroenterol Nutr 2014;58(5):666–8.

65. Honegger JR, Kim S, Price AA, et al. Loss of immune escape mutations during persistent HCV infection in pregnancy enhances replication of vertically transmitted viruses. Nat Med 2013;19(11):1529–33.

66. Mack CL, Gonzalez-Peralta RP, Gupta N, et al. NASPGHAN practice guidelines: diagnosis and management of hepatitis C infection in infants, children, and adolescents. J Pediatr Gastroenterol Nutr 2012;54(6):838–55.

67. Zibbell JE, Iqbal K, Patel RC, et al. Increases in hepatitis C virus infection related to injection drug use among persons aged ≤30 years - Kentucky, Tennessee, Virginia, and West Virginia, 2006-2012. MMWR Morb Mortal Wkly Rep 2015; 64(17):453–8.

68. Barritt AS, Lee B, Runge T, et al. Increasing prevalence of hepatitis C among hospitalized children is associated with an increase in substance abuse. J Pediatr 2018;192:159–64.

69. Beech BM, Myers L, Beech DJ. Hepatitis B and C infections among homeless adolescents. Fam Community Health 2002;25(2):28–36.

70. Murray KF, Richardson LP, Morishima C, et al. Prevalence of hepatitis C virus infection and risk factors in an incarcerated juvenile population. Pediatrics 2003;111(1):153–7.

71. Page K, Hahn JA, Evans J, et al. Acute hepatitis C virus infection in young adult injection drug users: a prospective study of incident infection, resolution, and reinfection. J Infect Dis 2009;200(8):1216–26.

72. Grebely J, Dore GJ, Morin S, et al. Elimination of HCV as a public health concern among people who inject drugs by 2030 - what will it take to get there? J Int AIDS Soc 2017;20(1):22146.

73. Martin NK, Hickman M, Hutchinson SJ, et al. Combination interventions to prevent HCV transmission among people who inject drugs: modeling the impact of antiviral teatment, needle and syringe programs, and opiate substitution therapy. Clin Infect Dis 2013;57(Suppl2):S39–45.

74. Indolfi G, Bailey H, Serranti D, et al. Treatment and monitoring of children with chronic hepatitis C in the Pre-DAA era: a European survey of 38 paediatric specialists. J Viral Hepat 2019;26(8):961–8.

75. Committee on Infectious Diseases, American Academy of Pediatrics. Red Book: 2021-2024 Report of the Committee on Infectious Diseases. 32nd edition. Itasca, IL: American Academy of Pediatrics; 2021.

76. Narkewicz MR, Horslen S, Hardison RM, et al. A Learning collaborative approach increases specificity of diagnosis of acute liver failure in pediatric patients. Clin Gastroenterol Hepatol 2018;16(11):1801–10.e3.

77. Squires JE, Balistreri WF. Hepatitis C virus infection in children and adolescents. Hepatol Commun 2017;1(2):87–98.

78. Jonas MM, Baron MJ, Bresee JS, Schneider LC. Clinical and virologic features of hepatitis C virus infection associated with intravenous immunoglobulin. Pediatrics 1996;98(2Pt1):211–5.

79. Squires RH, Shneider BL, Bucuvalas J, et al. Acute liver failure in children: the first 348 patients in the pediatric acute liver failure study group. J Pediatr 2006;148(5):652–8.

80. European Paediatric Hepatitis C Virus Network. Three broad modalities in the natural history of vertically acquired hepatitis C virus infection. Clin Infect Dis 2005;41(1):45–51.

81. Cesaro S, Bortolotti F, Petris MG, et al. An updated follow-up of chronic hepatitis C after three decades of observation in pediatric patients cured of malignancy. Pediatr Blood Cancer 2010;55(1):108–12.

82. Dyal HK, Aguilar M, Bhuket T, et al. Concurrent obesity, diabetes, and steatosis increase risk of advanced fibrosis among HCV patients: a systematic review. Dig Dis Sci 2015;60(9):2813–24.

83. Serra MA, Escudero A, Rodríguez F, et al. Effect of hepatitis C virus infection and abstinence from alcohol on survival in patients with alcoholic cirrhosis. J Clin Gastroenterol 2003;36(2):170–4.

84. Bortolotti F, Vajro P, Balli F, et al. Non-organ specific autoantibodies in children with chronic hepatitis C. J Hepatol 1996;25(5):614–20.

85. Gregorio GV, Pensati P, Iorio R, et al. Autoantibody prevalence in children with liver disease due to chronic hepatitis C virus (HCV) infection. Clin Exp Immunol 1998;112(3):471–6.

86. Indolfi G, Bartolini E, Olivito B, et al. Autoimmunity and extrahepatic manifestations in treatment-naïve children with chronic hepatitis C virus infection. Clin Dev Immunol 2012;2012:785627.

87. Bortolotti F, Verucchi G, Cammà C, et al. Long-term course of chronic hepatitis C in children: from viral clearance to end-stage liver disease. Gastroenterology 2008;134(7):1900–7.

88. Lee CK, Jonas MM. Hepatitis C: issues in children. Gastroenterol Clin North Am 2015;44(4):901–9.

89. Guido M, Bortolotti F, Leandro G, et al. Fibrosis in chronic hepatitis C acquired in infancy: is it only a matter of time? Am J Gastroenterol 2003;98(3):660–3.

90. González-Peralta RP, Langham MR, Andres JM, et al. Hepatocellular carcinoma in 2 young adolescents with chronic hepatitis C. J Pediatr Gastroenterol Nutr 2009;48(5):630–5.

91. Jara P, Resti M, Hierro L, et al. Chronic hepatitis C virus infection in childhood: clinical patterns and evolution in 224 white children. Clin Infect Dis 2003;36(3):275–80.

92. Mohan N, González-Peralta RP, Fujisawa T, et al. Chronic hepatitis C virus infection in children. J Pediatr Gastroenterol Nutr Feb 2010;50(2):123–31.

93. Barshes NR, Udell IW, Lee TC, et al. The natural history of hepatitis C virus in pediatric liver transplant recipients. Liver Transpl 2006;12(7):1119–23.

94. Malik S, Dekio F, Wen JW. Liver transplantation in a child with multifocal hepatocellular carcinoma hepatitis C and management of post-transplant viral recurrence using boceprevir. Pediatr Transplant 2014;18(2):E64–8.

95. Modin L, Arshad A, Wilkes B, et al. Epidemiology and natural history of hepatitis C virus infection among children and young people. J Hepatol 2019;70(3): 371–8.

96. Schwarz KB, Gonzalez-Peralta RP, Murray KF, et al. The combination of ribavirin and peginterferon is superior to peginterferon and placebo for children and adolescents with chronic hepatitis C. Gastroenterology 2011;140(2):450–8.e1.

97. Murray KF, Rodrigue JR, González-Peralta RP, et al. Design of the PEDS-C trial: pegylated interferon +/- ribavirin for children with chronic hepatitis C viral infection. Clin Trials 2007;4(6):661–73.

98. Indolfi G, Serranti D, Resti M. Direct-acting antivirals for children and adolescents with chronic hepatitis C. Lancet Child Adolesc Health 2018;2(4):298–304.

99. Zeng H, Li L, Hou Z, et al. Direct-acting antiviral in the treatment of chronic hepatitis C: bonuses and challenges. Int J Med Sci 2020;17(7):892–902.

100. Balistreri WF, Murray KF, Rosenthal P, et al. The safety and effectiveness of ledipasvir-sofosbuvir in adolescents 12-17 years old with hepatitis C virus genotype 1 infection. Hepatology 2017;66(2):371–8.

101. Wirth S, Rosenthal P, Gonzalez-Peralta RP, et al. Sofosbuvir and ribavirin in adolescents 12-17 years old with hepatitis C virus genotype 2 or 3 infection. Hepatology 2017;66(4):1102–10.

102. Rosenthal P, Schwarz KB, Gonzalez-Peralta RP, et al. Sofosbuvir and ribavirin therapy for children aged 3 to <12 Years with hepatitis C virus genotype 2 or 3 infection. Hepatology 2020;71(1):31–43.

103. Jonas MM, Rhee S, Kelly DA, et al. Pharmacokinetics, safety, and Efficacy of glecaprevir/pibrentasvir in children with chronic HCV: Part 2 of the DORA study. Hepatology 2021;74(1):19–27.

104. Sokal EM, Schwarz KB, Rosenthal P, et al. Safety and Efficacy of Sofosbuvir/Velpatasvir for the Treatment of Chronic Hepatitis C Infection in Children. and Adolescents Aged 3 to 17 Years Old Through 24 Weeks Posttreatment. Poster at AASLD: The Liver Meeting Digital Experience 2020. Held virtually Nov 2020; 13-16.

105. Ghany Marc G, Morgan Timothy R, AASLD-IDSA Hepatitis C Guidance Panel. Hepatitis C Guidance 2019 Update: American Association for the Study of Liver Diseases-Infectious Diseases Society of America Recommendations for Testing, Managing, and Treating Hepatitis C Virus Infection. Hepatology 2020;71(2): 686–721. https://doi.org/10.1002/hep.31060.

106. Global progress report on HIV, viral hepatitis and sexually transmitted infections, 2021. Accountability for the global health sector strategies 2016–2021: actions for impact. Geneva (Switzerland): World Health Organization; 2021.

107. Global Hepatitis Report 2017. Geneva (Switzerland): World Health Organization; 2017.

Mitochondrial Hepatopathy

Mary Ayers, MD, Simon P. Horslen, MB,ChB, FRCPCH,
Anna María Gómez, MD, PhD, James E. Squires, MD, MS*

KEYWORDS

- Mitochondrial disease • Acute liver failure • Children • Hepatocerebral dysfunction

KEY POINTS

- Alterations in mitochondrial structure and function are increasingly recognized as the cause for a wide range of pathologic conditions.
- Mitochondrial hepatopathies are a subset of mitochondrial diseases defined by primary dysfunction of hepatocyte mitochondria leading to a phenotype of hepatocyte cell injury, steatosis, or liver failure.
- Increasingly, diagnosis is established by new sequencing approaches that combine analysis of both nuclear DNA (nDNA) and mitochondrial DNA (mtDNA) and allow for timely diagnosis in most patients.
- Treatment remains mainly supportive; however, novel therapeutics and a more definitive role for liver transplantation hold promise for affected children.

INTRODUCTION

Mitochondria are dynamic bioenergetic organelles whose maintenance requires around 1500 proteins.[1] A unique feature of animal mitochondria is the contribution of both mitochondrial DNA (mtDNA) and nuclear DNA (nDNA) genes that encode the structural and functional proteome, which constitutes these complex organelles.[2,3] Alterations in mitochondrial structure and function are increasingly recognized as the cause for a wide range of pathologic conditions termed mitochondrial disorders (MDs).[4] As a group, they have been reported to affect ~1:5000 in the general population[5]; however, the prevalence is widely expected to increase as novel disease-causing defects in genes that affect oxidative phosphorylation (OXPHOS) and ATP synthesis are identified. The clinical spectrum of MD reflects the ubiquity of mitochondria throughout the body; however, the most common organs affected are those with high-energy requirements such as the brain, heart, muscle, and liver. The variability in disease presentation is complex due to the energy threshold of different cell types.[6]

University of Pittsburgh School of Medicine, Children's Hospital of Pittsburgh of UPMC, 4401 Penn Avenue, Pittsburgh, PA 15224, USA
* Corresponding author.
E-mail address: James.Squires2@chp.edu

Clin Liver Dis 26 (2022) 421–438
https://doi.org/10.1016/j.cld.2022.03.006
1089-3261/22/© 2022 Elsevier Inc. All rights reserved.

Hepatic disease is estimated to occur in up to 20% of patients with MD and is more commonly seen in early childhood.[7] These mitochondrial hepatopathies (MHs) are defined by primary dysfunction of hepatocyte mitochondria leading to cell injury, steatosis, or liver failure as major manifestations of disease.[3,8,9]

MITOCHONDRIAL STRUCTURE AND FUNCTION

Mitochondria are found in all nucleated human cells, including the hepatocyte, and function to generate most of a cell's energy needs via ATP production by the respiratory chain complex and OXPHOS (**Fig. 1**). Mitochondria are known to be more than isolated organelles and are often regarded as a dynamic network that move, fuse, and divide according to the needs of the cell.[10] In addition to energy production, mitochondria function to regulate calcium homeostasis, biosynthesize heme and steroid hormones, and modulate both apoptosis and cell cycle regulation.[11] In the liver, mitochondrial dysfunction results in the disruption of hepatocyte metabolic homeostasis, generation of injurious oxygen free radicals, and accumulation and export of potentially toxic metabolites to other organs.[12]

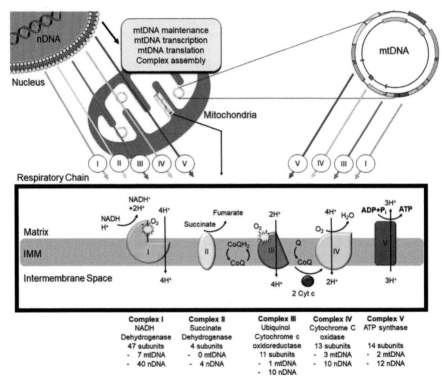

Fig. 1. Mitochondria and respiratory chain complex: The mitochondrial respiratory chain is the site of oxidative phosphorylation where NADH and succinate are oxidized, providing energy to power ATP synthase. In mammals, genes from both mitochondrial DNA (mtDNA) and nuclear DNA (nDNA) encode the functional protein complexes (I – V) that constitute the respiratory chain. There are additional nuclear-encoded proteins that function in various capacities to ensure mitochondrial assembly and mtDNA maintenance/processing. Genetic defects in any of the genes responsible for proper functioning and/or assembly result in mitochondrial disease. ATP, adenosine triphosphate; IMM, inner mitochondrial membrane; NADH, nicotinamide adenine dinucleotide + hydrogen.

DIAGNOSTIC EVALUATION

Establishing the diagnosis of primary MH requires a high index of suspicion. Traditionally, when an MH has been suspected, a "diagnostic odyssey" was undertaken whereby reaching a final diagnosis relied heavily on excluding other common metabolic disorders, and on subsequent biochemical and histochemical analysis of affected tissue, in particular muscle, skin, and liver.[4,13] Guidelines for the evaluation of the child with suspected mitochondrial liver disease are available and suggest that a comprehensive, tiered approach may be useful in establishing the diagnosis[13] (**Fig. 2**).

However, this traditional approach often results in an expensive, time-consuming, and invasive process that may ultimately fail to identify a conclusive diagnosis.[14] Although novel biomarkers such as FGF21 and GDF15 have demonstrated promise in certain clinical presentations such as myopathy,[15-18] they have shown overall poor specificity when used in general.[19] Furthermore, there remains ongoing debate as to whether an identifiable genetic basis for disease is required before establishing a diagnosis, to prevent misidentifying patients who may have phenotypic similarities but no true underlying MD or those with secondary mitochondrial dysfunction[20] (**Table 1**).

Thus, new sequencing approaches, particularly rapid, cost-effective whole-genome sequencing (WGS), are dramatically changing the landscape. These new technologies combine analysis of both nDNA and mtDNA and allow for timely diagnosis in most patients[26,27] while simultaneously eliminating the need for more invasive testing such as respiratory chain enzyme activity and mtDNA depletion assessment on biopsies of affected tissues. Tier-one use of WGS enables both definitive diagnosis when known disease-causing variants in established MH are identified and identification of novel

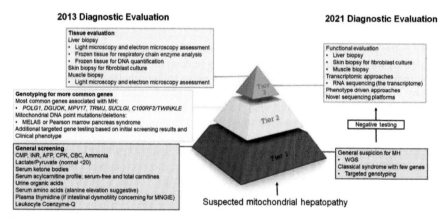

Fig. 2. Diagnostic approach of suspected mitochondrial disease. The diagnostic approach to patients with suspected MD, including MH, has evolved as new sequencing approaches such as whole-genome sequencing have become more accessible and cost effective. AFP, alpha-fetoprotein; CBC, complete blood cell count; CMP, complete metabolic panel; CPK, creatine phosphokinase; INR, international normalized ratio; MELAS, mitochondrial encephalopathy, lactic acidosis, and strokelike episodes; WGS, whole-genome sequencing. (*Adapted from* Schon KR, Ratnaike T, van den Ameele J, Horvath R, Chinnery PF. Mitochondrial Diseases: A Diagnostic Revolution. Trends Genet. 2020;36(9):702-17 and Molleston JP, Sokol RJ, Karnsakul W, Miethke A, Horslen S, Magee JC, et al. Evaluation of the child with suspected mitochondrial liver disease. J Pediatr Gastroenterol Nutr. 2013;57(3):269-76.)

Table 1
Possible secondary mitochondrial hepatopathies

Disorder	Mechanism/Agent	Characteristics of Mitochondrial Dysfunction
Wilson disease[21,22]	Disorder of Cu metabolism	• Abnormal mitochondrial morphology on EM • Increased mitochondrial Cu leads to oxidative stress and lipid peroxidation • Resultant abnormal respiratory chain dysfunction • Resultant mtDNA deletion has also been reported
Drugs and toxins[23]	Multiple offenders • Trovafloxacin • Sitaxentan • Valproate • Asparaginase • Salicylic acid • Linezolid • Amiodarone • APAP	Multiple defects that can interfere with: • fatty acid beta-oxidation • MPTP formation • oxidative phosphorylation • mtDNA replication
NAFLD/NASH[24]	Macrovesicular and microvesicular fat accumulation in hepatocytes	• Increased intracellular fat leads to respiratory chain deficiency • Increased ROS and lipid peroxidation • Positive feedback cycles leading to hepatocyte injury and damage
Ethanol[25]	Direct toxicity and hepatocellular steatosis	• Acquired respiratory chain defects • MPTP dysfunction

Abbreviations: APAP, *N*-acetyl-*p*-aminophenol; Cu, copper; EM, electron microscopy; MPTP, mitochondrial permeability transition pore; NAFLD, nonalcoholic fatty liver disease; NASH, nonalcoholic steatohepatitis; ROS, reactive oxygen species.

(likely pathogenic) variants in known MH genes.[4] Still, tier-one WGS is often supplemented by early screening tests, such as an acylcarnitine profile, serum lactate, or urine organic acid levels, which may provide clues to abnormalities in energy metabolism. Importantly, when the result of WGS is negative, both old (tissue functional assessment) and new (transcriptomic, biochemical, and long-read sequencing) approaches may ultimately be needed to enable a definitive diagnosis for patients and families (see **Fig. 2**).

In MH, genotype-phenotype correlations are challenging because the same pathogenic mutation can cause a range of different phenotypes across several organ systems. It is therefore a critical part of the evaluation of children with suspected and confirmed MH to have a systemic approach to assess for extrahepatic organ involvement[13] (**Fig. 3**); this is especially important for children presenting with acute liver failure in whom liver transplantation (LT) is being considered because the presence of multisystem disease portends worse outcomes (see next section).

CLINICAL PHENOTYPES

MDs comprise a group of clinically heterogeneous conditions with broad phenotypic manifestations ranging from multiorgan, life-threatening disease at birth to subtle, single-system symptoms with onset in middle age. In MH, while hepatic dysfunction represents a key driver of morbidity, liver involvement mirrors the diversity of MD

Multi-system Evaluation

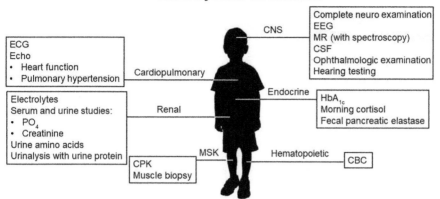

Fig. 3. Evaluation for disease in extrahepatic organ systems. Mitochondrial disease in childhood may affect any tissue or organ system in any combination. CBC, complete blood count; CNS, central nervous system; CPK, creatine phosphokinase; CSF, cerebrospinal fluid; ECG, electrocardiogram; EEG, electroencephalogram; HbA$_{1c}$, hemoglobin A$_{1c}$; MR, magnetic resonance; MSK, musculoskeletal; PO$_4$, phosphorus.

presentations, ranging from both neonatal and childhood acute liver failure (ALF) to later-onset disease, which may include hepatomegaly with elevated serum aminotransferase concentrations, hepatic steatosis, cholestasis, and cirrhosis.[3,28] Classically, MH may present in a patient with liver disease who has unexplained neuromuscular symptoms, including a seizure disorder, involvement of seemingly unrelated organ systems, a rapidly progressive course, or a chronic course that has proven to be a diagnostic dilemma.[13] In about 80% of patients, symptoms appear before age 2 years. Hypoketotic hypoglycemia, elevated lactate levels (>2.5 mmol/L), and a lactate to pyruvate ratio greater than 25 mol/mol may suggest mitochondrial distress and raise the clinician's suspicion for MH.[13,29] However, work from the Pediatric Acute Liver Failure Study Group (PALFSG) has demonstrated that lactate level elevations are common in all-cause PALF and may not be as specific to ALF secondary to MH as previously thought.[30] Notably, children with confirmed or suspected MD and ALF present a particular clinical challenge, given the still controversial role of LT in the management of MH[3] (see Treatment section).

Acute liver failure: MH as a cause of ALF in children is uncommon, reported in only 29 (2.5%) of 1144 participants enrolled into the PALFSG.[31] However, MHs are responsible for approximately 20% of infants younger than 2 years presenting with ALF, representing one of the most frequently identified causes in this age group.[32–34] Infantile liver failure has been reported in numerous MDs caused by mutations associated with MH[35–39] **(Table 2)**.

Liver biopsy: Liver biopsy specimens in MH typically show macrovesicular and microvesicular steatosis. Cholestasis may be present, and conditions associated with chronic liver disease can show micronodular cirrhosis. Other findings included hepatocyte hypereosinophilia and hemosiderosis. Immunohistochemical techniques can be used (eg, to diagnose cytochrome c oxidase deficiency). When needed, electron microscopy may show cytoplasmic crowding by atypical mitochondria[40] **(Fig. 4)**.

mtDNA depletion: The mitochondrial DNA depletion syndrome (MDS) is the most frequent subset of MH and is the final common phenotype resulting from multiple

Table 2
Genetic basis of mitochondrial hepatopathy

Syndrome	Gene	Defect/Complex Deficiency	Hepatic Presentation	ALF	Associated Symptoms	Defining Features
mtDNA depletion syndrome	DGUOK[32,50,51]	mtDNA depletion, complex I, III, IV	Hypoglycemia, cholestasis	Yes	Hypotonia; lactic acidosis; hypoglycemia	Hepatocerebral dysfunction, presents similar to GALD
	MPV17 (Navajo neurohepatopathy)[52]	mtDNA depletion, complex I, III, IV	Neonatal cholestasis	Yes	Myopathy, hypotonia, ophthalmoplegia	Hepatocerebral dysfunction
	POLG (Alpers-Huttenlocher syndrome)[53]	mtDNA depletion, complex I, III, IV	Neonatal liver failure; progressive seizures	Yes	Motor regression	Valproate-induced acute liver failure
	SUCLG1[54]	Abnormal succinate synthesis, complex I, III, IV	Episodic liver failure, steatosis	Yes	Hypotonia, progressive myopathy, hypertrophic cardiomyopathy	Elevated methylmalonic acid level
	QIL/MIC13[55,56]	Abnormal MICOS	Hypoglycemia, elevated levels of liver enzymes, neonatal liver failure	Yes	Progressive neurologic disease	Elevated 3-methylglutonic acid levels
	TWNK[57]	mtDNA replication defect due to helicase dysfunction, complex I, III, IV	Acute liver failure presentations	Yes	Progressive neurologic disease, renal tubulopathy	Infantile-onset spinocerebellar ataxia
Pearson syndrome[58]		mtDNA deletion, complex I, III, VI	Cirrhosis with hepatomegaly, cholestasis; progressive liver failure	Not reported	Bone marrow and exocrine pancreas insufficiency	Bone marrow failure and pancreatic insufficiency

Syndrome	Gene	Defect	Liver dysfunction		Key features	Notes
MNGIE syndrome	TYMP[59]	Thymidine phosphorylase deficiency, complex I, III, IV	Liver dysfunction macrovesicular steatosis, cirrhosis	Not reported	6 Key features: progressive external ophthalmoplegia, severe dysmotility of the gastrointestinal tract, cachexia, peripheral neuropathy, diffuse leukoencephalopathy, and mitochondrial dysfunction	Low thymidine level
	TRMU[60]	Mutation in translational RNA-modifying enzyme, complex I, III, IV	Neonatal liver failure, hypoglycaemia	Yes	Lactic acidosis with few extrahepatic manifestations[61]	Recover from ALF without need for liver transplant
GRACILE syndrome	BCS1L[62]	Complex III assembly deficiency	Neonatal liver failure, cholestasis	Yes	Growth failure, aminoaciduria, lactic acidosis	
	SCO1[46]	Complex IV deficiency	Neonatal liver failure, hepatomegaly	Yes	Hypotonia	Acidosis
MEGDEL syndrome	SERAC1[63]	SERAC1 involved in phospholipid exchange between ER and mitochondria	Reversible neonatal liver dysfunction, hypoglycemia	Yes	Progressive neurologic disease	
Mitochondrial aminoacyl-tRNA synthetase protein defects	LARS[38]	Defect in LARS which is responsible for leucine incorporation during polypeptide synthesis	Neonatal liver failure	Yes		Liver failure often associated with periods of illness or physiologic stress

(continued on next page)

Table 2
(continued)

Syndrome	Gene	Defect/Complex Deficiency	Hepatic Presentation	ALF	Associated Symptoms	Defining Features
	FARS2[47]	Encodes mtPheRS, which transfers phenylalanine to its cognate tRNA in mitochondria	Liver enzyme level elevations, hepatomegaly in most	No	Spectrum of disease severity with 2 phenotypes • Early-onset epileptic encephalopathy • Less severe phenotype characterized by spastic paraplegia	
	WARS2[48,64]	Encodes mtTrpRS. Complex I and IV	Liver involvement in minority but can be severe	Yes	Progressive neurologic disease	

Abbreviations: dystonia–deafness, hepatopathy, encephalopathy, Leigh-like syndrome; ER, endoplasmic reticulum; GALD, gestational alloimmune liver disease; GRACILE, growth retardation, aminoaciduria, cholestasis, iron, overload, lactic acidosis, and early death; LARS, leucyl-tRNA synthetase; MICOS, mitochondrial contact site and cristae organizing system; MEGDEL, 3-methylglutaconic aciduria; MNGIE, mitochondrial neurogastrointestinal encephalopathy; mtPheRS, mitochondrial phenylalanyl-tRNA synthetase; mtTrpRS, mitochondrial tryptophanyl-tRNA synthase.

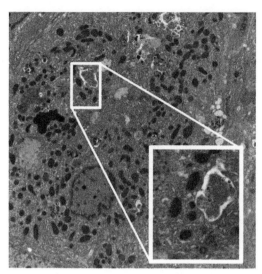

Fig. 4. Electron microscopy in mitochondrial hepatopathy. Cytoplasmic crowding by atypical mitochondria consistent with mitochondrial depletion syndrome.

gene defects (see **Table 2**). MDS, also classified as mitochondrial DNA maintenance defect, is heterogeneous and has been classified as myopathic, encephalomyopathic, neurogastrointestinal, or hepatocerebral.[41] In the hepatocerebral MDS involving the liver, identified genes have included *DGUOK, MPV17, SUCLGI, POLG1, QIL1,* and *TWNK*.[3,42] In this syndrome, nuclear gene mutations responsible for mtDNA replication and maintenance lead to impaired mtDNA synthesis or abnormally low amounts of mtDNA[3] (see **Fig. 1**). With reduced number of mtDNA, there is progressive impairment of respiratory chain complexes and increased oxidative stress.

Mitochondrial DNA deletion syndromes: mtDNA deletion syndromes occur when a large portion of the circular mtDNA is deleted. The most common phenotypes associated with mtDNA deletion are the Pearson syndrome, which is a multisystem respiratory chain disorder typically characterized by sideroblastic anemia and exocrine pancreatic insufficiency,[43] and the Kearns-Sayre syndrome, which manifests as progressive external ophthalmoplegia, hearing loss, cardiac dysfunction, renal tubular acidosis[44] (see **Table 1**). Both syndromes reflect a spectrum of disease resulting from single large-scale mtDNA deletions often found along a common stretch of mtDNA spanning bases 8471 to 13446,[45] although other less common deletions have been reported to be pathogenic.[43] When clinically suspected, newer technologies such as mtDNA sequencing and deletion analysis can be performed on affected tissue. Notably, in phenotypic Pearson syndrome with hematologic manifestations, the mtDNA deletion is detectable in the blood. However, because the hematologic manifestations of the disorder wane over the first years of life, analysis should be performed on other affected tissues such as liver or muscle.

Other MHs: Improved understanding of the genetic basis for proper mitochondrial functioning and maintenance has enabled additional gene defects to be identified where dysfunctional proteins result in the phenotype of MH. Examples include genes such as *SCO1,*[46] which encodes a critical copper chaperone protein needed for complex IV assembly and the mitochondrial aminoacyl-tRNA synthetase proteins, such as *LARS,*[38] *FARS2,*[47] and *WARS2,*[48] which are a group of nuclear-encoded enzymes that facilitate conjugation of amino acids to their cognate tRNA molecule[49] (see **Table 2**).

Table 3
Commonly avoided medications in mitochondrial hepatopathy

Medicine	MD-Related Complication
Valproic acid	Inhibit mitochondrial respiratory chain and beta-oxidation (common cause of ALF in *POLG*-related disorders)
Phenobarbital	Inhibit OXPHOS
Metformin	Exacerbates metabolic acidosis
Ringers lactate	Exacerbates poor handling of lactate
Propofol	Interferes with mitochondrial function
Chloramphenicol	Inhibits mitochondrial protein synthesis
Tetracyclines	Inhibits mitochondrial protein synthesis
Linezolid	Peripheral and optic neuropathy, lactic acidosis
Zidovudine	Interferes with mtDNA replication

TREATMENT

Treatment of MH remains supportive and is aimed at controlling the systemic, organ-specific complications that may define the disease. Antiepileptics are often used to manage concomitant seizure disorders and are supplemented by physical, occupational, and speech therapy when neurologic deficits are prevalent. Antioxidants and vitamin supplementation are often used to manage various aspects of systemic MD, although such therapies are not standardized, and multiple variations of treatment exist.[65] Common ingredients of such "mitochondrial cocktails" include coenzyme Q10, carnitine, citrulline, arginine, thiamine, riboflavin, and taurine. Although various other agents have been studied, to date little is known about the actual safety and

Table 4
Potential therapies for mitochondrial hepatopathy

Study Model	Condition	Intervention	Outcome Measure
Human clinical trial	*POLG*	Vatiquinone	Effect on seizure and seizure-related complication
	POLG	EPI-743	Effect on neuromuscular function
	POLG-TYMP	Cysteamine bitartrate	Change in NPMDS score
	TYMP	EETP	Preclinical safety and PK effect
	TYMP	Allogenic stem cells	Engraftment success, survival
	SUCLA2	Nebivolol	Cardiovascular effect (LVSD, RVEF)
Animal model	*Mpv17* (mouse)[69]	Gene therapy	Prevention of liver phenotype
Yeast-based screening assay	*POLG*[70]	Clofilium tosylate	Correct mtDNA instability
Human fibroblast culture	*POLG*[70]	Clofilium tosylate	Rescue mtDNA levels
iPSC-derived hepatocytes	*DGUOK*[71]	NAD	Improved mitochondrial function, improved ATP production

Abbreviations: ATP, adenosine triphosphate; iPSC, inducible pluripotent stem cell; LCSD, left ventricular systolic dysfunction; NAD, nicotinamide adenine dinucleotide; EETP, erythrocyte encapsulated thymidine phosphylase; NPMDS, Newcastle Pediatric Mitochondrial Disease scale; PK, pharmacokinetic; RVEF, right ventricular ejection fraction.

Table 5
Case series for liver transplantation and mitochondrial hepatopathy

Author	No. of Patients	Syndrome/ Protein/Complex	Clinical Course and Outcome
Sasaki et al,[29] 2017	9	• Co I (n = 4) • Co III (n = 1) • Co I, IV (n = 1) • MPV17 (n = 3)	• Median age at presentation 6 mo (1–26 mo) • 5 Of 9 presented with PALF • 3 Of 9 had diagnosis established before liver transplant • 9 Of 9 received living-donor LLS • 7 Of 9 alive at medial follow-up 17 mo
De Greef et al,[74] 2012	2	• Co I (n = 1) • DGUOK (n = 1)	• Median age at presentation 3 y (7 mo-6 y) • 0 Of 2 presented with PALF • 0 Of 2 with diagnosis established before liver transplant • 2 Of 2 received OLT • 1 Of 2 alive at median follow-up 3 y
Scheers et al,[75] 2005	2	• Co I, III, IV (n = 1) • Co IV (n = 1)	• 2 Of 2 developed HCC as the indication for liver transplant • 0 Of 2 presented with PALF • 2 Of 2 alive at median follow-up 2.5 y
Dubern et al,[76] 2001	5	• Co I, III, IV (n = 3) • Co IV (n = 1) • Co I, IV (n = 1)	• 1 Of 5 presented with PALF • 2 Of 5 died of progressive neurologic decline (n = 1) and MOSF (n = 1)
Durand et al,[77] 2001	5	• Not reported	• 3 Of 5 had known RC defect noted before liver transplant • 3 Of 5 died following transplant
Thomson et al,[78] 1998	2	• Co I (n = 1, second patient not reported)	• 1 Of 2 presented with PALF • 2 Of /2 died of neurologic decline and respiratory failure
Dimmock et al,[51] 2008	3	• DGUOK (n = 3)	• 1 Of 3 presented with PALF • 3 Of 3 established diagnosis after liver transplant • 3 Of 3 died (1 of progressive neurologic decline and cardiac arrest, 1 of transplant related complications, 1 not reported)
Tzoulis et al,[79] 2009	2	• POLG (n = 2)	• 1 Of 2 presented with PALF • 1 Of 2 died 1 mo posttransplant
Hynynen et al,[80] 2006	4	• POLG (n = 4)	• 4 Of 4 with valproate-induced ALF after neurologic symptom onset • OLT mean age 23 mo • 1 Sudden death at 2 y post-OLT • 3 Of 4 alive at mean 9 y post-LT

(continued on next page)

Table 5
(continued)

Author	No. of Patients	Syndrome/ Protein/Complex	Clinical Course and Outcome
Uchida et al,[81] 2021	13	• MPV17 (n = 6) • TRMU (n = 2) • MT-ND1 (n = 1) • NDUFA9 (n = 1) • Co I (n = 2) • Co III (n = 1)	• 10 Of 13 presented with ALF (3 non-ALF were all MPV17) • OLT mean 11 mo of life • 61.5% survival at median follow-up period of 1.8 y
Shimura et al,[56] 2020	12	• MPV17 (n = 9) • DGUOK (n = 2) • Not reported (n = 1)	• OLT mean 31 mo of life • 5 Of 12 alive after liver transplant at mean follow-up 42 mo
Jankowska et al,[72] 2021	2	• DGUOK (n = 2)	• Neonatal ALF • OLT mean 6.5 mo of life • 1 Of 2 alive after OLT
Grabhorn et al,[82] 2014	2	• DGUOK (n = 2)	• 2 Of 2 with ALF • OLT mean 8 mo • 2 Of 2 alive at mean follow-up 6.5 y post-LT

Abbreviations: Co, complex; LLS, left-lateral segment; MOSF, multi-organ system failure; OLT, orthotopic liver transplant; PALF, pediatric acute liver failure; HCC, hepatocellular carcinoma; RC, respiratory chain.

efficacy of any of these therapies.[2,66] Additional pharmacotherapy may be system specific,[2,10] and consensus-based recommendations for optimal management and care for patients with primary mitochondrial disease are available.[67]

Although the search to establish more definitive treatments for MH is critical, for most affected individuals their disorders are relentlessly progressive, and result is substantial morbidity and mortality. Therefore, where possible, preventative strategies may also be required.[2] In certain conditions, including mtDNA maintenance defects, medications may need to be avoided to mitigate MD-related complications[10] (**Table 3**).

Medical: Medical management of MH is aimed at avoiding mitochondrial crises and reducing toxic metabolites.[2] Few if any targeted medical therapies specifically treat the liver-related manifestations of mitochondrial dysfunction. An exception to this rule is the potential benefit of L-cysteine supplementation for patients with liver-related complications secondary to *TRMU* deficiency.[68] Nevertheless, there are numerous other therapeutic approaches that have been tested in human and animal populations where the genetic cause is known to contribute to the hepatopathy phenotype (**Table 4**). Ongoing and future efforts will be needed to quantify liver-related benefit from these potential interventions.

Transplant: Liver disease can be the driving cause of morbidity and mortality in MH. In some MDSs (*DGUOK, MPV17,* and others) LT has been considered; however, transplant as a therapeutic intervention remains controversial given the well-recognized extrahepatic progression of cardiac, neuromuscular, and central nervous system complications that can mitigate any liver-specific posttransplant benefits. Most reported experiences with LT in MH come from single-center experiences, and most patients presented with ALF (**Table 5**). This clinical scenario of a patient with ALF presents a unique challenge because even in those patients with a high clinical suspicion, transplant may be performed where a definitive contraindication is lacking.

Although more experience is needed, emerging data suggest that there may be a subset of patients (ie, *DGUOK*) with mitochondrial disease who may benefit from LT.[72] This fact is supported by experiences in other mitochondrial diseases with less severe or absent liver involvement, such as MNGIE syndrome, where LT may be the preferable therapy for select cases.[73]

PROGNOSIS

Hepatic involvement in primary MDs is well recognized; however, age-related prevalence, clinical presentation, and prognostic impact remain poorly understood. Certain clinical characteristics such as early age of onset, extrahepatic disease, and a rapidly progressive disease course portend poorer outcomes. Still, specific prognoses for patients affected by MH are challenging given the disease heterogeneity and interpatient variability.

SUMMARY

MH encompasses a growing population of heterogeneous diseases where liver complications may be the driving force leading to significant morbidity and mortality. Although collectively common, the incidence of each individual MH subtype is extremely rare. A complete diagnostic evaluation is needed to best understand the diagnosis, more often reliant on comprehensive genetic testing. Treatment remains mainly supportive; however, in rare circumstances LT may be considered, particularly when extrahepatic manifestations are minimal. Novel therapies currently under investigation may improve the therapeutic options afforded to these children.

CLINICS CARE POINTS

- A mitochondrial hepatopathy should be suspected in any child with liver abnormalities and unexplained neuromuscular symptoms, including a seizure disorder; involvement of seemingly unrelated organ systems; a rapidly progressive course; or a chronic course that has proven to be a diagnostic dilemma.

- A genetic basis for disease is increasingly recognized making timely investigation critical for optimal decision making.

- Treatment remains mainly supportive; however, in rare circumstances liver transplant may be considered, particularly when extrahepatic manifestations are minimal.

DISCLOSURE

M. Ayers: Nothing to disclose. S.P. Horslen: Nothing to disclose. A.M. Gómez: Nothing to disclose. J.E. Squires: Nothing to disclose.

REFERENCES

1. Rahman J, Rahman S. Mitochondrial medicine in the omics era. Lancet 2018; 391(10139):2560–74.
2. Gorman GS, Chinnery PF, DiMauro S, et al. Mitochondrial diseases. Nat Rev Dis Primers 2016;2:16080.
3. Lee WS, Sokol RJ. Mitochondrial hepatopathies: advances in genetics, therapeutic approaches, and outcomes. J Pediatr 2013;163(4):942–8.

4. Schon KR, Ratnaike T, van den Ameele J, et al. Mitochondrial diseases: a diagnostic Revolution. Trends Genet 2020;36(9):702–17.

5. Gorman GS, Schaefer AM, Ng Y, et al. Prevalence of nuclear and mitochondrial DNA mutations related to adult mitochondrial disease. Ann Neurol 2015;77(5): 753–9.

6. Koopman WJ, Willems PH, Smeitink JA. Monogenic mitochondrial disorders. N Engl J Med 2012;366(12):1132–41.

7. Cao J, Wu H, Li Z. Recent perspectives of pediatric mitochondrial diseases. Exp Ther Med 2018;15(1):13–8.

8. Lee WS, Sokol RJ. Liver disease in mitochondrial disorders. Semin Liver Dis 2007;27(3):259–73.

9. Lee WS, Sokol RJ. Mitochondrial hepatopathies: advances in genetics and pathogenesis. Hepatology 2007;45(6):1555–65.

10. El-Hattab AW, Craigen WJ, Scaglia F. Mitochondrial DNA maintenance defects. Biochim Biophys Acta Mol Basis Dis 2017;1863(6):1539–55.

11. Ylikallio E, Suomalainen A. Mechanisms of mitochondrial diseases. Ann Med 2012;44(1):41–59.

12. WR T. Mitochondrial Hepatopathies: disorders of fatty acid oxidation and the respiratory chain. In: Wyllie RHJ, Kay M, editors. Pediatric Gastrointestinal and liver disease. 4th edition. Elsevier Saunders; 2011. p. 767–85.

13. Molleston JP, Sokol RJ, Karnsakul W, et al. Evaluation of the child with suspected mitochondrial liver disease. J Pediatr Gastroenterol Nutr 2013;57(3):269–76.

14. Grier J, Hirano M, Karaa A, et al. Diagnostic odyssey of patients with mitochondrial disease: results of a survey. Neurol Genet 2018;4(2):e230.

15. Lovadi E, Csereklyei M, Merkli H, et al. Elevated FGF 21 in myotonic dystrophy type 1 and mitochondrial diseases. Muscle Nerve 2017;55(4):564–9.

16. Montero R, Yubero D, Villarroya J, et al. GDF-15 is elevated in children with mitochondrial diseases and is induced by mitochondrial dysfunction. PLoS One 2016; 11(2):e0148709.

17. Lehtonen JM, Forsstrom S, Bottani E, et al. FGF21 is a biomarker for mitochondrial translation and mtDNA maintenance disorders. Neurology 2016;87(22): 2290–9.

18. Morovat A, Weerasinghe G, Nesbitt V, et al. Use of FGF-21 as a biomarker of mitochondrial disease in clinical Practice. J Clin Med 2017;6(8).

19. Tsygankova PG, Itkis YS, Krylova TD, et al. Plasma FGF-21 and GDF-15 are elevated in different inherited metabolic diseases and are not diagnostic for mitochondrial disorders. J Inherit Metab Dis 2019;42(5):918–33.

20. Parikh S, Karaa A, Goldstein A, et al. Diagnosis of 'possible' mitochondrial disease: an existential crisis. J Med Genet 2019;56(3):123–30.

21. Sokol RJ, Twedt D, McKim JM Jr, et al. Oxidant injury to hepatic mitochondria in patients with Wilson's disease and Bedlington terriers with copper toxicosis. Gastroenterology 1994;107(6):1788–98.

22. Mansouri A, Gaou I, Fromenty B, et al. Premature oxidative aging of hepatic mitochondrial DNA in Wilson's disease. Gastroenterology 1997;113(2):599–605.

23. Shehu AI, Ma X, Venkataramanan R. Mechanisms of drug-induced hepatotoxicity. Clin Liver Dis 2017;21(1):35–54.

24. Begriche K, Igoudjil A, Pessayre D, et al. Mitochondrial dysfunction in NASH: causes, consequences and possible means to prevent it. Mitochondrion 2006; 6(1):1–28.

25. Ma L, Dong JX, Wu C, et al. Spectroscopic, polarographic, and microcalorimetric studies on mitochondrial dysfunction induced by Ethanol. J Membr Biol 2017; 250(2):195–204.

26. Pronicka E, Piekutowska-Abramczuk D, Ciara E, et al. New perspective in diagnostics of mitochondrial disorders: two years' experience with whole-exome sequencing at a national paediatric centre. J Transl Med 2016;14(1):174.

27. Dimmock D, Caylor S, Waldman B, et al. Project baby bear: rapid precision care incorporating rWGS in 5 California children's hospitals demonstrates improved clinical outcomes and reduced costs of care. Am J Hum Genet 2021;108(7): 1231–8.

28. Gibson K, Halliday JL, Kirby DM, et al. Mitochondrial oxidative phosphorylation disorders presenting in neonates: clinical manifestations and enzymatic and molecular diagnoses. Pediatrics 2008;122(5):1003–8.

29. Sasaki K, Sakamoto S, Uchida H, et al. Liver transplantation for mitochondrial respiratory chain disorder: a single-center experience and Excellent Marker of Differential diagnosis. Transplant Proc 2017;49(5):1097–102.

30. Feldman AG, Sokol RJ, Hardison RM, et al. Lactate and lactate: pyruvate ratio in the diagnosis and outcomes of pediatric acute liver failure. J Pediatr 2017;182: 217–222 e3.

31. Narkewicz MR, Horslen S, Hardison RM, et al. A Learning Collaborative approach increases specificity of diagnosis of acute liver failure in pediatric patients. Clin Gastroenterol Hepatol 2018;16(11):1801–18010 e3.

32. Al-Hussaini A, Faqeih E, El-Hattab AW, et al. Clinical and molecular characteristics of mitochondrial DNA depletion syndrome associated with neonatal cholestasis and liver failure. J Pediatr 2014;164(3):553–559 e1-2.

33. McKiernan P, Ball S, Santra S, et al. Incidence of primary mitochondrial disease in children younger than 2 Years presenting with acute liver failure. J Pediatr Gastroenterol Nutr 2016;63(6):592–7.

34. Taylor SA, Whitington PF. Neonatal acute liver failure. Liver Transpl 2016;22(5): 677–85.

35. Schara U, von Kleist-Retzow JC, Lainka E, et al. Acute liver failure with subsequent cirrhosis as the primary manifestation of TRMU mutations. J Inherit Metab Dis 2011;34(1):197–201.

36. Van Hove JL, Saenz MS, Thomas JA, et al. Succinyl-CoA ligase deficiency: a mitochondrial hepatoencephalomyopathy. Pediatr Res 2010;68(2):159–64.

37. Vedrenne V, Galmiche L, Chretien D, et al. Mutation in the mitochondrial translation elongation factor EFTs results in severe infantile liver failure. J Hepatol 2012; 56(1):294–7.

38. Hirata K, Okamoto N, Ichikawa C, et al. Severe course with lethal hepatocellular injury and skeletal muscular dysgenesis in a neonate with infantile liver failure syndrome type 1 caused by novel LARS1 mutations. Am J Med Genet A 2021; 185(3):866–70.

39. Goh V, Helbling D, Biank V, et al. Next-generation sequencing facilitates the diagnosis in a child with twinkle mutations causing cholestatic liver failure. J Pediatr Gastroenterol Nutr 2012;54(2):291–4.

40. Hazard FK, Ficicioglu CH, Ganesh J, et al. Liver pathology in infantile mitochondrial DNA depletion syndrome. Pediatr Dev Pathol 2013;16(6):415–24.

41. Invernizzi F, Legati A, Nasca A, et al. Myopathic mitochondrial DNA depletion syndrome associated with biallelic variants in LIG3. Brain 2021;144(9):e74.

42. Kishita Y, Shimura M, Kohda M, et al. A novel homozygous variant in MICOS13/QIL1 causes hepato-encephalopathy with mitochondrial DNA depletion syndrome. Mol Genet Genomic Med 2020;8(10):e1427.

43. Wild KT, Goldstein AC, Muraresku C, et al. Broadening the phenotypic spectrum of Pearson syndrome: five new cases and a review of the literature. Am J Med Genet A 2020;182(2):365–73.

44. Shemesh A, Margolin E. Kearns Sayre syndrome. Treasure Island (FL): StatPearls; 2021.

45. Broomfield A, Sweeney MG, Woodward CE, et al. Paediatric single mitochondrial DNA deletion disorders: an overlapping spectrum of disease. J Inherit Metab Dis 2015;38(3):445–57.

46. Valnot I, Osmond S, Gigarel N, et al. Mutations of the SCO1 gene in mitochondrial cytochrome c oxidase deficiency with neonatal-onset hepatic failure and encephalopathy. Am J Hum Genet 2000;67(5):1104–9.

47. Almannai M, Wang J, Dai H, et al. FARS2 deficiency; new cases, review of clinical, biochemical, and molecular spectra, and variants interpretation based on structural, functional, and evolutionary significance. Mol Genet Metab 2018; 125(3):281–91.

48. Vantroys E, Smet J, Vanlander AV, et al. Severe hepatopathy and neurological deterioration after start of valproate treatment in a 6-year-old child with mitochondrial tryptophanyl-tRNA synthetase deficiency. Orphanet J Rare Dis 2018; 13(1):80.

49. Fine AS, Nemeth CL, Kaufman ML, et al. Mitochondrial aminoacyl-tRNA synthetase disorders: an emerging group of developmental disorders of myelination. J Neurodev Disord 2019;11(1):29.

50. Spinazzola A, Invernizzi F, Carrara F, et al. Clinical and molecular features of mitochondrial DNA depletion syndromes. J Inherit Metab Dis 2009;32(2):143–58.

51. Dimmock DP, Zhang Q, Dionisi-Vici C, et al. Clinical and molecular features of mitochondrial DNA depletion due to mutations in deoxyguanosine kinase. Hum Mutat 2008;29(2):330–1.

52. El-Hattab AW, Wang J, Dai H, et al. MPV17-related mitochondrial DNA maintenance defect: new cases and review of clinical, biochemical, and molecular aspects. Hum Mutat 2018;39(4):461–70.

53. Wong LJ, Naviaux RK, Brunetti-Pierri N, et al. Molecular and clinical genetics of mitochondrial diseases due to POLG mutations. Hum Mutat 2008;29(9):E150–72.

54. Carrozzo R, Verrigni D, Rasmussen M, et al. Succinate-CoA ligase deficiency due to mutations in SUCLA2 and SUCLG1: phenotype and genotype correlations in 71 patients. J Inherit Metab Dis 2016;39(2):243–52.

55. Russell BE, Whaley KG, Bove KE, et al. Expanding and Underscoring the hepatoEncephalopathic phenotype of QIL1/MIC13. Hepatology 2019;70(3):1066–70.

56. Shimura M, Kuranobu N, Ogawa-Tominaga M, et al. Clinical and molecular basis of hepatocerebral mitochondrial DNA depletion syndrome in Japan: evaluation of outcomes after liver transplantation. Orphanet J Rare Dis 2020;15(1):169.

57. Sukhudyan B, Gevorgyan A, Sarkissian A, et al. Expanding phenotype of mitochondrial depletion syndrome in association with TWNK mutations. Eur J Paediatr Neurol 2019;23(3):537–40.

58. Kanungo S, Morton J, Neelakantan M, et al. Mitochondrial disorders. Ann Transl Med 2018;6(24):475.

59. Viscomi C, Zeviani M. MtDNA-maintenance defects: syndromes and genes. J Inherit Metab Dis 2017;40(4):587–99.

60. Murali CN, Soler-Alfonso C, Loomes KM, et al. TRMU deficiency: a broad clinical spectrum responsive to cysteine supplementation. Mol Genet Metab 2021; 132(2):146–53.

61. Sala-Coromina J, Miguel LD, de Las Heras J, et al. Leigh syndrome associated with TRMU gene mutations. Mol Genet Metab Rep 2021;26:100690.

62. Kotarsky H, Karikoski R, Morgelin M, et al. Characterization of complex III deficiency and liver dysfunction in GRACILE syndrome caused by a BCS1L mutation. Mitochondrion 2010;10(5):497–509.

63. Maas RR, Iwanicka-Pronicka K, Kalkan Ucar S, et al. Progressive deafness-dystonia due to SERAC1 mutations: a study of 67 cases. Ann Neurol 2017; 82(6):1004–15.

64. Wortmann SB, Timal S, Venselaar H, et al. Biallelic variants in WARS2 encoding mitochondrial tryptophanyl-tRNA synthase in six individuals with mitochondrial encephalopathy. Hum Mutat 2017;38(12):1786–95.

65. Parikh S, Goldstein A, Koenig MK, et al. Diagnosis and management of mitochondrial disease: a consensus statement from the Mitochondrial Medicine Society. Genet Med 2015;17(9):689–701.

66. Ramon J, Vila-Julia F, Molina-Granada D, et al. Therapy Prospects for mitochondrial DNA maintenance disorders. Int J Mol Sci 2021;22(12).

67. Parikh S, Goldstein A, Karaa A, et al. Patient care standards for primary mitochondrial disease: a consensus statement from the Mitochondrial Medicine Society. Genet Med 2017;19(12).

68. Soler-Alfonso C, Pillai N, Cooney E, et al. L-Cysteine supplementation prevents liver transplantation in a patient with TRMU deficiency. Mol Genet Metab Rep 2019;19:100453.

69. Bottani E, Giordano C, Civiletto G, et al. AAV-mediated liver-specific MPV17 expression restores mtDNA levels and prevents diet-induced liver failure. Mol Ther 2014;22(1):10–7.

70. Pitayu L, Baruffini E, Rodier C, et al. Combined use of Saccharomyces cerevisiae, Caenorhabditis elegans and patient fibroblasts leads to the identification of clofilium tosylate as a potential therapeutic chemical against POLG-related diseases. Hum Mol Genet 2016;25(4):715–27.

71. Jing R, Corbett JL, Cai J, et al. A screen using iPSC-Derived hepatocytes Reveals NAD(+) as a potential treatment for mtDNA depletion syndrome. Cell Rep 2018; 25(6):1469–14684 e5.

72. Jankowska I, Czubkowski P, Rokicki D, et al. Acute liver failure due to DGUOK deficiency-is liver transplantation justified? Clin Res Hepatol Gastroenterol 2021;45(1):101408.

73. Hirano M, Carelli V, De Giorgio R, et al. Mitochondrial neurogastrointestinal encephalomyopathy (MNGIE): Position paper on diagnosis, prognosis, and treatment by the MNGIE International Network. J Inherit Metab Dis 2021;44(2):376–87.

74. De Greef E, Christodoulou J, Alexander IE, et al. Mitochondrial respiratory chain hepatopathies: role of liver transplantation. A case series of five patients. JIMD Rep 2012;4:5–11.

75. Scheers I, Bachy V, Stephenne X, et al. Risk of hepatocellular carcinoma in liver mitochondrial respiratory chain disorders. J Pediatr 2005;146(3):414–7.

76. Dubern B, Broue P, Dubuisson C, et al. Orthotopic liver transplantation for mitochondrial respiratory chain disorders: a study of 5 children. Transplantation 2001;71(5):633–7.

77. Durand P, Debray D, Mandel R, et al. Acute liver failure in infancy: a 14-year experience of a pediatric liver transplantation center. J Pediatr 2001;139(6):871–6.

78. Thomson M, McKiernan P, Buckels J, et al. Generalised mitochondrial cytopathy is an absolute contraindication to orthotopic liver transplant in childhood. J Pediatr Gastroenterol Nutr 1998;26(4):478–81.

79. Tzoulis C, Engelsen BA, Telstad W, et al. The spectrum of clinical disease caused by the A467T and W748S POLG mutations: a study of 26 cases. Brain 2006; 129(Pt 7):1685–92.

80. Hynynen J, Komulainen T, Tukiainen E, et al. Acute liver failure after valproate exposure in patients with POLG1 mutations and the prognosis after liver transplantation. Liver Transpl 2014;20(11):1402–12.

81. Uchida H, Sakamoto S, Shimizu S, et al. Outcomes of liver transplantation for mitochondrial respiratory chain disorder in children. Pediatr Transpl 2021;25(8): e14091.

82. Grabhorn E, Tsiakas K, Herden U, et al. Long-term outcomes after liver transplantation for deoxyguanosine kinase deficiency: a single-center experience and a review of the literature. Liver Transpl 2014;20(4):464–72.

Nonalcoholic Steatohepatitis in Children

Stavra A. Xanthakos, MD, MS

KEYWORDS

- Nonalcoholic fatty liver disease • Cirrhosis • Vitamin E • Liraglutide
- Bariatric surgery

KEY POINTS

- Nonalcoholic fatty liver disease (NAFLD) is currently the leading cause of chronic liver disease in children.
- While environmental exposures are major contributors to the earlier onset in childhood, children may also have unique genetic risk alleles, compared with adults with NAFLD.
- NAFLD in childhood is associated with increased risk of incident diabetes and other cardiovascular risk factors.
- Reducing modifiable risk factors that contribute to obesity and associated metabolic dysregulation is the primary and first-line approach for treating NAFLD in children.
- Long term follow-up is needed to determine if children with NAFLD will have increased risk of hepatic and non-hepatic morbidity and mortality in adulthood.

INTRODUCTION

Nonalcoholic fatty liver disease (NAFLD) encompasses a spectrum of fatty liver that ranges from mild steatosis to more severe nonalcoholic steatohepatitis (NASH). NASH with fibrosis carries a higher risk for progression to cirrhosis and end-stage liver disease over time, although the disease usually progresses slowly over a decade or more. NAFLD affects both children and adults and is strongly associated with excess adiposity, in particular visceral adiposity, and insulin resistance.

NAFLD shares many histologic findings with alcohol-associated fatty liver disease; thus, excess alcohol intake (>2 units of 28 g per day in women, >3 units or 42 g per day in men) is considered exclusionary for a diagnosis of NAFLD but rarely a concern among children.[1] Historically, the diagnosis of NAFLD required excluding other concomitant liver diseases, such as chronic viral hepatitis. However, with the global increase in obesity and other environmental risk factors, NAFLD can co-occur in the

Professor of Pediatrics, Division of Gastroenterology Hepatology and Nutrition, Cincinnati Children's, Department of Pediatrics, Director, Nonalcoholic Steatohepatitis Center, University of Cincinnati College of Medicine, 3333 Burnet Avenue, Cincinnati, OH 45229, USA
E-mail address: stavra.xanthakos@cchmc.org

Clin Liver Dis 26 (2022) 439–460
https://doi.org/10.1016/j.cld.2022.05.001
1089-3261/22/© 2022 Elsevier Inc. All rights reserved.

setting of other liver or systemic diseases. Assessing children with NAFLD for other liver diseases or contributing factors remains important, as coexisting conditions may affect treatment recommendations.

Nomenclature and Histologic Characteristics

Recently, multidisciplinary proposals have emerged to modify the current nomenclature of NAFLD to *metabolic-associated fatty liver disease* (MAFLD) to better reflect the positive diagnostic criteria of hepatic steatosis in the setting of excess adiposity and related metabolic dysregulation.[2] In addition, there is some concern that "nonalcoholic" overemphasizes alcohol, which may carry a stigma and is not as applicable in children.[2] However, full consensus is still lacking because of concern that prematurely changing the terminology without fully understanding the molecular basis or risk stratification of the disease could heighten confusion among the public and clinicians and impede ongoing research focused on drug and biomarker development.[2] In children, several other genetic conditions can cause metabolic liver disease; thus, a change to "MAFLD" could also trigger confusion. Thus, NAFLD remains the most accepted terminology at this time, until a multidisciplinary consensus with all stakeholders is reached.

Suspected NAFLD should be considered in a child or adolescent with chronically elevated liver enzymes and known risk factors, such as overweight or obesity, central adiposity, insulin resistance, and dyslipidemia. *Presumed NAFLD* is defined as the presence of fatty liver (confirmed on imaging) and the exclusion of other causes of chronic hepatitis or liver disease (see the section "Evaluation of Children with Suspected NAFLD"). *Confirmed NAFLD* requires liver biopsy assessment. On histologic assessment, the presence of greater than 5% predominantly macrovesicular hepatocellular steatosis is the minimum criterion for NAFLD, but there are several distinct histologic subtypes based on pattern and severity of injury (**Table 1**).[1]

The NAFLD activity score (NAS) is a validated and very commonly reported measure of histologic disease activity, which was initially designed to assess endpoints in clinical trials. The NAS (range 0–8) is an unweighted composite of semiquantitative scores for steatosis (0–3), lobular inflammation (0–3), and hepatocellular ballooning severity (0–2).[1] Fibrosis severity is staged separately (stages 0–4). The NAS was neither designed to, nor should it be used to diagnose NASH. The NAS score also does not adequately capture the full spectrum of histologic disease activity in children, who often have more prominent portal inflammation, but minimal or no ballooning degeneration. In addition, the prognostic significance of the NAS score in predicting the long-term risk of fibrosis progression or adverse outcomes in children with NAFLD is unknown. The European Consortium for the Study of Fatty Liver Disease has also developed an alternate method of grading NAFLD activity that includes scores for steatosis, activity, and fibrosis, termed the SAF score.[3] Although similar to the NAS score, the SAF assesses ballooning and lobular inflammation differently. It is also insufficiently validated in children.

Epidemiology of Nonalcoholic Fatty Liver Disease in Children

Although initially reported in children in North America and Europe, NAFLD has been increasingly described in all regions of the globe, particularly in South America, Asia, and the Middle East. A 2015 pediatric meta-analysis of epidemiologic studies estimated a global pooled prevalence of 7.6% (95% confidence interval [CI]: 5.5% to 10.3%) in the general pediatric population. Among children with obesity, the estimated prevalence increased to 34.2% (95% CI: 27.8% to 41.2%).[4] Male sex was associated with a higher odds ratio of NAFLD (OR 1.63, 95% CI: 1.10–2.41).[4]

Table 1
Histologic phenotypes of nonalcoholic fatty liver disease

NAFLD Phenotype	Key Characteristics
Nonalcoholic fatty liver (NAFL)	Hepatocellular steatosis (>5%, predominantly macrovesicular) without sufficient inflammation and hepatocellular injury to establish the diagnosis of NASH • May include foci of mild lobular or portal inflammation • Fibrosis typically not present
Nonalcoholic steatohepatitis (NASH)	Zone 3 (centrilobular) predominant pattern of injury More common in adults • Hepatocellular steatosis • Ballooning degeneration, ± Mallory–Denk bodies (zone 3) • Inflammation (predominantly lobular, ± portal) • ± fibrosis (zone 3 in early stages)
Borderline zone 3 NASH	Some criteria of NASH, but not meeting all criteria Mainly zone 3 (centrilobular) pattern of injury in adults • Ballooning degeneration may be absent or rare • Centrilobular fibrosis Less prevalent among children
Borderline zone 1 NASH (portal predominant)	Some criteria of NASH, but not meeting all criteria Mainly zone 1 (periportal) pattern of steatosis and injury • Mild-to-moderate portal inflammation, rare lobular foci • Absent ballooning • ± Portal/periportal fibrosis More common in pre- or peripubertal children
NASH-related cryptogenic cirrhosis	Cirrhosis in absence of >5% hepatic steatosis (steatosis can diminish as cirrhosis develops) • In the setting of clinical risk factors (obesity, type 2 diabetes) or prior history of known NAFLD or NASH • May have some evidence of steatosis or ballooning

Prevalence also varies by ethnicity and race. In a population-based autopsy study, children of Hispanic ethnicity and Asian race had a higher prevalence of NAFLD compared with White children, whereas children of Black, non-Hispanic race and ethnicity had the lowest prevalence (**Fig. 1**).[5] Ethnic and racial variation may in part

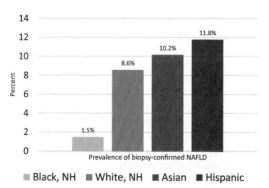

Fig. 1. Racial and ethnic prevalence of biopsy-confirmed NAFLD in a population-based autopsy study conducted in San Diego County. NH = non-Hispanic.[5]

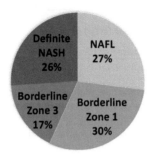

Fig. 2. Histologic NAFLD phenotypes in children at the time of enrollment into a multicenter observational cohort study in the NASH Clinical Research Network in the United States ($N = 675$)[7]

be due to different frequency of a key genetic risk allele (discussed in the section "Pathogenesis").

Estimating the true prevalence of NASH is challenging due to the need for biopsy confirmation. Variation in screening and clinical practice may lead to referral or selection bias in undergoing a liver biopsy and estimates of histologic disease severity can vary widely depending on center and sample size. Among large multicenter cohort studies of children ($n = 358–665$) in the United States with biopsy-confirmed NAFLD, the prevalence of NASH ranges from 26% to 46% (**Fig. 2**), whereas advanced fibrosis ($\geq$stage 3) is present in 10% to 15% and cirrhosis is rare.[5–7]

Serial US National Health and Nutrition Examination Survey (NHANES) analyses have reported a doubling in suspected NAFLD prevalence, based on serum alanine aminotransferase (ALT) elevation, in overweight or obese children, ages 12 to 19 years old—from 3.9% to 10.7%—over a 20-year period ending in 2007 to 2010.[8] Importantly, the prevalence of NAFLD is often lower in studies that rely on abnormal ALT for detection because an estimated 20% to 25% of children with NAFLD can have normal levels ($\leq$25–30 U/L).[9]

Although strongly associated with overweight and obesity, NAFLD can be present in children and adolescents with normal body mass index (BMI $\leq$ 85th percentile for age and sex). In an NHANES analysis (2005–2014), an estimated 8% of lean adolescents with normal BMI had suspected NAFLD as defined by elevated serum ALT level.[10] The affected lean adolescents had a higher prevalence of risk factors, including low high-density lipoprotein (HDL) cholesterol, elevated triglycerides, and insulin resistance compared with lean adolescents without NAFLD.

The mean age at the time of diagnosis of NAFLD is typically around the onset of puberty, ~age 12 to 13 years. This may be due to transient insulin resistance that occurs around the time of puberty but could also be influenced by selection bias. Most current pediatric obesity guidelines recommend initial screening for cardiometabolic comorbidities, including NAFLD, starting at age 9 to 10 years of age.[7] Historically, autopsy-based studies suggested low rates of presumed NAFLD in the general population of children ages 2 to 5 years of age (<1%), and slightly higher prevalence (3.3%) at ages 5 to 9 years.[11,12] However, obesity may also increase the risk of NAFLD in young prepubertal children. Among 73 children 2 to 5 years old (45% men and 70% Hispanic) who were attending a tertiary obesity clinic, 26% had elevated liver enzymes (>30 IU/L) concerning NAFLD.[13]

Rarely, children are at increased risk for NAFLD or NASH due to systemic or syndromic conditions. These include children with congenital or acquired lipodystrophy and children with pituitary or hypothalamic dysfunction that can result in growth hormone (GH) deficiency or severe obesity.[14,15]

Pathogenesis of Nonalcoholic Fatty Liver Disease in Children

Multiple environmental exposures are driving the onset of NAFLD in childhood, in large part due to a rising rate of pediatric obesity across all age groups, including in very young children. An estimated 26% of 2 to 5 year olds in the United States are overweight and 14% are obese.[16] Even before birth, there may be factors associated with the increase in NAFLD prevalence among children. With the increase in adult obesity, there has been increasing *in utero* exposure to maternal obesity and insulin resistance, including gestational diabetes, which may alter placental signaling and function, leading to fetal epigenetic changes that promote hepatic steatosis.[17] Microbial gut dysbiosis, linked to NAFLD pathogenesis in children and adults, can begin in early infancy and continue in childhood, in response to caesarian section delivery, maternal and childhood dietary factors, and frequent antibiotic and antacid medication exposure.[17,18]

One of the key dietary risk factors that has been linked to NAFLD pathogenesis, and its more severe form of NASH, is high intake of fructose, both in the form of added sugars and high-fructose corn syrup. Dietary fructose, absorbed via the portal vein, is delivered in higher concentrations to the liver, where it directly upregulates enzymes that drive hepatic de novo lipogenesis.[19] This promotes hepatic steatosis and subsequent hepatic insulin resistance. Fructose metabolism is not inhibited by insulin and continues to upregulate de novo lipogenesis even in the setting of systemic insulin resistance.[19] In addition, fructose metabolism impairs mitochondrial function by depleting adenosine triphosphate and suppressing fatty-acid oxidation, promoting oxidative stress.[19] Diets high in fructose, saturated fat, and cholesterol also can promote intestinal dysbiosis, which has been associated with a risk of more severe NASH.[20]

Children often become less physically active as they enter adolescence, which is another contributing factor in NAFLD development. Adolescents with greater physical activity measured by accelerometry at age 12 and 14 years of age had reduced odds of developing fatty liver in later adolescence in a prospective study.[21]

Prenatal and postnatal exposure to endocrine-disrupting chemicals has also increased worldwide in the past 50 years, and several of these chemicals have been linked to the development of NAFLD. Higher maternal levels of perfluoroalkyl substances, for example, correlated with increased serum aminotransferase levels in offspring[22] and higher serum levels of perfluoroalkyl substances have been linked to more severe histologic NAFLD in children.[23] Several other chemical exposures potentially linked to the childhood development of NAFLD include arsenic and mercury, which can contaminate the food supply.[24,25] Compared with adults, children are at heightened risk for metabolic perturbations from endocrine-disrupting chemical exposure during development and also due to their smaller body size.

In addition to environmental factors, children carry specific genetic polymorphisms that have been associated with an increased risk of NAFLD (**Table 2**). The most prominent risk allele in both children and adults is the PNPLA3 I148 M variant, which is associated with increased susceptibility to NAFLD and greater histologic severity.[26,27] In children, the PNPLA3 variant interacts with increased dietary sugar and carbohydrate consumption to strengthen the association with the severity of hepatic steatosis.[28,29] A higher frequency of PNPLA3 risk alleles has been reported in children of Hispanic heritage, a demographic group with a high prevalence of NAFLD.[4] In

Table 2
Genes associated with histologic characteristics in children with nonalcoholic fatty liver disease

Histologic Characteristic	Gene
↑ Hepatic steatosis	PNPLA3
	PNPLA3 + GCKR
↑ NAS	PNPLA3
	NCAN
	LCP1
	TRAPPC9[a]
	IL17RA
↓ NAS and ↓ fibrosis	LPIN1[a]
↑ Fibrosis	NCAN
	PNPLA3
	TM6SF2
	ACTR5[a]
	IL17RA

Abbreviations: ACTR5, ARP5 actin-related protein 5 homolog; GCKR, glucokinase regulatory protein; IL17RA, interleukin 17 receptor A; NAS, NAFLD activity score; NCAN, neurocan; LCP1, lymphocyte cytosolic protein-1; TM6SF2, transmembrane 6 superfamily member 2; TRAPPPC9, C8orf17/potassium channel, subfamily K, member 9.
[a] Novel allele identified in pediatric cohorts.

contrast, populations with sub-Saharan African heritage have a lower frequency of the PNPLA3 risk allele.[30,31]

Several other variants have been associated with histologic features of NAFLD in children (see **Table 2**).[27,32] Several novel genetic loci, not previously reported in adults, have also been associated with histologic features of NAFL in some cohorts of children with NAFLD.[32]

Natural History of Nonalcoholic Fatty Liver Disease in Children

Long-term outcomes studies are limited in children with NAFLD. A retrospective cohort study of 66 children with biopsy-confirmed NAFLD, followed for up to 20 years, reported progression to liver transplantation in two children and the other two who died from non-liver-related causes. However, only five children had serial liver biopsies.[33] A more recent and larger multicenter study evaluated the progression of biopsy-confirmed NAFLD in children enrolled in placebo arms of two clinical trials. Over a period of 1 to 2 years of follow-up, 36% of those with baseline NAFL or borderline NASH progressed to definite NASH and/or advanced in fibrosis severity, despite receiving standard of care lifestyle counseling.[34] In combination, 11% either progressed to definite NASH or had worsening fibrosis, but no child progressed to cirrhosis. By the end of follow-up, eight children had incident type 2 diabetes, with a cumulative incidence of 36.8/1000 person-years. Other single-center case series have documented that some children are at risk of rapid progression, with advanced fibrosis or even cirrhosis developing more than 2 to 5 years.[35–37]

Because children develop the disease at a much younger age, with longer potential exposure to environmental risk factors, and the hepatic lipotoxic and inflammatory milieu that drives fibrogenesis, longer-term prospective cohort studies are needed to determine the natural history of NAFLD in children, including the risk of liver-related and non-liver-related adverse outcomes as they progress into adulthood. Outcomes derived from adult cohorts who had onset of disease much later in life may not extrapolate to youth-onset NAFLD.

Screening for Nonalcoholic Fatty Liver Disease in Children

Serologic biomarkers: Screening for NAFLD in children remains reliant on elevated ALT levels, as current serum-based noninvasive tests perform poorly in children.[38] Various thresholds for biologically-derived upper limits of normal (ULN) for ALT have been proposed in children based on large population-based pediatric cohort studies. In the United States, > 22 U/L for women and >26 U/L for men are often used cut-points to define abnormal liver enzymes in children, but these thresholds were derived from an NHANES analysis in healthy, non-overweight adolescents and may be less applicable to younger children.[18] Similar studies in North America and Europe have found comparable cut-points in the mid-20 U/L range for healthy non-overweight adolescents, but a slightly higher ULN of <30 U/L for ALT in children younger than 12 years.[39,40]

The current Endocrine Society Clinical Practice Guideline for pediatric obesity recommends using the stringent biologically-derived cut-points of >22 U/L for girls and >25 U/L for boys for screening for NAFLD in overweight children (BMI ≥85th percentile for age and sex).[41] In contrast, to increase specificity, the North American Society for Pediatric Gastroenterology, Hepatology and Nutrition (NASPGHAN) clinical practice guideline recommends using an ALT cut-off twice the ULN (approximately 45–50 U/L, depending on sex) to screen for NAFLD in overweight children with metabolic risk factors and all obese children (BMI ≥95th percentile for age and sex).[42] Using this twice the ULN cut-off estimated a 26% prevalence of NAFLD in a cohort of 344 children being evaluated for suspected NAFLD, compared with 54% prevalence if using the lower biological ULN of 22 U/L for girls and 26 U/L for boys.[43] Using an ALT > 45 U/L plus presence of increased hepatic echogenicity on ultrasound resulted in a comparable prevalence of suspected NAFLD (58%). Of note, 25% of those with fatty infiltration found on ultrasound had normal liver enzyme levels. The NASPGHAN guideline recommends using a higher cut-off of ≥ 80 U/L to identify children who are at higher risk of NASH and expedite referral.[38]

Novel noninvasive serologic diagnosis of NAFLD is limited in children. A recent study in a cohort of children, adolescents, and young adults, aged 2 to 25 year old, with NAFLD (n = 222) and without NAFLD (n = 337) used a machine learning approach to develop a novel metabolomic-based panel that detected NAFLD with a sensitivity of 73% and specificity of 84%.[44] With the addition of selected clinical phenotype variables, waist circumference, homeostasis model assessment of insulin resistance, and blood triglycerides, the specificity for NAFLD increased to 97%. This promising approach requires further external validation.

Imaging biomarkers: Routine abdominal ultrasound lacks sensitivity and may not detect lower degrees of steatosis, but is often part of the initial evaluation of a child with persistently elevated liver enzymes to evaluate for abnormalities of the liver or gallbladder, and increased hepatic echogenicity supports a diagnosis of NAFLD.[45] A measure of the controlled attenuation parameter (CAP) can be simultaneously obtained during vibration-controlled transient elastography (VCTE) assessment with the Fibroscan device. Increasing mean values of CAP are associated with increasing grades of steatosis severity on liver biopsy in children and adults with NAFLD,[46] but have not been sufficiently validated in children to provide specific cut-offs for detection of NAFLD or to enable noninvasive grading of steatosis in children. Magnetic resonance spectroscopy and MRI-proton density fat fraction (MRI-PDFF) are more sensitive and accurate methods of quantifying hepatic steatosis in children compared with ultrasound and the CAP measures.[45,47,48] However, owing to the high cost and limited availability, the use of MRI is not recommended for routine NAFLD screening in children.

Clinical Presentation

Generally, children with NAFLD are asymptomatic at presentation, with the incidental finding of elevated liver enzymes or as a result of screening guidelines. However, some children may complain of right upper quadrant or generalized abdominal pain or fatigue.[42] Children rarely present with signs of advanced liver disease, because progression to decompensated cirrhosis is rare during childhood.

Most children with NAFLD are overweight or obese, though children may have normal or low BMI in the setting of other causes of insulin resistance, such as lipodystrophy or genetic disorders such as lysosomal acid lipase deficiency. Unusual symptoms such as short stature, decline in height velocity, developmental delay, or hypogonadism raise concern for a potential endocrine or genetic cause of obesity.[41]

Elevated blood pressure can be present in about a third of children at the time of diagnosis.[49] Common physical examination findings include central adiposity and acanthosis nigricans. Striae can occur in the setting of rapid weight gain, but if very prominent and violaceous should prompt further examination for signs of Cushing's syndrome.[41] Hepatomegaly and splenomegaly may be present but can be challenging to detect on examination when significant abdominal adiposity is present.

Laboratory testing usually includes elevations in ALT and aspartate aminotransferase (AST). ALT is typically greater than AST elevation. A real-world longitudinal observational cohort study was conducted in 660 children with NAFLD (median age 13 years, 30% women, 60% Hispanic) receiving care in both academic and community gastroenterology, hepatology, and endocrinology clinics. The median ALT was 103 U/L (range 10–929) and the median AST was 59 U/L (range 18–486). Gamma glutamyl-peptidase (GGT) may be normal or elevated. Isolated elevations of GGT can indicate an alternate etiology such as primary sclerosing cholangitis, excess alcohol intake, or a medication side effect, most commonly antiepileptic medications.

Owing to the strong association with obesity, numerous associated comorbidities are often present in children with NAFLD, and routine screening for these conditions is recommended, as some require specific therapy that may also benefit NAFLD (eg, type 2 diabetes) (**Box 1**). Several of these conditions are also associated with more severe NAFLD histology (**Table 3**).[42]

Prediabetes and Type 2 Diabetes

NAFLD is associated with both prediabetes and type 2 diabetes in children in cross-sectional cohort studies.[50,51] The first study to examine the prevalence of abnormal glucose metabolism in a large multicenter cohort of children with biopsy-proven NAFLD was performed by the National Institute of Health-funded NASH-Clinical

---

Box 1
Recommended comorbidity assessment in children with suspected nonalcoholic fatty liver disease

- Fasting lipid profile
- Fasting glucose and insulin
- Hemoglobin A1C
- Blood pressure with an appropriately sized cuff
- Symptoms of sleep apnea, with follow-up testing if indicated
- Menstrual history, hirsutism, severe acne in women (suggestive of polycystic ovary syndrome)
- Thyroid function (TSH, with free T4 if indicated)

Table 3
Prevalence of cardiometabolic comorbid conditions and associations with histologic disease severity in children with nonalcoholic fatty liver disease

Risk Factor	Reported Prevalence	Phenotypic Association	N (Source)
Prediabetes	23%	1.9 OR of NASH	675 (NASH CRN)[1]
Diabetes	6.5%	3.1 OR of NASH	675 (NASH CRN)[1]
High blood pressure	36%	More severe steatosis	484 (NASH CRN)[2]
Sleep Apnea	60%	More severe fibrosis[4] 4.9 OR of NASH[5] 5.9 OR of significant fibrosis[5]	25 (United States, single site)[4] 65 (Italy, single site)[5]
Dyslipidemia	14% elevated LDL 51% high triglycerides	Unclear	585 (NASH CRN)[6]

Abbreviations: NASH CRN, NASH clinical research network; OR, odds ratio.

Research Network (NASH CRN), which includes a broad geographic representation of children with histologically-characterized NAFLD enrolled across 10 clinical centers in the United States.[7] At the time of enrollment, nearly 30% of children had abnormal glucose metabolism with 6.5% satisfying the criteria for type 2 diabetes. Of note, independent of age and BMI, girls with NAFLD were more likely to have diabetes than boys. Finally, children with prediabetes and diabetes had significantly higher odds of having NASH compared with those with normal glucose (see **Table 3**).

Another recent study validated these findings in a cohort of 599 Caucasian children/adolescents with biopsy-proven NAFLD compared with 118 children/adolescents without NAFLD but similar age, sex, BMI, and waist circumference.[52] The children with NAFLD had a significantly higher prevalence of prediabetes or diabetes than those without NAFLD (20.6% vs 11%, $P = .02$). Abnormal glucose tolerance was also associated with a higher risk of NASH.[52]

NAFLD may also be an early predictor and determinant of subsequent development of T2D and cardiovascular disease.[53] Hepatic steatosis correlates with both hepatic and adipose tissue insulin resistance and may drive the development of impaired glucose tolerance.[54,55]

Atherogenic Risk Factors

About one-third of children have elevated blood pressure at the time of diagnosis, and this has also been associated with more severe steatosis in a large NASH CRN pediatric cohort study.[49] Lipid abnormalities are also common among children with NAFLD, particularly elevated triglyceride levels. Among 585 children with NAFLD enrolled in the NASH CRN cohort, more than half met the criteria for intervention for either LDL-C or TG elevation based on the 2011 National Heart, Lung and Blood Institute guidelines.[6] Elevated triglyceride concentration (41%) was the most common. Following 1 year of standard of care lifestyle recommendations, only half of children in the target LDL-C group and one-fourth of children in the target TG group reached the recommended lipid level as per the NHLBI guidelines, indicating the need for close follow-up and management of lipid abnormalities in children with NAFLD. In another study of children with confirmed NAFLD, increased histologic disease activity and fibrosis stage were independently associated with a more pro-atherogenic lipid profile including TG/HDL, TC/HDL, and LDL/HDL ratios.[56] More recently, changes in plasma lipidomic profiles have been noted in obese children with hepatic steatosis versus obese controls.[57]

Hypothyroidism

Thyroid hormones play a key role in regulating whole-body metabolism and lipid utilization by the liver. Thyroid hormones bind to thyroid hormone receptors α and β, which interact with other transcription factors to either activate or inhibit the transcription of genes in numerous target tissues, including adipose tissue and the liver.[58] Murine models suggest that mild hypothyroidism promotes the development of fatty liver, by impaired suppression of adipose tissue lipolysis.[58] This increases the delivery of fatty acids to the liver where they are esterified and stored as triglycerides, promoting hepatic insulin resistance.[58] In adults, hypothyroidism has been associated with NAFLD, including with increased histologic severity of the disease.[59,60] In children, elevated TSH levels have been associated with increasing ALT and severity of steatosis by ultrasound.[61–63] More recently, mediation analysis in children with biopsy-confirmed NAFLD suggested an obesity-independent effect of TSH on NAFLD, when compared with age-matched controls without liver disease.[64] However, the study was too small to detect associations with histologic severity. Further research is ongoing in this area.

Polycystic Ovarian Syndrome

Polycystic ovary syndrome (PCOS) is an endocrine syndrome common in young women of childbearing age (prevalence 6% to 15%), characterized by androgen excess, irregular menses, and higher rates of infertility. A diagnosis of PCOS can be challenging in adolescents because irregular menses and mildly elevated serum androgen concentrations can occur during normal pubertal development; therefore, formal diagnosis is often deferred until at least 2 years after menarche.[65] In adult women, PCOS has been associated with a more severe feature of NAFLD, including ballooning and advanced fibrosis.[66] Data in children are less robust, but a higher prevalence of MRI-assessed NAFLD (50%) has been reported in adolescent girls with obesity and PCOS compared with obese adolescents without PCOS (13%).[67] Alterations in sex hormones, particularly testosterone, may mediate this relationship. In an analysis of 573 children, mean age 13 years, with biopsy-confirmed NAFLD, higher testosterone levels were positively associated with increased steatosis severity among girls, whereas higher testosterone levels were associated with lower stages of fibrosis in boys.[68] Further research is needed to elucidate the role of sex hormones in the development of NAFLD, including in the pediatric transgender population, where cross-sex hormones may be administered to adolescent children and continued into adulthood.

Obstructive Sleep Apnea

Obstructive sleep apnea (OSA) has an estimated prevalence of 6% in the general pediatric population but can increase steeply to up to 78% in children with severe obesity.[69] OSA has been correlated with a higher risk of NAFLD in children in several studies, including an association with more severe liver histology.[70–72] Further supporting a mechanistic relationship, treatment of OSA with continuous positive airway pressure in children with biopsy-confirmed NAFLD improved ALT and cardiometabolic measures.[73] All children with NAFLD should be screened for OSA symptoms and referred for sleep evaluation if concerns are identified.[24,42]

Growth Hormone Deficiency

In addition to promoting linear growth in childhood, GH is a key regulator of metabolism, body composition, strength, and aerobic capacity. Children with hypothalamic or pituitary dysfunction and resultant GH deficiency have a higher risk of progressive NASH.[14] Case reports indicate improvement in NASH with GH treatment in children with panhypopituitarism.[74] In children without known GH deficiency, peak GH levels after stimulation test were negatively associated with NAFLD among 84 obese children with and without NAFLD.[75] A recent open-label study randomizing 44 obese boys with NAFLD to 6-month treatment with recombinant human GH found significant benefits in reducing BMI, ALT, AST, GGT, c-reactive protein, and LDL levels in the GH-treated group.[76] However, further research and clinical trials are needed before recommending routine testing or treatment with GH in children with NAFLD.

Evaluation of Children with Suspected Nonalcoholic Fatty Liver Disease

The formal diagnosis of NAFLD in children is like adults: confirmation of abnormal hepatic steatosis by imaging or histology, with the absence of significant alcohol consumption (in adolescents), and no alternative causes of hepatic steatosis or chronic liver disease (**Box 2**).

In a single-center study of 347 predominantly Hispanic children being evaluated for suspected NAFLD, 18% had alternate causes of liver disease, primarily autoimmune liver disease.[38] However, in a more recent retrospective, multicenter cohort study of 900 children evaluated for suspected NAFLD, only 2% had alternate causes, with hypothyroidism the leading cause, and no cases of viral hepatitis or Wilson disease.[77] Although 13% had elevated autoantibodies, no children met clinical or histologic criteria for autoimmune hepatitis. Although very rare, inborn errors of metabolism or genetic causes of hepatic steatosis must also be considered in young children presenting with hepatic steatosis and other systemic abnormalities. Although alternate conditions are much less common than NAFLD in children with chronically elevated liver enzymes, testing is still recommended because some alternate conditions require specific treatments or can increase the risk of progression to cirrhosis.

Risk Stratification of Children with Nonalcoholic Fatty Liver Disease

Risk stratification in children is limited by the lack of long-term longitudinal outcome studies in children with NAFLD. Extrapolating from risk factors for disease progression

---

Box 2
Recommended evaluation for causes of chronic liver disease in children with suspected nonalcoholic fatty liver disease

Standard screening:
- Chronic viral hepatitis (hepatitis B, C)
- Autoimmune hepatitis
- Alpha-1 antitrypsin deficiency
- Celiac disease
- Hypothyroidism
- Wilson disease
- Hemochromatosis
- Alcohol intake (age 12 years and above)
- Medications (exogenous estrogen, glucocorticoids, valproic acid, methotrexate, most commonly)

Additional testing if clinical concern:
- Lysosomal acid lipase deficiency
- Lipodystrophy
- Hypobetalipoproteinemia
- Abetalipoproteinemia
- Fatty acid oxidation defects
- Glycogen storage diseases
- Mitochondrial hepatopathy
- Cystic fibrosis

and adverse outcomes in adults, children with NASH and/or fibrosis are anticipated to be at higher risk of developing complications earlier in life, including liver-related complications and non-liver-related complications of diabetes and cardiovascular disease. For example, children with biopsy-confirmed NAFLD enrolled in the placebo arms of clinical trials had a nearly 300-fold high risk of developing incident type 2 diabetes over a period of 1 to 2 years of follow-up compared with the general pediatric population. Also, having or developing diabetes during the period of observation was associated with a higher risk of progression to NASH or in fibrosis.[34] Other factors associated with progression in histologic severity included adolescent (vs preadolescent) age, higher waist circumference, ALT, AST, total and LDL cholesterol at the time of initial biopsy, as well as increasing ALT, HbA1C, and particularly GGT over the 1 to 2 year period of follow-up. However, additional longer term natural history studies are needed to determine the rate of liver and non-liver-related complications as they progress into adulthood and to identify factors that predict which children will be at the highest risk of developing complications.

Unfortunately, most current noninvasive fibrosis prediction scores incorporating clinical and/or serologic markers were developed and validated in adults and performed poorly when applied to children, including Fibrosis-4, AST/ALT ratio, and AST to platelet ratio index.[38,78] Although some specific pediatric NAFLD fibrosis prediction scores have been developed in single-center cohort studies (pediatric NAFLD fibrosis index and pediatric NAFLD fibrosis score), they were also found to perform poorly in external validation in independent cohorts of children.[38,78]

Liver elastography, a measure of tissue stiffness, positively correlates with liver fibrosis and can be assessed using several different modalities: VCTE, US-based shear wave elastography (SWE), or MRI-based elastography (MRE). All these techniques have been most extensively validated in adults, including comparative studies. However, studies in children with a variety of chronic liver diseases, including NAFLD, also show a significant correlation between increasing liver stiffness and worsening fibrosis. Each technique is best at detecting advanced fibrosis/cirrhosis, but they cannot reliably discriminate between early stages of fibrosis.[79,80] Both US-SWE and VCTE are less reliable in children with severe obesity. Moreover, VCTE, and to some degree US-SWE have less validated cutoffs for detecting advanced fibrosis stages in children with NAFLD. VCTE is very attractive in its speed, relatively lower cost and point-of-care testing, and has become more widespread in the assessment of NAFLD in some pediatric centers but requires further validation against liver biopsy assessment in children to increase confidence in findings, particularly in severely obese children.

MRE has more rigorous data in children with biopsy-confirmed NAFLD as well as normative reference data in healthy lean children without evidence of liver disease.[81,82] In a multicenter study of 90 children with biopsy-confirmed NAFLD, two-dimensional MRE had an overall cross-validated accuracy of 72.2% for detecting any fibrosis.[83] For detecting advanced fibrosis, accuracy ranged between 86.7% and 89% across two centers and by an automated analysis. However, owing to high expense and more limited availability, MRE is not a practical first-line method for assessing advanced fibrosis in NAFLD.

A recent meta-analysis of diagnostic accuracy of various fibrosis screening tests in children with NAFLD included 20 studies that evaluated three prediction scores, five simple biomarkers, two combined biomarkers, and six imaging techniques.[84] Most studies lacked external validation and there was substantial heterogeneity, limiting the ability to assess the accuracy and clinical utility in detecting fibrosis in children with NAFLD. There is an urgent need for more robust studies, including comparative analyses to determine optimal implementation in the clinical care of children with NAFLD.

Currently, liver biopsy remains the only way to definitively diagnose and stage NASH severity in children and assess for progression of the disease, before the onset of clinically evident hepatic decompensation. In children who are not improving with initial lifestyle counseling, a liver biopsy can guide escalation of therapy, which may range from intensification of lifestyle intervention to adolescent bariatric surgery or enrollment in pharmacotherapy trials when available. In addition, liver biopsy remains essential to exclude other liver diseases such as autoimmune hepatitis. As discussed, younger children with NAFLD have a unique periportal pattern of steatosis, inflammation, and fibrosis, and lack of ballooning.[85] Interestingly, about a quarter of these children already demonstrate bridging fibrosis.[85] In children enrolled in the placebo arms of clinical trials in the NASH CRN, the zone 1 pattern of injury decreased in prevalence over a 1- to 2-year period of follow-up, but persisted in some with unknown long-term clinical significance.[34]

Longitudinal studies of elastography in children are also scant. Whether changes in liver stiffness will correlate with progression in NASH or fibrosis severity, or with adverse clinical outcomes in youth with NAFLD is unknown. One study of 65 children with NAFLD who had to repeat MRI assessments over a mean of 27 ± 14 months found that there was no correlation between change in liver stiffness and change in ALT and only a weak positive correlation between change in MRI-PDFF and ALT.[86] Additional longitudinal studies are needed to determine the role of elastography in assessing the progression of disease in children and correlation with clinical endpoints.

Treatment of Nonalcoholic Fatty Liver Disease in Children

Lifestyle modification

Lifestyle modifications to reduce excess adiposity or visceral adiposity remain the first-line treatment for children with NAFLD.[42] Current recommendations for lifestyle interventions in children with NAFLD mirror those recommended for children with obesity (**Table 4**).[42]

Studies of the efficacy of specific lifestyle interventions in children with NAFLD are limited. A randomized controlled study in 40 Hispanic boys showed that those assigned to a reduction in added sugar intake over an 8-week period had significant improvement in MRI-assessed hepatic steatosis and serum ALT level compared with controls following their usual diet.[87] Another controlled study showed a significant reduction in hepatic steatosis by ultrasound after a 12 weeks of either Mediterranean diet or conventional low-fat diet in children with NAFLD.[88] Further, rigorous and randomized controlled studies of different dietary interventions with rigorous endpoints are needed to determine optimal dietary approaches.

Robust evidence to support specific physical activity interventions (eg, type, duration, intensity of exercise) is likewise lacking in children.[89] Studies in adults have found that aerobic exercise, particularly when combined with resistance training, can reduce intrahepatic lipid, even in the absence of reduction in visceral adiposity and BMI.[90,91] A recent study in adolescents with NAFLD found that children assigned to a school-based exercise program or to a high-intensity interval training had similar and significant improvement in levels of insulin resistance, dyslipidemia, ALT, and AST levels. Until more evidence is available, current guidelines recommend daily moderate to high-intensity activity in children with NAFLD, but do not endorse specific types of exercise.[42]

Pharmacotherapy

There are no regulatory-approved pharmacotherapies for children with NAFLD. Only two randomized placebo-controlled trials with histologic outcomes have been conducted in youth to date.[92] The first 2-year study found no benefit to metformin

---

Table 4
Summary of current therapeutic options for children and adolescents with nonalcoholic fatty liver disease

Lifestyle Recommendations	• No sweetened foods/drinks per day • 5 Servings fruits/vegetables per day • Screen time ≤ 2 h per day • Physical activity ≥ 1 h per day • Reduce highly processed food intake More frequent follow-up and multidisciplinary support are associated with greater improvement in weight and cardiometabolic outcomes in pediatric weight management studies.
Medications	No FDA-approved medications specifically for NASH Consider high-dose vitamin E (400 IU orally twice daily if < 18 y of age, or 800 IU daily if 18 y or older) if biopsy-confirmed NASH Use FDA-approved medications for obesity (liraglutide, topiramate/phentermine) or type 2 diabetes (metformin, GLP1) in adolescents, if clinically indicated and available (in the United States, insurance coverage can be limited for some options)
Bariatric surgery	Medical criteria in adolescents: • Class 2 severe obesity BMI ≥120% of the 95th percentile or BMI ≥ 35 kg/m² (whichever is lower), with significant comorbid conditions (type 2 diabetes, pseudotumor cerebri, obstructive sleep apnea, and severe NASH) • Class 3 severe obesity BMI ≥140% of the 95th percentile or BMI ≥ 40 kg/m² (whichever is lower) irrespective of comorbid conditions Vertical sleeve gastrectomy is currently preferred over Roux-en-Y gastric bypass due to greater safety and comparable efficacy. Intragastric balloons are not currently approved by the FDA for use in adolescents. Insufficient evidence to recommend endoscopic sleeve gastrectomy over laparoscopic sleeve gastrectomy in adolescents currently.

500 mg orally twice daily or high-dose vitamin E 400 IU orally twice daily for a primary outcome of achieving a reduction in NAS of ≥2 in children compared with placebo. However, secondary analyses found significantly greater resolution of NASH in the group receiving high dose vitamin E versus placebo. Because this was a secondary outcome and the long-term efficacy and long-term safety of high dose vitamin E in children are not known, there is no consensus on using vitamin E in children with NASH, though it is an accepted treatment in adults with NASH.

A 1-year-long, double-blind randomized placebo-controlled trial of cysteamine bitartrate versus placebo in children also did not achieve the primary histologic outcome of NAS of ≥2 and no worsening in fibrosis.[93] However, there was a significant reduction in ALT in those receiving cysteamine versus placebo.[93] Subgroup analysis suggested a benefit in younger children and there was concern that older children may have had lower adherence because of a much higher number of daily oral pills required due to weight-based dosing. Losartan, an angiotensin II receptor antagonist, was recently also studied in a randomized placebo-controlled study of children with biopsy-confirmed NAFLD due to preliminary studies suggesting anti-fibrogenic effect. Treatment with 100 mg orally over a 6-month period was not found to result in significant improvement in ALT compared with placebo.[94] Similarly, randomized pediatric trials of other off-label agents, such as omega-3 fatty acid supplements or probiotics, have had negative or inconclusive results.

Although there are no approved therapies for NAFLD, some medications that are approved for the treatment of diabetes or obesity in children may hold promise in the treatment of NAFLD. Glucagon-like peptide-1 (GLP1) receptor agonists have been approved for use in adolescents for the treatment of diabetes (age ≥ 10 years) or severe obesity (age ≥ 12 years).[95] Although not studied specifically for NAFLD outcomes in children, recent GLP1 trials in adults showed significantly greater NASH resolution (approximately 40%) versus placebo (9%–18%).[96,97] Pioglitazone, another diabetes medication that has shown histologic benefit in adults with NASH, could potentially be used off-label in older adolescents and young adults ≥ 18 years of age but has the undesirable side effect of weight gain.[98] There are insufficient data to determine whether other novel diabetes medications (sodium-glucose co-transporter 2 inhibitors, etc.) will be beneficial in children with NAFLD, but these medications, like the GLP1 receptor agonists, are increasingly being used in older adolescents with type 2 diabetes, a group at higher risk for NAFLD.

Two other obesity medications are approved by the Food and Drug Administration (FDA) for use in adolescents ≥16 years of age: combined phentermine/topiramate (an appetite suppressant) and orlistat (lipoprotein lipase inhibitor), but direct studies on outcomes in children with NAFLD are lacking.[99] Orlistat is not used often in clinical care due to undesirable side effects of steatorrhea, whereas topiramate is sometimes used as off-label monotherapy in children as an anti-obesity medication. Metformin is also sometimes used off-label as an anti-obesity medication and can have modest benefits on weight and insulin resistance in adolescents, particularly when given at the recommended dose of up to 2000 mg daily.[92,100] However, at the lower dose studied in the randomized clinical trial in children with NAFLD (1000 mg total per day), it did not provide any significant benefit over placebo for histologic liver outcomes.

Bariatric surgery

Bariatric surgery is an accepted and highly effective treatment for youth with class 2 severe obesity with significant comorbid conditions and those with class 3 severe obesity with or without comorbid conditions.[101] One small single-center study of 20 adolescents showed 90% resolution rates of NASH at 1 year after sleeve gastrectomy but did not include children with advanced fibrotic NASH or with type 2 diabetes.[102] Risks of surgery in adolescents in general are comparable to those in adults, but with the potential for nutritional complications long term.[103] Safety in children with cirrhosis has not been established. Endoscopic bariatric procedures, including intragastric balloons and endoscopic sleeve gastrectomy, offer less invasive treatment options for obesity in adults, but the efficacy and outcome data in children are still emerging.[104,105] One study of intragastric balloons in children with severe obesity showed modest benefit in weight loss, with improvement in mean liver enzymes at 6 months, but no sustained benefit at 2-year follow-up.[105] A recent large cohort study of endoscopic sleeve gastrectomy in children in Saudi Arabia did not include hepatic outcomes.[106] Further research will be helpful in determining the role of these endoscopic approaches in the management of children with NAFLD.

CLINICS CARE POINTS

- Nonalcoholic fatty liver disease (NAFLD) should be suspected in a child or adolescent with chronically elevated liver enzymes and known risk factors, such as overweight or obesity, central adiposity, insulin resistance, and/or dyslipidemia, but other causes of chronic hepatitis must also be evaluated as they may require specific treatment or increase risk of disease progression.

- Confirmation of nonalcoholic steatohepatitis requires liver biopsy assessment, as there are no reliable biomarkers that can reliably assess for nonalcoholic steatohepatitis.
- Liver elastography methods can be helpful in detecting advanced fibrosis but most require further validation in children with NAFLD to determine sensitivity and specificity and identify optimal cut points.
- The first-line treatment of NAFLD in children is lifestyle modification to reduce excess adiposity and insulin resistance. Significantly reducing added sugar intake has shown benefits in children with NAFLD.
- Although there are no approved therapies for NAFLD, some medical and surgical treatments for pediatric obesity or diabetes may have beneficial hepatic outcomes and should be considered in children who meet clinical criteria.

CONFLICTS OF INTEREST

Dr. S.A. Xanthakos has received restricted research funding related to NAFLD from the National Institutes of Health and Target RWE. She receives royalties from UpToDate for articles related to pediatric NAFLD.

REFERENCES

1. Brunt EM, Kleiner DE, Carpenter DH, et al. NAFLD: reporting histologic findings in clinical practice. Hepatology 2021;73:2028–38.
2. Younossi ZM, Rinella ME, Sanyal AJ, et al. From NAFLD to MAFLD: implications of a premature change in terminology. Hepatology 2021;73:1194–8.
3. Bedossa P, Consortium FP. Utility and appropriateness of the fatty liver inhibition of progression (FLIP) algorithm and steatosis, activity, and fibrosis (SAF) score in the evaluation of biopsies of nonalcoholic fatty liver disease. Hepatology 2014;60:565–75.
4. Anderson EL, Howe LD, Jones HE, et al. The prevalence of non-alcoholic fatty liver disease in children and adolescents: a systematic review and meta-analysis. PLoS One 2015;10:e0140908.
5. Schwimmer JB, Deutsch R, Kahen T, et al. Prevalence of fatty liver in children and adolescents. Pediatrics 2006;118:1388–93.
6. Harlow KE, Africa JA, Wells A, et al. Clinically actionable hypercholesterolemia and hypertriglyceridemia in children with nonalcoholic fatty liver disease. J Pediatr 2018;198:76–83 e2.
7. Newton KP, Hou J, Crimmins NA, et al. Prevalence of prediabetes and type 2 diabetes in children with nonalcoholic fatty liver disease. JAMA Pediatr 2016; 170:e161971.
8. Welsh JA, Karpen S, Vos MB. Increasing prevalence of nonalcoholic fatty liver disease among United States adolescents, 1988-1994 to 2007-2010. J Pediatr 2013;162:496–500 e1.
9. Molleston JP, Schwimmer JB, Yates KP, et al. Histological abnormalities in children with nonalcoholic fatty liver disease and normal or mildly elevated alanine aminotransferase levels. J Pediatr 2014;164:707–713 e3.
10. Conjeevaram Selvakumar PK, Kabbany MN, Lopez R, et al. Prevalence of suspected nonalcoholic fatty liver disease in lean adolescents in the United States. J Pediatr Gastroenterol Nutr 2018;67:75–9.
11. Yuksel F, Turkkan D, Yuksel I, et al. Fatty liver disease in an autopsy series of children and adolescents. Hippokratia 2012;16:61–5.

12. Rorat M, Jurek T, Kuchar E, et al. Liver steatosis in Polish children assessed by medicolegal autopsies. World J Pediatr 2013;9:68–72.

13. Beacher DR, Ariza AJ, Fishbein MH, et al. Screening for elevated risk of liver disease in preschool children (aged 2-5 years) being seen for obesity management. SAGE Open Med 2014;2. 2050312114555211.

14. Adams LA, Feldstein A, Lindor KD, et al. Nonalcoholic fatty liver disease among patients with hypothalamic and pituitary dysfunction. Hepatology 2004;39:909–14.

15. Polyzos SA, Perakakis N, Mantzoros CS. Fatty liver in lipodystrophy: a review with a focus on therapeutic perspectives of adiponectin and/or leptin replacement. Metabolism 2019;96:66–82.

16. Skinner AC, Ravanbakht SN, Skelton JA, et al. Prevalence of obesity and severe obesity in US children, 1999-2016. Pediatrics 2018;141(3):e20173459.

17. Wesolowski SR, Kasmi KC, Jonscher KR, et al. Developmental origins of NAFLD: a womb with a clue. Nat Rev Gastroenterol Hepatol 2017;14:81–96.

18. Schwimmer JB, Dunn W, Norman GJ, et al. SAFETY study: alanine aminotransferase cutoff values are set too high for reliable detection of pediatric chronic liver disease. Gastroenterology 2010;138:1357–64, 64 e1-2.

19. Softic S, Cohen DE, Kahn CR. Role of dietary fructose and hepatic de novo lipogenesis in fatty liver disease. Dig Dis Sci 2016;61:1282–93.

20. Rahman K, Desai C, Iyer SS, et al. Loss of Junctional Adhesion Molecule A promotes severe steatohepatitis in mice on a diet high in saturated fat, fructose, and cholesterol. Gastroenterology 2016;151:733–746 e12.

21. Anderson EL, Fraser A, Howe LD, et al. Physical activity is prospectively associated with adolescent nonalcoholic fatty liver disease. J Pediatr Gastroenterol Nutr 2016;62:110–7.

22. Stratakis N, Conti DV, Jin R, et al. Prenatal exposure to perfluoroalkyl substances associated with increased susceptibility to liver injury in children. Hepatology 2020;72:1758–70.

23. Jin R, McConnell R, Catherine C, et al. Perfluoroalkyl substances and severity of nonalcoholic fatty liver in Children: an untargeted metabolomics approach. Environ Int 2020;134:105220.

24. Chen R, Xu Y, Xu C, et al. Associations between mercury exposure and the risk of nonalcoholic fatty liver disease (NAFLD) in US adolescents. Environ Sci Pollut Res Int 2019;26:31384–91.

25. Frediani JK, Naioti EA, Vos MB, et al. Arsenic exposure and risk of nonalcoholic fatty liver disease (NAFLD) among U.S. adolescents and adults: an association modified by race/ethnicity, NHANES 2005-2014. Environ Health 2018;17:6.

26. Valenti L, Alisi A, Galmozzi E, et al. I148M patatin-like phospholipase domain-containing 3 gene variant and severity of pediatric nonalcoholic fatty liver disease. Hepatology 2010;52:1274–80.

27. Namjou B, Lingren T, Huang Y, et al. GWAS and enrichment analyses of nonalcoholic fatty liver disease identify new trait-associated genes and pathways across eMERGE Network. BMC Med 2019;17:135.

28. Nobili V, Liccardo D, Bedogni G, et al. Influence of dietary pattern, physical activity, and I148M PNPLA3 on steatosis severity in at-risk adolescents. Genes Nutr 2014;9:392.

29. Davis JN, Le KA, Walker RW, et al. Increased hepatic fat in overweight Hispanic youth influenced by interaction between genetic variation in PNPLA3 and high dietary carbohydrate and sugar consumption. Am J Clin Nutr 2010;92:1522–7.

30. Fernandes DM, Pantangi V, Azam M, et al. Pediatric nonalcoholic fatty liver disease in New York city: an autopsy study. J Pediatr 2018;200:174–80.
31. Samji NS, Snell PD, Singal AK, et al. Racial disparities in diagnosis and prognosis of nonalcoholic fatty liver disease. Clin Liver Dis (Hoboken) 2020;16:66–72.
32. Wattacheril J, Lavine JE, Chalasani NP, et al. Genome-wide associations related to hepatic histology in nonalcoholic fatty liver disease in hispanic boys. J Pediatr 2017;190:100–107 e2.
33. Feldstein AE, Charatcharoenwitthaya P, Treeprasertsuk S, et al. The natural history of non-alcoholic fatty liver disease in children: a follow-up study for up to 20 years. Gut 2009;58:1538–44.
34. Xanthakos SA, Lavine JE, Yates KP, et al. Progression of fatty liver disease in children receiving standard of care lifestyle advice. Gastroenterology 2020;159:1731–1751 e10.
35. Molleston JP, White F, Teckman J, et al. Obese children with steatohepatitis can develop cirrhosis in childhood. Am J Gastroenterol 2002;97:2460–2.
36. HH AK, Henderson J, Vanhoesen K, et al. Nonalcoholic fatty liver disease in children: a single center experience. Clin Gastroenterol Hepatol 2008;6:799–802.
37. Kohli R, Boyd T, Lake K, et al. Rapid progression of NASH in childhood. J Pediatr Gastroenterol Nutr 2010;50:453–6.
38. Schwimmer JB, Newton KP, Awai HI, et al. Paediatric gastroenterology evaluation of overweight and obese children referred from primary care for suspected non-alcoholic fatty liver disease. Aliment Pharmacol Ther 2013;38:1267–77.
39. Bussler S, Vogel M, Pietzner D, et al. New pediatric percentiles of liver enzyme serum levels (alanine aminotransferase, aspartate aminotransferase, gamma-glutamyltransferase): effects of age, sex, body mass index, and pubertal stage. Hepatology 2018;68:1319–30.
40. Shaw JL, Cohen A, Konforte D, et al. Validity of establishing pediatric reference intervals based on hospital patient data: a comparison of the modified Hoffmann approach to CALIPER reference intervals obtained in healthy children. Clin Biochem 2014;47:166–72.
41. Styne DM, Arslanian SA, Connor EL, et al. Pediatric obesity-assessment, treatment, and prevention: an endocrine society clinical practice guideline. J Clin Endocrinol Metab 2017;102:709–57.
42. Vos MB, Abrams SH, Barlow SE, et al. NASPGHAN Clinical practice guideline for the diagnosis and treatment of nonalcoholic fatty liver disease in children: recommendations from the expert committee on NAFLD (ECON) and the North American society of pediatric gastroenterology, hepatology and nutrition (NASPGHAN). J Pediatr Gastroenterol Nutr 2017;64:319–34.
43. Ezaizi Y, Kabbany MN, Conjeevaram Selvakumar PK, et al. Comparison between non-alcoholic fatty liver disease screening guidelines in children and adolescents. JHEP Rep 2019;1:259–64.
44. Khusial RD, Cioffi CE, Caltharp SA, et al. Development of a plasma screening panel for pediatric nonalcoholic fatty liver disease using metabolomics. Hepatol Commun 2019;3:1311–21.
45. Awai HI, Newton KP, Sirlin CB, et al. Evidence and recommendations for imaging liver fat in children, based on systematic review. Clin Gastroenterol Hepatol 2014;12:765–73.
46. Desai NK, Harney S, Raza R, et al. Comparison of controlled attenuation parameter and liver biopsy to assess hepatic steatosis in pediatric patients. J Pediatr 2016;173:160–164 e1.

47. Jia S, Zhao Y, Liu J, et al. Magnetic resonance imaging-proton density fat fraction vs. transient elastography-controlled attenuation parameter in diagnosing non-alcoholic fatty liver disease in children and adolescents: a meta-analysis of diagnostic accuracy. Front Pediatr 2021;9:784221.

48. Middleton MS, Van Natta ML, Heba ER, et al. Diagnostic accuracy of magnetic resonance imaging hepatic proton density fat fraction in pediatric nonalcoholic fatty liver disease. Hepatology 2018;67:858–72.

49. Schwimmer JB, Zepeda A, Newton KP, et al. Longitudinal assessment of high blood pressure in children with nonalcoholic fatty liver disease. PLoS One 2014;9:e112569.

50. Cali AM, De Oliveira AM, Kim H, et al. Glucose dysregulation and hepatic steatosis in obese adolescents: is there a link? Hepatology 2009;49:1896–903.

51. D'Adamo E, Cali AM, Weiss R, et al. Central role of fatty liver in the pathogenesis of insulin resistance in obese adolescents. Diabetes Care 2010;33:1817–22.

52. Nobili V, Mantovani A, Cianfarani S, et al. Prevalence of prediabetes and diabetes in children and adolescents with biopsy-proven non-alcoholic fatty liver disease. J Hepatol 2019;71:802–10.

53. Li WD, Fu KF, Li GM, et al. Comparison of effects of obesity and non-alcoholic fatty liver disease on incidence of type 2 diabetes mellitus. World J Gastroenterol 2015;21:9607–13.

54. Samuel VT, Shulman GI. Nonalcoholic fatty liver disease as a nexus of metabolic and hepatic diseases. Cell Metab 2018;27:22–41.

55. Kim JY, Bacha F, Tfayli H, et al. Adipose tissue insulin resistance in youth on the spectrum from normal weight to obese and from normal glucose tolerance to impaired glucose tolerance to type 2 diabetes. Diabetes Care 2019;42:265–72.

56. Nobili V, Alkhouri N, Bartuli A, et al. Severity of liver injury and atherogenic lipid profile in children with nonalcoholic fatty liver disease. Pediatr Res 2010;67:665–70.

57. Draijer LG, Froon-Torenstra D, van Weeghel M, et al. Lipidomics in Nonalcoholic fatty liver disease: exploring serum lipids as biomarkers for pediatric nonalcoholic fatty liver disease. J Pediatr Gastroenterol Nutr 2020;71:433–9.

58. Ferrandino G, Kaspari RR, Spadaro O, et al. Pathogenesis of hypothyroidism-induced NAFLD is driven by intra- and extrahepatic mechanisms. Proc Natl Acad Sci U S A 2017;114:E9172–80.

59. Kim D, Kim W, Joo SK, et al. Subclinical hypothyroidism and low-normal thyroid function are associated with nonalcoholic steatohepatitis and fibrosis. Clin Gastroenterol Hepatol 2018;16:123–131 e1.

60. Guo Z, Li M, Han B, et al. Association of non-alcoholic fatty liver disease with thyroid function: a systematic review and meta-analysis. Dig Liver Dis 2018;50:1153–62.

61. Torun E, Ozgen IT, Gokce S, et al. Thyroid hormone levels in obese children and adolescents with non-alcoholic fatty liver disease. J Clin Res Pediatr Endocrinol 2014;6:34–9.

62. Bilgin H, Pirgon O. Thyroid function in obese children with non-alcoholic fatty liver disease. J Clin Res Pediatr Endocrinol 2014;6:152–7.

63. Pacifico L, Bonci E, Ferraro F, et al. Hepatic steatosis and thyroid function tests in overweight and obese children. Int J Endocrinol 2013;2013:381014.

64. Nichols PH, Pan Y, May B, et al. Effect of TSH on non-alcoholic fatty liver disease (NAFLD) independent of obesity in children of predominantly Hispanic/Latino ancestry by causal mediation analysis. PLoS One 2020;15:e0234985.

65. Witchel SF, Burghard AC, Tao RH, et al. The diagnosis and treatment of PCOS in adolescents: an update. Curr Opin Pediatr 2019;31:562–9.
66. Sarkar M, Terrault N, Chan W, et al. Polycystic ovary syndrome (PCOS) is associated with NASH severity and advanced fibrosis. Liver Int 2020;40:355–9.
67. Cree-Green M, Bergman BC, Coe GV, et al. Hepatic steatosis is common in adolescents with obesity and pcos and relates to de novo lipogenesis but not insulin resistance. Obesity (Silver Spring) 2016;24:2399–406.
68. Mueller NT, Liu T, Mitchel EB, et al. Sex hormone relations to histologic severity of pediatric nonalcoholic fatty liver disease. J Clin Endocrinol Metab 2020; 105(11):3496–504.
69. Chen LD, Chen MX, Chen GP, et al. Association between obstructive sleep apnea and non-alcoholic fatty liver disease in pediatric patients: a meta-analysis. Pediatr Obes 2021;16:e12718.
70. Kheirandish-Gozal L, Sans Capdevila O, Kheirandish E, et al. Elevated serum aminotransferase levels in children at risk for obstructive sleep apnea. Chest 2008;133:92–9.
71. Sundaram SS, Sokol RJ, Capocelli KE, et al. Obstructive sleep apnea and hypoxemia are associated with advanced liver histology in pediatric nonalcoholic fatty liver disease. J Pediatr 2014;164:699–706 e1.
72. Nobili V, Cutrera R, Liccardo D, et al. Obstructive sleep apnea syndrome affects liver histology and inflammatory cell activation in pediatric nonalcoholic fatty liver disease, regardless of obesity/insulin resistance. Am J Respir Crit Care Med 2014;189:66–76.
73. Sundaram SS, Halbower AC, Klawitter J, et al. Treating obstructive sleep apnea and chronic intermittent hypoxia improves the severity of nonalcoholic fatty liver disease in children. J Pediatr 2018;198:67–75 e1.
74. Gilliland T, Dufour S, Shulman GI, et al. Resolution of non-alcoholic steatohepatitis after growth hormone replacement in a pediatric liver transplant patient with panhypopituitarism. Pediatr Transplant 2016;20:1157–63.
75. Liang S, Yu Z, Song X, et al. Reduced growth hormone secretion is associated with nonalcoholic fatty liver disease in obese children. Horm Metab Res 2018; 50:250–6.
76. Xue J, Liang S, Ma J, et al. Effect of growth hormone therapy on liver enzyme and other cardiometabolic risk factors in boys with obesity and nonalcoholic fatty liver disease. BMC Endocr Disord 2022;22:49.
77. Yodoshi T, Orkin S, Arce-Clachar AC, et al. Alternative etiologies of liver disease in children with suspected NAFLD. Pediatrics 2021;147(4). e2020009829.
78. Jackson JA, Konomi JV, Mendoza MV, et al. Performance of fibrosis prediction scores in paediatric non-alcoholic fatty liver disease. J Paediatr Child Health 2018;54:172–6.
79. Tutar O, Beser OF, Adaletli I, et al. Shear wave elastography in the evaluation of liver fibrosis in children. J Pediatr Gastroenterol Nutr 2014;58:750–5.
80. Farmakis SG, Buchanan PM, Guzman MA, et al. Shear wave elastography correlates with liver fibrosis scores in pediatric patients with liver disease. Pediatr Radiol 2019;49:1742–53.
81. Goyal NP, Sawh MC, Ugalde-Nicalo P, et al. Evaluation of quantitative imaging biomarkers for early-phase clinical trials of steatohepatitis in adolescents. J Pediatr Gastroenterol Nutr 2020;70:99–105.
82. Trout AT, Anupindi SA, Gee MS, et al. Normal liver stiffness measured with MR elastography in children. Radiology 2020;297:663–9.

83. Schwimmer JB, Behling C, Angeles JE, et al. Magnetic resonance elastography measured shear stiffness as a biomarker of fibrosis in pediatric nonalcoholic fatty liver disease. Hepatology 2017;66:1474–85.
84. Draijer LG, van Oosterhout JPM, Vali Y, et al. Diagnostic accuracy of fibrosis tests in children with non-alcoholic fatty liver disease: a systematic review. Liver Int 2021;41(9):2087–100.
85. Brown GT, Kleiner DE. Histopathology of nonalcoholic fatty liver disease and nonalcoholic steatohepatitis. Metabolism 2016;65:1080–6.
86. Mouzaki M, Trout AT, Arce-Clachar AC, et al. Assessment of nonalcoholic fatty liver disease progression in children using magnetic resonance imaging. J Pediatr 2018;201:86–92.
87. Schwimmer JB, Ugalde-Nicalo P, Welsh JA, et al. Effect of a low free sugar diet vs usual diet on nonalcoholic fatty liver disease in adolescent boys: a randomized clinical trial. JAMA 2019;321:256–65.
88. Yurtdas G, Akbulut G, Baran M, et al. The effects of Mediterranean diet on hepatic steatosis, oxidative stress, and inflammation in adolescents with non-alcoholic fatty liver disease: a randomized controlled trial. Pediatr Obes 2022; 17:e12872.
89. Katsagoni CN, Papachristou E, Sidossis A, et al. Effects of dietary and lifestyle interventions on liver, clinical and metabolic parameters in children and adolescents with non-alcoholic fatty liver disease: a systematic review. Nutrients 2020;12.
90. Winn NC, Liu Y, Rector RS, et al. Energy-matched moderate and high intensity exercise training improves nonalcoholic fatty liver disease risk independent of changes in body mass or abdominal adiposity - a randomized trial. Metabolism 2018;78:128–40.
91. Babu AF, Csader S, Lok J, et al. Positive effects of exercise intervention without weight loss and dietary changes in nafld-related clinical parameters: a systematic review and meta-analysis. Nutrients 2021;13(9):3135.
92. Lavine JE, Schwimmer JB, Van Natta ML, et al. Effect of vitamin E or metformin for treatment of nonalcoholic fatty liver disease in children and adolescents: the TONIC randomized controlled trial. JAMA 2011;305:1659–68.
93. Schwimmer JB, Lavine JE, Wilson LA, et al. In children with nonalcoholic fatty liver disease, cysteamine bitartrate delayed release improves liver enzymes but does not reduce disease activity scores. Gastroenterology 2016;151: 1141–11454 e9.
94. Vos MB, Van Natta ML, Blondet NM, et al. Randomized placebo-controlled trial of losartan for pediatric NAFLD. Hepatology 2022.
95. Kelly AS, Auerbach P, Barrientos-Perez M, et al. A randomized, controlled trial of liraglutide for adolescents with obesity. N Engl J Med 2020;382:2117–28.
96. Newsome PN, Buchholtz K, Cusi K, et al. A placebo-controlled trial of subcutaneous semaglutide in nonalcoholic steatohepatitis. N Engl J Med 2021;384: 1113–24.
97. Armstrong MJ, Gaunt P, Aithal GP, et al. Liraglutide safety and efficacy in patients with non-alcoholic steatohepatitis (LEAN): a multicentre, double-blind, randomised, placebo-controlled phase 2 study. Lancet 2016;387:679–90.
98. Sanyal AJ, Chalasani N, Kowdley KV, et al. Pioglitazone, vitamin E, or placebo for nonalcoholic steatohepatitis. N Engl J Med 2010;362:1675–85.
99. Jebeile H, Kelly AS, O'Malley G, et al. Obesity in children and adolescents: epidemiology, causes, assessment, and management. Lancet Diabetes Endocrinol 2022;10(5):351–65.

100. Masarwa R, Brunetti VC, Aloe S, et al. Efficacy and safety of metformin for obesity: a systematic review. Pediatrics 2021;147(3):e20201610.

101. Pratt JSA, Browne A, Browne NT, et al. ASMBS pediatric metabolic and bariatric surgery guidelines, 2018. Surg Obes Relat Dis 2018;14:882–901.

102. Nobili V, Carpino G, De Peppo F, et al. Laparoscopic sleeve gastrectomy improves nonalcoholic fatty liver disease-related liver damage in adolescents by reshaping cellular interactions and hepatic adipocytokine production. J Pediatr 2018;194:100–108 e3.

103. Xanthakos SA, Khoury JC, Inge TH, et al. Nutritional risks in adolescents after bariatric surgery. Clin Gastroenterol Hepatol 2020;18:1070–10781 e5.

104. Nobili V, Della Corte C, Liccardo D, et al. Obalon intragastric balloon in the treatment of paediatric obesity: a pilot study. Pediatr Obes 2015;10:e1–4.

105. Sachdev P, Reece L, Thomson M, et al. Intragastric balloon as an adjunct to lifestyle programme in severely obese adolescents: impact on biomedical outcomes and skeletal health. Int J Obes (Lond) 2018;42:115–8.

106. Alqahtani A, Elahmedi M, Alqahtani YA, et al. Endoscopic sleeve gastroplasty in 109 consecutive children and adolescents with obesity: two-year outcomes of a new modality. Am J Gastroenterol 2019;114:1857–62.

An Update on Pediatric Acute Liver Failure

Emerging Understanding of the Impact of Immune Dysregulation and Novel Opportunities for Intervention

Sakil Kulkarni, MD[a,1], Catherine A. Chapin, MD, MS[b,1],
Estella M. Alonso, MD[b], David A. Rudnick, MD, PhD[a,c],*

KEYWORDS

- Pediatric acute liver failure • Indeterminate diagnosis • Immune dysregulation

KEY POINTS

- Prospective study of pediatric acute liver failure (PALF) by the PALF study group (PALFSG) revealed the higher rates of liver transplantation in PALFSG subjects diagnosed as "indeterminate" etiology.
- Diagnosis with "indeterminate" PALF declined over the course of PALFSG studies coincident with the implementation of standardized, electronic medical record-based, age-specific order sets. Nevertheless, many PALF subjects are still diagnosed with indeterminate etiology.
- Subsequent work by PALFSG investigators identified specific immune activation markers associated with PALF, particularly in subjects with indeterminate etiology.
- The TRIUMPH study is a new NIH-funded intervention trial to test the hypothesis that specific immunosuppressive therapies will improve outcomes in PALF subjects diagnosed as indeterminate even after comprehensive, algorithm-based testing for age-related etiologies.

[a] Department of Pediatrics, St. Louis Children's Hospital, One Children's Place, St Louis, MO 63110, USA; [b] Department of Pediatrics, Ann and Robert H. Lurie Children's Hospital of Chicago, Northwestern University Feinberg School of Medicine, Box 65, 225 E Chicago Avenue, Chicago, IL 60611, USA; [c] Department of Developmental Biology, Washington University School of Medicine, 3105 McDonnell Pediatric Research Building, 660 S Euclid Avenue, Campus Box 8208, St Louis, MO 63110, USA
[1] These authors contributed equally to this work.
* Corresponding author.
E-mail address: rudnick_d@wustl.edu

Clin Liver Dis 26 (2022) 461–471
https://doi.org/10.1016/j.cld.2022.03.007
1089-3261/22/© 2022 Elsevier Inc. All rights reserved.

liver.theclinics.com

INTRODUCTION

Pediatric acute liver failure (PALF) is a complex, unpredictable, often rapidly progressive, potentially devastating clinical syndrome that occurs in infants, children, and adolescents without preexisting liver disease.[1] PALF is characterized by the acute onset of hepatocellular injury and liver-based coagulopathy, frequently accompanied by hepatic encephalopathy (HE). Etiologies include drug and toxin exposures, metabolic and genetic disorders, infections, and immune-mediated disease. However, prospective studies have found that a specific etiologic diagnosis is not identified in 30% to 50% of cases.[2,3] PALF management primarily involves early contact with the consideration of transfer to a pediatric liver transplant center and intensive supportive multidisciplinary clinical care, with targeted therapies available for a subset of causes.[4] Outcomes include survival with native liver, death, and liver transplantation. Efforts to develop reliable clinical prognostic tools to predict PALF outcomes early in the course of disease have not yet been fulfilled, and the possibility remains that some transplanted PALF patients might have survived without transplantation.

Recent and prior publications have addressed PALF issues including historical considerations, clinical characteristics, medical history and examination findings, standardized order set-based diagnostic testing, general- and etiology-specific management considerations, complications, and outcomes.[1–4] In this update, we summarize more recently published contributions to the PALF literature, with particular emphasis on the role of immune dysregulation in PALF of indeterminate etiology and their relevance to new opportunities for identification of novel treatments.

THE PEDIATRIC ACUTE LIVER FAILURE STUDY GROUP

The National Institutes of Health (NIH)-funded PALF study group (PALFSG, 1UO1DK072146) was the first multicenter, multinational collaboration established to identify, characterize, and develop management strategies for infants, children, and adolescents with acute liver failure (ALF). From 1999 to 2015, the PALFSG enrolled and prospectively collected clinical and outcomes data on 1144 children with ALF as defined by the criteria listed in **Box 1**.[5]

The initial report describing the first 348 cases enrolled in the PALFSG enumerated the range of specific causes and also revealed that a definitive etiologic diagnosis was lacking in approximately half of those cases.[2] This publication also reported that ultimate outcomes (ie, alive or dead with or without liver transplantation) differed significantly between indeterminate PALF cases and those cases in which a specific etiology was identified, with higher than expected rates of liver transplantation in the indeterminate group. A subsequent PALFSG study showed that implementation of electronic medical record (EMR)-based age-specific diagnostic testing reduced the percentage of subjects with an indeterminate diagnosis and such reduction correlated with reduced liver transplantation rates without increased mortality.[3] More recent studies have identified specific, unique inflammatory signatures in biosamples from

---

Box 1
Criteria for PALFSG enrollment

- No underlying chronic liver disease
- INR greater than 1.5, uncorrectable by vitamin K, and clinical hepatic encephalopathy (HE), or
- INR greater than 2, uncorrectable by vitamin K, with or without HE

indeterminate PALF subjects and have begun to characterize those patterns at histopathological, cellular, and molecular levels.[6–9] Together, the results of these studies have led to the hypothesis that a dysregulated immune response represents a potentially treatable cause of liver injury in at least a subset of patients with indeterminate PALF. This review summarizes the studies published to date in support of this hypothesis and briefly discusses a new NIH-funded PALF intervention trial (ie, The PALF Immune Response Network: Treatment for Immune Mediated Pathophysiology [TRIUMPH], U01DK127995) based on this hypothesis.

RECENT INSIGHTS INTO THE NATURE OF INDETERMINATE PEDIATRIC ACUTE LIVER FAILURE

As mentioned above, many PALF patients do not receive a specific etiologic diagnosis. In the initial, 348 patient PALFSG cohort 49% of subjects carried a diagnosis of indeterminate, and indeterminate subjects were more likely to have the outcome of liver transplantation (46%) compared with PALFSG subjects in the known diagnoses group (19%).[2] Subsequent review of diagnostic evaluations performed within the PALFSG revealed that such workups were not complete in a significant percentage of patients, suggesting the possibility that a diagnosis could have been determined in some cases if a more extensive, age-appropriate evaluation was completed.[10] Ensuing efforts were made to adjudicate etiology considerations in those indeterminate PALFSG study subjects with incomplete diagnostic evaluations by using expert consensus and selected retrospective analyses of banked biosamples. The results identified a subset of study subjects with previously undiagnosed viral infections, including herpes simplex virus and others,[11] or with elevated acetaminophen adducts.[12] Nevertheless, most of the indeterminate PALFSG subjects remained unexplained with respect to current etiologic understanding of disease mechanism. The PALFSG also subsequently investigated the influence of incomplete diagnostic workup on the prevalence of indeterminate PALF. That analysis examined PALFSG subjects by the three phases of study group enrollment, with phase 3 notable for implementation of age-specific diagnostic testing using EMR-based order sets among all participating study group centers.[3] The results showed that the proportion of study subjects with an indeterminate diagnosis decreased between phases 1 to 2 and phase 3 (from 48% to 31%, **Fig. 1**) and the overall liver transplantation rates also declined over this interval (from 35% to 20%) without an increase in mortality (18% in phase 1, 11% in phase 3).

Relevant to these considerations, another study of clinical course among 380 PALFSG subjects with indeterminate diagnosis revealed distinct disease trajectories identifiable within the first 7 days that correlated with 21-day outcomes. Although a subset of indeterminate subjects displayed mild, quickly improving trajectories, the majority (57%) had disease trajectories that worsened over time.[13] Also pertinent, a different recent study independently compared all 1144 PALFSG subjects to define clinical features associated with listing for liver transplant.[5] Consistent with prior findings, the cumulative incidences of listing for and receiving a liver transplant decreased over the three phases of the PALFSG study (**Fig. 2**) without an increase in the cumulative incidence of death. This analysis also showed that an indeterminate diagnosis was more common in subjects listed for liver transplantation, and most listed subjects proceeded to liver transplant. The authors concluded that the diagnosis of indeterminate etiology correlated with and perhaps influenced the likelihood of being listed for liver transplant. Consistent with these considerations, a more recent independent assessment of liver transplantation practices in PALF using the

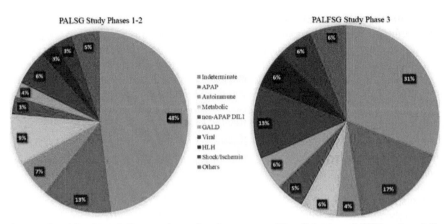

Fig. 1. Algorithm-based diagnostic testing for age-specific etiologies of PALF reduced the proportion of indeterminate diagnoses. The distribution of diagnoses is from PALFSG study phases 1 to 2 (*left*) and study phase 3 (*right*), respectively. Numerical data from Table 4 in Ref[3] were used to generate the pie chart data illustrated here. The distributions are significantly different. APAP, acetaminophen; DILI, drug-induced liver injury; GALD, gestational alloimmune liver disease; HLH, hemophagocytic lymphohistiocytosis.

Scientific Registry of Transplant Recipients database[14] revealed that two-thirds of the transplanted PALF patients had indeterminate etiology (Kulkarni et al., Outcomes analyses of Pediatric Acute Liver Failure Subjects Listed for Transplantation, PMID 35442235).

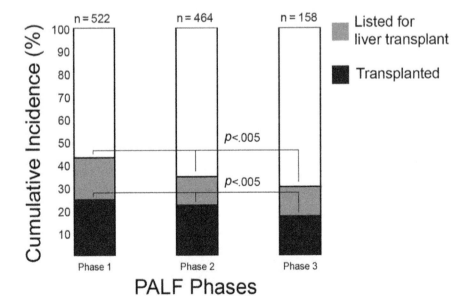

Fig. 2. Cumulative incidences of listing for and receiving liver transplantation over the three phases of PALF. (*From* Squires et al., Liver Transplant Listing in Pediatric Acute Liver Failure: Practices and Participant Characteristics, Hepatology, 68, 2018, 2338-2347. Reused with permission.)

EMERGING UNDERSTANDING OF THE ROLE OF IMMUNE DYSREGULATION IN INDETERMINATE PEDIATRIC ACUTE LIVER FAILURE

More than 20 years ago, Rolando and colleagues[15] reported the first analysis of the relationship between the systemic inflammatory response syndrome (SIRS) and ALF in adult subjects. Those investigators compared measures of SIRS (including white blood cell count, heart rate, and temperature) to clinical course and outcomes in 887 ALF patients and concluded that SIRS worsens the risk of progression of HE, reduces the chance of transplantation, and confers an overall poorer prognosis in ALF. Since that time, support has been growing for the hypothesis that many ALF patients have liver injury secondary to a hyper-inflammatory immune response.

More than a decade later, Taylor and colleagues[16] reported the outcomes after administration of immunosuppressive therapy (antithymocyte globulin (ATG), methylprednisolone, and cyclosporine) to two pediatric patients presenting with acquired aplastic anemia that occurred coincidentally with acute severe liver injury, with those subjects completely recovering from both processes. Hepatitis-associated aplastic anemia (HAAA) is a well-recognized clinical syndrome, in which acute hepatitis occurs before or concurrently with bone marrow failure.[17] Another single-center report described four patients diagnosed with HAAA that also improved with ATG.[18]

A PALFSG analysis of the association between peripheral blood immune activation markers (IAMs) and 21-day outcome in 77 PALF patients found that patients with higher soluble interleukin 2 receptor alpha (sIL2Rα) levels were more likely to die or undergo liver transplantation.[6] Of note, subjects with the highest sIL2Rα levels (>5000 IU/mL) were more likely to have an indeterminate diagnosis (67%). Taken together, these studies established a foundation for targeted PALF clinical intervention trials with immunomodulatory drugs.

Based on these considerations, in 2017, a NIH/National Institute of Diabetes and Digestive and Kidney Diseases-sponsored workshop was held, entitled PALF of undetermined cause, with the goal to better understand the basis for PALFSG outcome studies showing lower rates of spontaneous survival and higher rates of transplantation and death in children with PALF of indeterminate etiology compared with other diagnostic groups and to develop a foundation for future mechanistic studies and treatment trials based on such undertanding.[19] Presentations at the workshop considered that the clinical phenotype of indeterminate PALF shares features with hyper-inflammatory syndromes, including hemophagocytic lymphohistiocytosis (HLH) and macrophage activation syndrome (MAS). Based on the data presented in this forum, the authors proposed a model of liver injury progression in indeterminate PALF (**Fig. 3**) and speculated that existing pediatric HLH and MAS therapies might inform development of an intervention trial for treatment of indeterminate PALF.[19]

Subsequent studies by Zamora and colleagues[8] sought to discover novel predictors of PALF outcomes by comparing circulating levels of 27 inflammatory mediators over time to 21-day outcomes in a cohort of 101 PALFSG subjects. Using dynamic network analysis and other sophisticated data analysis algorithms, distinct patterns of change in circulating inflammatory mediators were identified in PALFSG subjects who died compared with those who survived or underwent liver transplantation. The results suggested that this approach might be developed into a tool for improved PALF outcomes prognostication. These investigators went on to assess those inflammatory mediator networks in a subset of non-transplanted PALFSG subjects that received N-acetylcysteine (NAC), either for acetaminophen-induced ALF or as part of the PALFSG NAC intervention trial for non-acetaminophen-induced ALF.[20] The results were compared

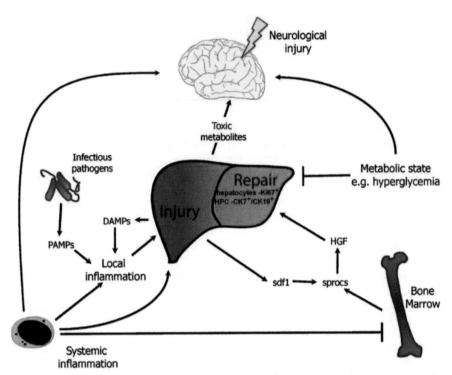

Fig. 3. Proposed model of liver injury progression in indeterminate pediatric ALF. See original reference[19] for detailed summary of model. CK7+, cytokeratin 7 positive; CK19+, cytokeratin 19 positive; DAMPs, damage-associated molecular patterns; HGF, hepatocyte growth factor; HPC, hepatic progenitor cell; PAMPs, pathogen-associated molecular patterns. (*From* Alonso et al., Pediatric Acute Liver Failure of Undetermined Cause: A Research Workshop, Hepatology, 65, 2017, 1026–1037; with permission.)

with parallel analyses of PALF caused by other (ie, non-acetaminophen-induced) etiologies in subjects who did not receive NAC or who did not survive. This analysis revealed strong correlations between inflammatory mediator networks and clinical outcomes in PALFSG subjects and implicated the "alarmin" high-mobility group B1 as a key regulator of these networks.[21] More recently, this group reexamined the relationships between study subject age, patient etiology, and ultimate outcome on these inflammatory mediator networks and concluded that this approach could inform PALF patient selection for novel therapeutic intervention studies.[22]

While Zamora and colleagues were defining the molecular basis for immune dysregulation in PALF with the studies described above, other investigators sought to characterize the histologic and cellular features of such pathology. A pilot study compared histopathological patterns of hepatic inflammation in liver biopsies from PALF patients with indeterminate etiology ($n = 33$) versus autoimmune hepatitis ($n = 9$) or other diagnoses ($n = 14$).[23] The liver tissue sections were assessed for immunohistochemical markers of cytotoxic T cells (ie, CD8+[Cluster of Differentiation (CD)]), perforin, and tissue resident memory T cells (ie, CD103+), and hepatic lymphocytes were evaluated by T-cell receptor beta (TCRβ) sequencing and flow cytometry. Significantly increased hepatic CD8+ T-cell infiltrates and perforin and CD103+ staining were found in samples from the indeterminate PALF patients versus those with specific, non-

---

Box 2
Biomarkers of immune activation in indeterminate PALF

- From Chapin and colleagues[23]:
  - Increased CD8+ T-cell infiltrates
  - Increased perforin and CD103+ staining
  - Increased TCRβ clonality
  - Predominance of memory CD8+ T cells

- From Leonis and colleagues[27]:
  - % perforin+ CD8 cells
  - % granzyme+ CD8 cells
  - Absolute number of CD8 cells
  - sIL2Rα levels

---

autoimmune-hepatitis PALF etiologies (**Box 2, Fig. 4**). TCRβ sequencing also demonstrated increased T-cell clonality, and flow cytometry showed a predominance of memory CD8+ T cells in indeterminate versus other study subjects. Those findings were subsequently validated in an independent multicenter PALFSG study-derived cohort.[24] Available PALFSG biosamples from 37 subjects with indeterminate PALF and 18 with known causes of PALF were analyzed by blinded investigators. Again, increased CD8+ T cell infiltrates and increased TCRβ clonality were found in livers from PALFSG subjects with indeterminate versus other (non-autoimmune hepatitis) etiologies. The investigators concluded that increased TCR clonality raised the possibility of antigen-driven T-cell expansion and proposed CD8 liver tissue staining as a new biomarker of this novel activated CD8 T-cell PALF phenotype. These findings

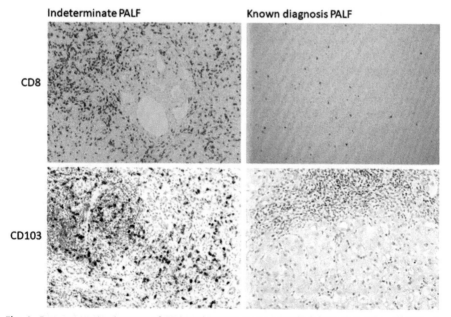

Fig. 4. Representative images of CD8 and CD103 immunohistochemical staining patterns in liver from PALF subjects with indeterminate (*left*) and known (*right*) disease etiology.

agree with those of McKenzie and colleagues who reported prominent CD8+ staining on liver biopsies from a case series of indeterminate PALF and acute hepatitis patients who were thought to have immune dysregulation and treated with immunomodulating therapies.[25] Several other reports have described CD8+ staining of liver tissue specimens as a frequent finding in patients with HAAA both with and without ALF.[18,26] Together these studies implicate CD8+ T cells as a novel biomarker of immune dysregulation in PALF of indeterminate etiology that may be used to better identify and define this group and could lead to the development of targeted therapies for these patients.

Also coincident with these studies implicating immune activation in the pathogenesis of indeterminate PALF, Leonis and colleagues[27] sought to identify specific IAMs in PALFSG subjects with indeterminate versus specific etiologies associated with clinical features and outcomes. Their analyses of blood natural killer and CD8+ lymphocyte samples from 47 PALFSG study subjects identified 4 IAMs (% perforin+ CD8 cells, % granzyme+ CD8 cells, absolute number of CD8 cells, and sIL2Rα levels) that defined cohorts of subjects with "high" ($n = 10$), "medium" ($n = 15$), and "low" ($n = 22$) immune activation patterns (see **Box 2**). High IAM levels were significantly more common in patients with indeterminate etiology (80%) than in those with defined diagnoses (20%) and were associated with higher peak serum bilirubin levels and peak coma grades compared with subjects with low IAM levels. The 21-day outcomes also differed between groups, with liver transplantation significantly more frequent in subjects with high IAMs (62.5%) compared with those with medium (28.2%) or low (4.8%) IAMs. An independent validation cohort of 71 subjects from a prior study was subsequently reanalyzed and showed trends of segregation between high, medium, and low IAM groups by etiology, initial biochemistries, and short-term outcomes, although those differences were not statistically significant. High serum aminotransferases, total bilirubin levels, and leukopenia at study entry predicted a high immune activation profile. These investigators concluded that the four circulating T-lymphocyte activation markers identified by this research define a subgroup of PALF patients with immune activation associated with a distinct clinical phenotype and increased likelihood of liver transplantation and that these biomarkers could be used to identify PALF participants for future clinical trials of early targeted immunosuppression.

In more recent work, Chapin and colleagues[28] sought to further characterize biomarkers of immune dysregulation in PALF of indeterminate etiology by characterizing hepatic cytokine profiles and transcriptional signatures in liver tissue from those subjects. Available liver tissue samples from 17 pediatric patients with indeterminate PALF were analyzed and compared with samples from 6 PALF subjects with known diagnoses. The results showed most livers from patients with indeterminate PALF exhibited evidence of Th1-mediated inflammation with higher levels of immune analytes including TNFα, IFNγ, and IL-1β. Transcriptional analyses identified a subset of indeterminate PALF cases with a more inflammatory phenotype characterized by increased expression of genes related to innate inflammation, T-cell activation, and antigen stimulation. To explore the evidence for immunosuppressive therapy in PALF to date, a four-center retrospective review of corticosteroid therapy in patients with indeterminate PALF or HAAA between 2009 and 2018 was performed.[29] The results showed that many steroid-treated patients improved but also almost half of the steroid-treated PALF patients underwent liver transplantation, and survival with native liver in this cohort was not different than historical reports. The study investigators recommended the consideration of a randomized controlled trial studying the effects of steroid therapy in PALF of indeterminate etiology.

TREATMENT FOR IMMUNE MEDIATED PATHOPHYSIOLOGY IN PEDIATRIC ACUTE LIVER FAILURE: THE TRIUMPH STUDY

These recent and prior studies led PALFSG investigators to propose the theory that many indeterminate PALF patients have liver injury that results from a dysregulated, hyper-inflammatory immune response. The studies that endorse this hypothesis have also implicated CD8$^+$ T lymphocytes as central regulators of this immune response and led to the consideration of targeted T-cell suppressing therapies. Clinical experiences in children with abnormal hyper-inflammatory immune responses associated with other diseases (ie, systemic juvenile idiopathic arthritis and acquired aplastic anemia) have demonstrated that both high-dose corticosteroids and equine ATG can suppress immune responses and reverse progressive tissue damage in those diseases. The PALF Immune Response Network (IRN) was thus established. The goal of this network was to develop and support a treatment trial of immunosuppressive therapy to reverse harmful inflammatory immune responses in children with PALF to prevent further disease progression and reduce mortality and liver transplantation.[19] The TRIUMPH trial (ie, ClinicalTrials.gov identifier NCT04862221) emerged from that effort as a recent, NIH-funded (U01-DK127995), double-blind, randomized, placebo controlled trial of high-dose methylprednisolone or equine ATG that will test the hypothesis that survival with native liver will be significantly higher in patients that receive immunosuppressive therapy compared with controls that receive supportive care alone. The trial will also assess the safety of immunosuppressive therapy in PALF patients and seek to define the balance between the risk of side-effects and treatment benefit. Outcomes will include both clinical end points such as patient survival, time to resolution of disease and adverse health events, and measures of patient-reported outcomes during rehabilitation from the illness. Trial participants will provide biosamples that will be examined to better understand their immune responses, especially that of T lymphocytes, in both the circulation and the liver. Samples will be stored in a repository to support future studies exploring new aspects of this rare disease.

In summary, PALF is a rare and devastating clinical syndrome that may result from many different etiologies. Despite significant advances in supportive care, mortality, and liver transplantation rates have remained relatively static over time. A clear diagnosis is lacking in up to 30% of PALF cases, and mounting evidence over the past 5 years implicates immune-mediated liver injury as a primary feature in many of these patients. Many studies to date have found evidence for a unique pattern of T-cell predominant inflammation in the indeterminate PALF group. The multicenter TRIUMPH treatment trial has been developed to test the hypothesis that immunosuppressive therapies will improve outcomes in these patients. This study is expected to significantly advance the care of PALF patients and will provide valuable insights into the pathophysiologic mechanisms driving inflammation in this group.

SUMMARY

- Prospective study of PALF by the PALFSG identified many subjects with indeterminate PALF and showed that liver transplantation rates is higher in those subjects than in PALFSG subjects with identified disease etiologies.

- Subsequent PALFSG studies have also characterized specific patterns of immune activation in biosamples collected from those subjects.

- ATG and steroids reverse inflammatory injury in other conditions, such as juvenile rheumatoid arthritis and aplastic anemia.

- The TRIUMPH study was recently funded by the NIH to test whether such interventions can also reverse progressive disease in indeterminate PALF.

ACKNOWLEDGMENT

The authors received no funding for the authorship and publication of this article.

REFERENCES

1. Squires JE, McKiernan P, Squires RH. Acute liver failure: an update. Clin Liver Dis 2018;22(4):773–805.
2. Squires RH Jr, Shneider BL, Bucuvalas J, et al. Acute liver failure in children: the first 348 patients in the pediatric acute liver failure study group. J Pediatr 2006; 148(5):652–8.
3. Narkewicz MR, Horslen S, Hardison RM, et al. A learning collaborative approach increases specificity of diagnosis of acute liver failure in pediatric patients. Clin Gastroenterol Hepatol 2018;16(11):1801–10.e3.
4. Squires JE, Alonso EM, Ibrahim SH, et al. North american society for pediatric gastroenterology, hepatology, and nutrition position paper on the diagnosis and management of pediatric acute liver failure. J Pediatr Gastroenterol Nutr 2021.
5. Squires JE, Rudnick DA, Hardison RM, et al. Liver transplant listing in pediatric acute liver failure (PALF): practices and participant characteristics. Hepatology 2018;68(6):2338–47.
6. Bucuvalas J, Filipovich L, Yazigi N, et al. Immunophenotype predicts outcome in pediatric acute liver failure. J Pediatr Gastroenterol Nutr 2013;56(3):311–5.
7. Azhar N, Ziraldo C, Barclay D, et al. Analysis of serum inflammatory mediators identifies unique dynamic networks associated with death and spontaneous survival in pediatric acute liver failure. PLoSOne 2013;8(11):e78202.
8. Zamora R, Vodovotz Y, Mi Q, et al. Data-driven modeling for precision medicine in pediatric acute liver failure. Mol Med 2017;22:821–9.
9. Narkewicz MR, Horslen S, Belle SH, et al. Prevalence and significance of autoantibodies in children with acute liver failure. J Pediatr Gastroenterol Nutr 2017; 64(2):210–7.
10. Narkewicz MR, Dell OD, Karpen SJ, et al. Pattern of diagnostic evaluation for the causes of pediatric acute liver failure: an opportunity for quality improvement. JPediatr 2009;155(6):801–6.
11. Schwarz KB, Dell Olio D, Lobritto SJ, et al. Analysis of viral testing in nonacetaminophen pediatric acute liver failure. J Pediatr Gastroenterol Nutr 2014;59(5): 616–23.
12. Alonso EM, James LP, Zhang S, et al. Pediatric acute liver failure study G. Acetaminophen adducts detected in serum of pediatric patients with acute liver failure. J Pediatr Gastroenterol Nutr 2015;61(1):102–7.
13. Li R, Belle SH, Horslen S, et al. Clinical course among cases of acute liver failure of indeterminate diagnosis. J Pediatr 2016;171:163–170 e161.
14. Leppke S, Leighton T, Zaun D, et al. Scientific registry of transplant recipients: collecting, analyzing, and reporting data on transplantation in the United States. Transpl Rev (Orlando) 2013;27(2):50–6.
15. Rolando N, Wade J, Davalos M, et al. The systemic inflammatory response syndrome in acute liver failure. Hepatology 2000;32(4 Pt 1):734–9.

16. Taylor S, Hu C, Pan DH, et al. Treatment of acquired aplastic anemia in patients with acute liver failure occurring concurrently: a case series. J Pediatr Hematol Oncol 2012;34(8):e349–52.
17. Brown KE, Tisdale J, Barrett AJ, et al. Hepatitis-associated aplastic anemia. N Engl J Med 1997;336(15):1059–64.
18. Kemme S, Stahl M, Brigham D, et al. Outcomes of severe seronegative hepatitis-associated aplastic anemia: a pediatric case series. J Pediatr Gastroenterol Nutr 2021;72(2):194–201.
19. Alonso EM, Horslen SP, Behrens EM, et al. Pediatric acute liver failure of undetermined cause: a research workshop. Hepatology 2017;65(3):1026–37.
20. Squires RH, Dhawan A, Alonso E, et al. Intravenous N-acetylcysteine in pediatric patients with nonacetaminophen acute liver failure: a placebo-controlled clinical trial. Hepatology 2013;57(4):1542–9.
21. Zamora R, Barclay D, Yin J, et al. HMGB1 is a central driver of dynamic pro-inflammatory networks in pediatric acute liver failure induced by acetaminophen. Sci Rep 2019;9(1):5971.
22. Vodovotz Y, Barclay D, Yin J, et al. Dynamics of systemic inflammation as a function of developmental stage in pediatric acute liver failure. Front Immunol 2020; 11:610861.
23. Chapin CA, Burn T, Meijome T, et al. Indeterminate pediatric acute liver failure is uniquely characterized by a CD103(+) CD8(+) T-cell infiltrate. Hepatology 2018; 68(3):1087–100.
24. Chapin CA, Melin-Aldana H, Kreiger PA, et al. Activated CD8 T-cell hepatitis in children with indeterminate acute liver failure: results from a multicenter cohort. J Pediatr Gastroenterol Nutr 2020;71(6):713–9.
25. McKenzie RB, Berquist WE, Nadeau KC, et al. Novel protocol including liver biopsy to identify and treat CD8+ T-cell predominant acute hepatitis and liver failure. Pediatr Transplant 2014;18(5):503–9.
26. Patel KR, Bertuch A, Sasa GS, et al. Features of hepatitis in hepatitis-associated aplastic anemia: clinical and histopathologic study. J Pediatr Gastroenterol Nutr 2017;64(1):e7–12.
27. Leonis MA, Miethke AG, Fei L, et al. Four biomarkers linked to activation of cluster of differentiation 8-positive lymphocytes predict clinical outcomes in pediatric acute liver failure. Hepatology 2021;73(1):233–46.
28. Chapin CA, Taylor SA, Malladi P, et al. Transcriptional analysis of liver tissue identifies distinct phenotypes of indeterminate pediatric acute liver failure. Hepatol Commun 2021;5(8):1373–84.
29. Chapin CA, Horslen SP, Squires JE, et al. Corticosteroid therapy for indeterminate pediatric acute liver failure and aplastic anemia with acute hepatitis. J Pediatr 2019;208:23–9.

Wilson Disease in Children

Nanda Kerkar, MD, MRCPCH, FAASLD*, Ajay Rana, MD, MCTR

KEYWORDS

- Wilson disease • *ATP7B* • Copper metabolism • Cirrhosis • Acute liver failure
- Chelating agents

KEY POINTS

- Wilson disease is an autosomal recessive inherited disease with protean manifestations primarily in the liver, neurologic system and kidney where a mutation in the *ATP7B* gene causes a defect in copper transportation resulting in excessive copper deposition.
- The disease is seen both in childhood where hepatic manifestations prevail ranging from "silent" disease to liver failure and in adults where neurologic presentation is more frequent.
- Molecular diagnosis is becoming increasingly possible and management with chelators, zinc, liver transplantation, as well as genetic counseling is included in standard care.
- Newer therapies including gene therapy and newer preparations of chelating agents are being used in clinical trials.

INTRODUCTION

Wilson disease (WD) also known as "hepatolenticular degeneration" occurs secondary to accumulation of excess copper in the body, particularly in the liver, brain, and kidney. This disease was first described by Kinnear Wilson in 1912, and timeline in the discovery of WD is summarized in **Table 1** below.

This autosomal recessively inherited disease is caused by mutations in the*ATP7B* gene. More than 500 pathogenic variants and more than 500 polymorphisms have been identified in *ATP7B*, with most affected individuals being compound heterozygotes, possessing one copy each of 2 different mutations.[2] The worldwide prevalence of WD is one in 30,000 with a carrier frequency of one in 90.[3]

ATP7B

In 1993, the gene for WD *ATP7B*, was identified on the long arm of chromosome 13 using genetic linkage analysis in families with multiple members who had WD. Previously, in 1985 the same *ATP7B* had been linked to another gene encoding enzyme esterase D, the latter subsequently became useful in the diagnosis of retinoblastoma. The discovery

University of Rochester Medical Center, Pediatric Liver Disease and Liver Transplant Program, Division of Pediatric Gastroenterology, Hepatology and Nutrition, Golisano Childrens Hospital, 601 Elmwood Avenue Box 667, Rochester, NY 14642, USA
* Corresponding author.
E-mail address: nanda_kerkar@urmc.rochester.edu
Twitter: @KerkarNanda (N.K.); @ascleppios (A.R.)

Clin Liver Dis 26 (2022) 473–488
https://doi.org/10.1016/j.cld.2022.03.008
1089-3261/22/© 2022 Elsevier Inc. All rights reserved.
liver.theclinics.com

of the gene causing Menkes disease, a P-type ATPase involved in copper transport, now known as *ATP7A*, in early 1993, led to a lot of interest in cloning the gene for WD. Menkes disease is a rare X-linked disorder where a defect in copper transport causes a deficiency of copper in enzymes but there is an accumulation of copper in tissues. Sequences from the "Menkes gene" were used to probe liver complementary DNA (cDNA) libraries by 2 groups, whereas another group used brain cDNA library to isolate the gene mutation. In the second half of 1993, the discovery of ATP7B was published separately from New York, Toronto, and Washington, respectively.[4–6]

The *ATP7B* is localized in the trans-Golgi apparatus of the hepatocytes. The protein Wilson ATPase contains 6 metal binding domains, 3 cytoplasmic ATPase domains of P-type, and 8 transmembrane helices.[5] This protein is expressed mainly in the liver and promotes binding of copper to apoceruloplasmin to produce ceruloplasmin that is then secreted into the circulation. It also sequesters excess copper and facilitates excretion of copper from hepatocytes into bile. The copper is transported to a cytoplasmic vesicular component located near the biliary canaliculus, and the copper-containing vesicle is then released into bile via exocytosis, whereas the ATP7B returns to the trans-Golgi network. Apart from the liver, there is abundant ATPase in the locus ceruleus of the brainstem, Purkinje cells in the cerebellum and the crypts of the small intestine.

COPPER METABOLISM

Copper is an essential micronutrient and a cofactor of several enzymes. The daily requirement of copper is estimated to be 0.9 to 1.7 mg.[7] High copper-containing foods include shellfish (oysters), chocolates, mushrooms, kale, nuts, liver, and kidney. The average diet contains 2 to 5 mg of copper, and because the amount ingested exceeds the amount of copper required by the body, it is usually excreted in bile to maintain copper homeostasis. An adult contains 1.2 to 2.2 mg of copper per kilogram body weight and accumulates mainly in the liver, brain, and kidney.[8] Ingested copper is absorbed in the small intestine, mediated by human copper transport protein 1 and stored with metallothionein and copper chaperones. Metallothionein also binds to other metals such as zinc and cadmium. Zinc stimulates synthesis of metallothionein and increasing zinc ingestion can lead to retention of copper in the enterocytes and subsequent shedding in the feces when the enterocytes desquamate. This is the rationale of using Zinc as a therapeutic agent in WD. The absorbed copper is then secreted by the enterocytes into the blood, complexed with albumin and amino acids and rapidly goes to the liver in the portal circulation by the copper transporting enzyme ATP7A.[9] The copper entry into the hepatocytes is mediated by human copper transport protein 1. The copper is then bound to proteins that act as chaperones to allow secretion of ceruloplasmin and excretion in bile. Copper regulates several cellular processes and is also a regulator of cell-signaling pathways. Copper-containing metallothionine include Cu/Zn superoxide dismutase, cytochrome oxidase, dopamine beta-hydroxylase, and lysyl oxidase, the latter with a role in cross-linking collagen in extracellular matrix and connective tissue.[10]

PATHOGENESIS

Copper homeostasis in the body is dependent on Wilson ATPase. Depending on the amount of copper in the system, this protein can switch from its function of "metallating" ceruloplasmin to upregulating trafficking of copper from hepatocytes into bile. Ceruloplasmin is a "sky blue protein" that has been associated with WD even before the identification of the ATP7B gene. Ceruloplasmin belongs to a family of multicopper oxidases that is not involved in the transport of copper but incorporates 95% of

Table 1		
Milestones in the discovery of Wilson Disease[a]		
Year	**Name**	**Clinical or Genetic Event**
1888	Gowers	"tetanoid chorea with cirrhosis"
1902–03	Kayser and Fleischer	Corneal pigmented ring described separately by both, now known as Kayser-Fleischer (KF) ring
1912	Wilson	Published "progressive lenticular degeneration: a familial nervous disease associated with cirrhosis of the liver" in Brain, based on his MD thesis dissertation
1916	Bramwell	First description in children—"familial cirrhosis of the liver"
1945	Glazebook	Raised copper in basal ganglia of a patient dying of WD
1947	Laurell	Ceruloplasmin discovered
1948	Cumings	Proposed that copper toxicity causes tissue damage
1951	Denny-Brown and Cumings	British anti-lewisite (dimercaprol) as chelating agent used for treating WD
1955	Walshe	Penicillamine given to first patient with WD
1961	Schouwink	Zinc used for treating WD
1970	Walshe	Trientine used as alternative to Penicillamine
1984	Walshe	Tetrathiomolybdenate
1985	Frydman	WD gene locus on chromosome 13
1993	3 groups	Menkes disease gene
1993	3 groups	Wilson disease gene

[a] Adapted from: Kerkar and Roberts (Eds) Clinical and Translational Perspectives in Liver Disease 2019: 1-11. Elsevier, with permisssion.[1]

copper found in serum. Mutation in the ceruloplasmin gene including aceruloplasminemia not only prevents copper incorporation in ceruloplasmin but also impact iron metabolism causing iron deposition in liver, spleen, and can lead to severe neurologic disease, retinal degeneration, and diabetes mellitus.

Mutations in the Wilson ATPase result in lack of copper trafficking in the trans-Golgi network and impair incorporation of copper in ceruloplasmin.[11] As a result, there is a low level of ceruloplasmin in the plasma of most patients with WD but this is not universal as ceruloplasmin is an acute phase reactant and may be increased to normal range in up to a third of WD patients. Excess copper is deposited in the liver and also goes via the blood stream to the eyes KF rings and brain (neurologic WD). Mitochondria, which are regarded as the powerhouse of cells, require adequate copper for synthesis of enzymes that are essential for ATP production. Excessive copper as seen in WD leads to structural and functional impairment of mitochondria. Several animal models with ATP7B defects have been described—inbred such as the Long Evans Cinnamon rat and toxic milk mouse models and genetically generated such as the ATP7B knockout mouse. These rodent models of WD have been helpful in developing better understanding of the relationship between copper overload and its effect on different metabolic pathways.

Epigenetics is the study of the way environment can affect the function of genes. Gene expression refers to creation of proteins based on instructions encoded within the gene. Epigenetics can affect gene expression such that genes can be switched "on" and "off." Epigenetic changes are reversible and do not change DNA sequences but can change how our body reads that DNA sequence. Epigenetic changes include DNA methylation, histone modification, and noncoding RNA.[12] In WD, although the gene has been identified, there is a wide spectrum of clinical presentations. This lack of genotype–phenotype correlation suggests that other factors including epigenetic mechanisms may be at work. Methionine metabolism in the liver regulates DNA methylation reactions. In animal models of WD, adult livers as well as fetal livers show changes in enzymes involved in hepatic methionine metabolism and in enzymes involved in DNA methylation reactions that are responsive to dietary methyl donor supplementation. Additionally, maternal supplementation with methyl donor choline was associated with improvement in DNA methylation and several mitochondrial metabolic pathways in fetal livers. This may have implication in the development of newer therapies for WD starting very early in life.

CLINICAL FEATURES

The clinical manifestations of WD are most common between the age of 3 and 40 years (mean age of diagnosis is 13 years) but may occur earlier or later.[13] Children most often present with hepatic manifestations and older patients (teenagers and adults) often tend to present with neuropsychiatric manifestations.[14–17]

The hepatic manifestations are quite varied and may range from asymptomatic biochemical abnormalities and steatosis to acute hepatitis, acute liver failure (ALF), chronic hepatitis, and cirrhosis. Common signs and symptoms may include abdominal pain, anorexia, clubbing, jaundice, hepatosplenomegaly, ascites, caput medusae, spider angioma, and upper gastrointestinal bleeding. The jaundice is worse than in other causes of chronic liver disease, and this may be secondary to the concomitant intravascular hemolysis in addition to liver decompensation. About 40% of pediatric WD patients with hepatic disease have KF rings. The hepatic involvement in WD may mimic nonalcoholic fatty liver disease, autoimmune hepatitis, and/or acute infectious hepatitis. The ALF presentation in WD—Wilsonian ALF—is usually associated with Coombs-negative hemolytic anemia, aspartate aminotransferase (AST) to alanine aminotransferase (ALT) ratio that is often greater than 2, normal or subnormal alkaline phosphatase (ALP) with an ALP to total bilirubin ratio typically less than 4, coagulopathy that is unresponsive to vitamin K, encephalopathy, and renal failure. This is seen more commonly in women and despite the acute presentation, it is not uncommon to see cirrhosis on histology. Occasionally, in a completely asymptomatic patient there may be biochemical or genetic evidence of WD and this is deemed to be "silent" WD.

The neurologic manifestations of WD, predominantly extrapyramidal, may develop insidiously or precipitously and the severity of symptoms often fluctuates, sometimes during the same day. Although neurologic involvement is more common in adults, it has been described in early childhood and can also develop in a WD patient with hepatic disease who is nonadherent. Difficulty with speech (dysathria) is the most common initial manifestation (85%–97%).[18] Other common neurologic manifestations include bradykinesia, facial grimacing, dystonia, tremor, rigidity (lead pipe and not clasp-knife or cogwheel), intentional tremors, urinary incontinence, hyperreflexia, and cognitive impairment.[19] In adults, psychiatric disturbance may be the earliest feature and the most common psychiatric symptoms include depression, acute personality changes, aggressiveness, and irritability. In teenagers, these symptoms are often confused with normal adolescence behavior or substance abuse. In children, changes may be very subtle, falling under the diagnostic umbrella of "learning difficulties."

Ocular manifestations—KF rings are the classic ocular feature. KF rings are seen as a gray brown opacity in the peripheral cornea (deposits of copper-rich and sulfur-rich granules in the Descemet membrane). KF ring first develops superiorly, then inferiorly and finally in the lateral and medial areas of cornea. These occur in approximately 50%

of patients with hepatic manifestations and in about 95% of patients with neurologic manifestations.[7,18,20,21] They are reversible and dissipate over time with the treatment of WD. Patients should be referred to an ophthalmologist for slit-lamp examination. Other findings at later stages may include sunflower cataracts (copper deposits under the lens capsule and not within), loss of accommodation, and apraxia of eyelid. Other clinical manifestations of WD are described in **Box 1**.

DIAGNOSIS

Diagnosis of WD is based on clinical findings as well as biochemical and genetic tests. Patients suspected to have WD (hepatic, neurologic, psychiatric abnormalities or in a first-degree relative of a patient) should undergo serologic testing (complete blood count, comprehensive metabolic panel, serum ceruloplasmin), 24-h urinary copper excretion as well as ocular slit-lamp examination for the detection of KF rings.

AST and ALT are often elevated in hepatic disorders resulting in parenchymal damage. ALT is often more elevated than AST in hepatitis secondary to infections, autoimmune hepatitis, or drug-induced hepatotoxicity. In WD, the serum aminotransferases are usually mildly elevated, and the AST is often higher than ALT with an AST-to-ALT ratio usually greater than 2. A ratio greater than 1 may also be seen in other conditions such as liver failure, cirrhosis, alcoholic hepatitis, cardiac, and skeletal muscle disorders. However, compared with other causes of liver failure, the serum ALP is low in WD (usually <40 IU/L). An ALP to total bilirubin ratio less than 2 has good discriminative power and helps to differentiate WD from other causes of liver failure.[22,23] The complete blood count may show anemia and thrombocytopenia, indicatinge hypersplenism due to portal hypertension. The anemia in WD could also be secondary to Coombs-negative hemolytic anemia.

As mentioned earlier, ceruloplasmin is an α_2-globulin that binds more than 95% of plasma copper. In hepatocytes, *ATP7B* helps incorporate copper ions into apoceruloplasmin resulting in holoceruloplasmin or ceruloplasmin. Apoceruloplasmin, devoid of copper has a short half-life (about 5 hours) compared with ceruloplasmin (5.5 days). In WD, due to the defective *ATP7B*, apoceruloplasmin without copper incorporation, is rapidly cleared from circulation, resulting in low serum ceruloplasmin.[24–26] Ceruloplasmin is often the first-line screening test for WD. A normal ceruloplasmin level is more than 20 mg/dL. A serum level less than 10 mg/dL is suggestive of WD but a normal value does not exclude WD. Of note, a low-ceruloplasmin concentration may also be seen in other conditions such as malnutrition, protein-losing enteropathy, healthy neonates, Menkes disease, nephrotic syndrome, hereditary aceruloplasminemia, and acquired copper deficiency states.

Urinary copper excretion during 24 hours reflects nonceruloplasmin bound copper in the plasma and is elevated in most WD patients. To assess the completeness of urine collection, often urine volume and total creatinine excretion in the 24-h urine collection are also measured. In the presence of KF rings, a 24-h urinary copper excretion greater than 40 mcg (0.64 μmol) is considered diagnostic of WD, and if the levels are 40 mcg or lesser, a liver biopsy should be considered for assessing the hepatic copper concentration. If KF rings are absent, a 24-h urinary copper excretion greater than 100 mcg (1.6 μmol) is considered highly suggestive of WD. In the past, when genetic tests were not so readily available, Penicillamine challenge test was used in equivocal cases. It should be noted that high excretion of copper may be seen in other chronic cholestatic disease including MDR3 deficiency.

Liver biopsy is important in the work-up of a child with WD. Light microscopy may show microvesicular or macrovesicular steatosis as well as glycogen deposits in the

---

Box 1
Clinical manifestations of Wilson disease

Asymptomatic (detected during screening)
  Hepatic
  - Asymptomatic (elevated aspartate aminotransferase, alanine aminotransferase, hepatomegaly)
  - Nonalcoholic fatty liver disease/Nonalcoholic steatohepatitis (NAFLD/NASH)
  - Acute hepatitis
  - Acute liver failure
  - Chronic hepatitis
  - Chronic liver failure/cirrhosis
  Neuropsychiatric
  - Dysarthria, drooling
  - Ataxia
  - Parkinsonism
  - Emotional lability
  - Depression
  - Acute personality changes
  - Tremor
  - Dystonia
  - Chorea, athetosis
  - Seizures
  - Dementia and cognitive impairment
  - Autonomic dysfunction
  Ocular
  - Kayser-Fleischer rings
  - Sunflower cataracts
  Hematologic
  - Coombs-negative hemolytic anemia
  Renal
  - Fanconi syndrome
  - Nephrolithiasis
  Endocrinologic
  - Hypothyroidism
  - Hypoparathyroidism
  - Amenorrhea
  - Infertility
  - Gigantism
  Skeletal
  - Arthritis
  - Osteopenia
  - Osteoporosis
  Cardiac
  - Cardiomyopathy
  - Arrhythmias
  Cutaneous
  - Jaundice
  - Lunulae ceruleae
  Other
  - Pancreatitis
  - Myopathy

---

nuclei of the periportal hepatocytes. Later in the disease course, the histologic picture may resemble autoimmune hepatitis or chronic viral hepatitis with a predominance of lymphocytic portal infiltration, periportal interface activity, and ductular reaction. Cirrhotic changes marked by nodular appearance and septal fibrosis may also be seen in untreated WD. For assessing hepatic copper concentrations, rhodanine stain is often used. A hepatic copper concentration greater than 250 μg/g dry weight in the absence of cholestasis is diagnostic of WD (a liver tissue biopsy core of at least 1 cm should be obtained).[27] Normal levels less than 50 µg/g exclude WD in untreated symptomatic patients.[28] For equivocal levels between 50 and 250 µg/g, molecular genetic testing for *ATP7B* mutations should be considered.

Although imaging modalities are not suitable diagnostic methods for confirmation of WD due to their low specificity, cranial MRI has high sensitivity (90%–95%)[29] and should be considered before treatment in all patients with neurologic WD. The morphologic and pathophysiological changes in the central nervous system are primarily related to copper toxicity on the nerve cells.

GENETIC DIAGNOSIS AND COUNSELING

Molecular diagnosis of WD is made when both copies of *ATP7B* gene are noted to be pathogenic variants. Screening of siblings involves liver chemistries, ceruloplasmin, 24-hour urine copper, and ocular examination for KF rings. If genotype of the proband is known, genetic testing of siblings is best to establish a diagnosis. Genotyping allows diagnostic testing in a simple, rapid, and economical manner. It is most useful when there is a "known" mutation. There have been up to 800 different pathogenic variants reported in WD. DNA Sanger sequencing can interrogate the entire sequence of the gene and is able to identify the rarer pathogenic variants with a sensitivity of 98%. Next generation sequencing allows many genes to be sequenced at the same time and is more economical than Sanger sequencing.

Given WD is autosomal recessive, each child has a 25% chance of being affected if both parents are carriers, and this risk is increased to 50% if one parent has WD and the other is a carrier. In consanguineous marriages (where parents are related to each other), with family history of WD, there is a likelihood that each parent is a carrier of an identical (homozygous) pathogenic variant on ATP7B. In contrast, when parents are unrelated and each has WD, it is very likely, that both will carry a different pathogenic ATP7B variant. If their child inherits both the pathogenic variants, he/she will be a "compound heterozygote" and develop WD. Depending on the laboratory used, genetic diagnosis of WD is possible in up to 98% of symptomatic individuals. Genetic counseling should be offered before and after testing, and using the services of a genetic counselor is valuable. Once a child is diagnosed, other family members also need to undergo screening and genetic testing. Trio-analysis is when parental samples are added to that of the proband because this improves interpretation of variants that are discovered particularly during whole genome or exome sequencing and allows more accurate identification of the variant being inherited or sporadic. Genetic counsellors are important not only in helping to share the genetic information with families but also to empower them to move forward with their genetic diagnosis integrated in their lives and not be stigmatized. If other significant results, unrelated to WD are revealed on genetic testing, it is important to ensure that the family is referred appropriately early.

SCORING SYSTEMS

The diagnosis of WD may often be confounded secondary to variable clinical presentations and laboratory test results. Given the lack of diagnostic criteria, the Leipzig scoring system was established based on clinical symptoms, available laboratory tests, and mutation analysis. The Leipzig score has also been referred to as the Ferenci score and a score of 4 and above is considered diagnostic of Wilson disease (**Table 2**). This scoring system has been validated based on both adult and pediatric studies. Based on a retrospective study by Koppiker and colleagues, the scores had a sensitivity of 98.14%, specificity of 96.59%, positive predictive value (PPV) of 94.64%, and negative predictive value of 98.83%.[30]

Prognostic criteria for WD with liver failure but without encephalopathy were developed by the King's College group.[32,33] The modified prognostic score, known as the New Wilson Index score or Dhawan score is based on serum bilirubin levels, international normalized ratio (INR), AST, white cell count, and serum albumin with 1 to 4 points allocated to each variable (**Table 3**). Based on the New Wilson Index, a score of 11 or greater predicts mortality without liver transplantation. This translates into a sensitivity of 93%, a specificity of 98%, and a PPV of 88%.[33]

TREATMENT

The treatment strategies for WD are aimed at decreasing copper load in the body. This is usually achieved by reducing the dietary copper intake, decreasing copper absorption from the digestive tract by using zinc salts and/or by increasing the copper excretion in urine by using chelators including D-penicillamine and trientine. In the following sections, we will discuss the various pharmacologic interventions available for the treatment of WD.

D-Penicillamine is one of the first oral chelating agents used to treat WD.[34,35] It is a monothiol that binds nonceruloplasmin bound copper in the plasma and forms penicillamine–Cu complexes that are water soluble and easily excreted in urine.[3,20,36] Due to its high affinity for copper, it also strips peptide and tissue complexes bound copper. D-penicillamine is available as a capsule or tablet (125 or 250 mg). The dose for adults is typically 1000 to 1500 mg/d and for children, it is 20 mg/kg/d (maximum 1000–1500 mg/d), given in 2 to 3 doses per day. Because food, milk, zinc, or iron preparations can decrease the absorption of D-penicillamine, it needs to be taken on an empty stomach at least 1 hour before meals or 2 hours postprandial. Due to concerns for paradoxic neurologic deterioration during treatment, it should be introduced at a low dose and advanced slowly. The initial dose is 125 to 250 mg/d, with a 125 to 250 mg/d increase every 4 to 7 days.[7,20] The maintenance dose is approximately 1000 mg/d. Because penicillamine can inactivate and result in vitamin B6 (pyridoxine) deficiency, vitamin B6 should be supplemented (25 mg daily).

D-penicillamine is associated with numerous adverse events. The early adverse events tend to occur during the first 3 weeks of treatment and include hypersensitivity reactions (eg, fever, rash, urticarial, pruritis), arthralgia, proteinuria, leukopenia, and/or thrombocytopenia. The late adverse events can occur anywhere from after 3 weeks to a few years of treatment. Based on the organ system involved, these may include paradoxic neurologic worsening, nephrotoxicity, lupus-like syndrome, bone marrow failure, myasthenia-like syndrome, hair loss, gastrointestinal symptoms (nausea, vomiting, diarrhea, cholestatic jaundice), immunoglobulin deficiency, and breast enlargement.[7,20,37]

Paradoxic neurologic deterioration (worsening of neurologic status after starting D-penicillamine) is one of the most frequent adverse events and can be irreversible in 33% of the cases.[20,35,38,39] It has been linked to rapid introduction of D-penicillamine resulting in transient increase in nonceruloplasmin bound copper in serum and cerebrospinal fluids causing oxidative stress and brain damage. Therefore, when starting treatment with D-penicillamime, the recommended practice is to "start low and go slow" with strict dose titration.[40] The nephrotoxic effects may include proteinuria, hematuria, nephrotic syndrome, Goodpasture syndrome, or renal vasculitis. Lupus-like syndromes tend to occur 6 to 12 months after starting treatment and are more common in women and in older age groups. Common symptoms may include pleurisy, polyarthritis, leukopenia, and thrombocytopenia.

Table 2
Leipzig score[a]

Kayser-Fleischer Rings	Neuropsychiatric Symptoms	Coombs-Negative Hemolytic Anemia	Serum Ceruloplasmin, mg/dL	Urinary Copper*	Liver Copper**	Mutation Analysis
Absent (0)	Absent (0)	Absent (0)	Normal (0)	Normal-0	Normal (−1)	No mutation (0)
Present (2)	Present (2)	Present (2)	10–20 (1)	1–2 xULN (1)	Up to 5 xULN (1)	Mutation on one chromosome (1)
			<10 (2)	>2 xULN (2)	>5 xULN (2)	Mutation on both chromosomes (4)

*If urinary copper is normal but greater than 5 xULN 1 d after ᴅ-penicillamine challenge, a score of 2 is assigned.

**If quantitative hepatic copper measurement is not available, then scores can be assigned based on the presence of rhodanine-positive hepatocytes (0 if absent and 1 if present).

Assessment of the Leipzig score.

4 or more: diagnosis of Wilson disease highly likely.

2 to 3: diagnosis of Wilson disease probable, more investigations needed.

0 to 1: diagnosis of Wilson disease unlikely.

[a] Adapted from: Kerkar and Roberts (Eds) Clinical and Translational Perspectives in Liver Disease 2019: 279-285. Elsevier, with permission.[31]

Table 3
New Wilson index for predicting mortality[a]

Laboratory Values	Score
Bilirubin (mg/dL)	
0–5.8	0
5.9–8.8	1
8.8–11.7	2
11.8–17.5	3
>17.5	4
INR	
0–1.29	0
1.3–1.6	1
1.7–1.9	2
2.0–2.4	3
>2.5	4
AST (IU/L)	
0–100	0
101–150	1
151–300	2
301–400	3
>401	4
White cell count (10⁹/L)	
0–6.7	0
6.8–8.3	1
8.4–10.3	2
10.4–15.3	3
>15.4	4
Albumin (g/dL)	
>4.5	0
3.4–4.4	1
2.5–3.3	2
2.1–2.4	3
<2.0	4

[a] Adapted from: Kerkar and Roberts (Eds) Clinical and Translational Perspectives in Liver Disease 2019: 279-285. Elsevier, with permission.[31]

Given the nephrotoxic adverse effects, patient should be screened for proteinuria before initiating treatment and at least every 6 months thereafter. During treatment, clinical markers of liver diseases such as jaundice, coagulopathy, and ascites should be monitored. Moreover, complete blood count, serum aminotransferases, coagulation profile, serum copper, ceruloplasmin, nonceruloplasmin bound copper should be checked at least twice a year. The adequacy of therapy as well as medication adherence can be determined by monitoring 24-hour urinary copper excretion, serum nonceruloplasmin bound copper levels, urinary copper excretion at baseline and then 48 hours after cessation of D-penicillamine.[41] Estimated levels of nonceruloplasmin bound copper (normal range 5–15 μg/dL) may assist in determining treatment adequacy. Levels less than 5 μg/dL suggest overtreatment, and levels greater than

15 μg/dL indicate nonadherence. Basal 24-hour urinary copper excretion should be measured at least once a year. Physical and neurologic examination should be performed at least twice a year. Although D-penicillamine can be used during pregnancy, its dose should be decreased by 25% to 50%. Mother treated with anticopper agents should avoid breastfeeding because these drugs can pass into milk and can result in copper deficiency in the newborn.

Trientine was first introduced as an alternative oral chelator in WD patients who were not tolerating or responding to D-penicillamine. It is the dihydrochloride salt of triethylenetetramine. It is a copper chelator and forms a stable complex with nonceruloplasmin bound copper in the plasma compartment, and the complex is excreted by the kidneys.[42–44] Trientine was approved by the US Food and Drug Administration in 1985.[45] It was initially approved for patients intolerant to penicillamine but given its superior safety profile, it has become the first-line chelator in the United States.[7] It is available as 250 mg capsules (Syprine)in the United States and as 300 mg capsules in the Europe. The dose in adults is 750 to 1500 mg daily in 2 to 4 divided doses and 750 to 1000 mg daily for maintenance therapy.[9] In children, 20 mg/kg/d (up to 1500 mg daily) is recommended. Higher doses may increase the adverse events in the pediatric population.[46] Urinary copper excretion should be monitored during treatment. The urinary copper excretion increases more than 1000 μg/24 h at the start of therapy and should be approximately 200 to 500 μg/24 h during maintenance treatment. A level less than 200 μg/24 h suggests overtreatment or noncompliance.[44]

Mineral supplementation should be avoided during treatment with trientine. Avoid iron supplementation because it forms toxic complexes with trientine, and patients should be evaluated for iron deficiency anemia before starting trientine. Zinc, if used as combination therapy with trientine, should not be administered simultaneously, and the 2 drugs should be given at least 6 hours apart from each other.[47] The most common adverse event associated with trientine is nausea. Paradoxic worsening of neurologic symptoms has been reported in treatment naïve patients but is not as frequent as with D-penicillamine.[48] Other less common adverse events include aplastic anemia, iron deficiency anemia, rash, pruritus, leukopenia, lupus erythematous, colitis, arthralgia, myalgia, nephropathy, and hirsutism. Similar to D-penicillamine, the dose of trientine should be reduced by 25% to 50% during pregnancy. No major teratogenic effect has been associated with trientine.[49]

Zinc (Zn) is a transition metal that interferes with the uptake of copper from the diet and reuptake from body fluids (saliva, gastric juice, and pancreatic fluid).[50] In large oral doses, it induces metallothionein in enterocytes that preferentially binds copper, and the complexes are excreted in feces. Zn may also enhance hepatocellular physiology by improving nuclear receptor function (farsenoid X and retinoid X receptor).[51] Zn is available as zinc salt, and the amount of elemental Zn varies based on the salt. The standard adult dose is 50 mg elemental Zn 3 times daily. For school-aged children, the dose is 25 mg elemental Zn 3 times daily, and for children aged younger than 5 years, the recommended dose is 25 mg elemental Zn twice daily.[52,53] Zn should be taken at least an hour apart from food. Care should be taken to instruct families to also keep Zinc at least an hour apart from the chelator if both drugs are being used.

Compared with D-penicillamine, Zn is better tolerated but it is not the best choice as primary therapy for hepatic WD. Zn monotherapy is preferred for silent WD (asymptomatic). Zinc monotherapy may also be considered in patients with predominantly neurologic symptoms as the worsening neurologic status seen with oral chelators is less common with Zn therapy. To assess the clinical efficacy and adherence to Zn therapy, monitor 24-hour urinary copper and Zn excretion. Copper excretion of 50 to 125 μg/d shows good dose effect, and Zn excretion greater than 2 mg/d marks good adherence.[54] Serum transaminases, amylase, lipase, lipid profile, and renal status should be checked annually. The most common adverse effect of Zn therapy is gastritis. Less common side effects that may result from copper deficiency state may include anemia, neutropenia, ataxia, neuropathy, and myopathy. Hyperlipidemia as well as asymptomatic elevation of amylase and lipase levels may also occur. Zn is a good therapeutic option during pregnancy and is also believed to be safe for breastfeeding.

LIVER TRANSPLANTATION

Although medical therapy tends to stabilize most patients, some may have progressive liver disease resulting in cirrhosis and liver failure. Classic Wilsonian ALF-WD often requires liver transplantation.[55] ALF-WD is often characterized by low serum transaminases and ALP levels, elevated bilirubin, acute intravascular hemolysis, and renal Fanconi syndrome. An acute decompensated WD patient is prioritized to the top of the regional transplant list (United Network for Organ Sharing with a status 1 designation). The 1-year and 5-year patient survival rates are 90.1% and 89% in children and 88.3% and 86% in adults, respectively, as per United Network of Organ Sharing (UNOS) analysis.[55] Liver transplantation helps to restore normal biliary copper excretion. As far as neurologic deficits are concerned, minimal improvement is noted in case of patients with severe neurologic complications.[56] Moreover, liver transplant may result in neurologic worsening by rapidly restoring biliary copper excretion in WD and accelerating total body copper depletion. Therefore, liver transplantation is a relative contraindication for active neurologic WD. Postliver transplantation, patients have to take immunosuppressive agents to prevent rejection and often require antibiotics for prophylaxis. Transplant recipients on chronic immunosuppression often develop hypertension, weight gain, diabetes, chronic kidney disease, and are also at the risk for de novo malignancy, especially skin cancer. Long-term posttransplant outcomes in WD are extremely good especially in younger patients who do not have medical comorbidities.

NEW THERAPIES

Medications (D-penicillamine, trientine, and zinc salts) currently used in the management of WD have several limitations, including neurologic worsening, that may be occasionally irreversible. There is a significant adverse event profile associated particularly with D-penicillamine therapy that can contribute to poor adherence. Thus, there is a need to develop new therapies that have better safety and efficacy, particularly for neurologic WD. Tetrathiomolybdenate has been used since the 1980s by Brewer and works by complexing circulating copper with albumin and increasing hepatic excretion of copper in bile.[57] It has been shown to have a more favorable neurologic outcome compared with trientine but use in the past had been limited by need for frequent dosing and unstable formulation. The development of a stable form of this drug (WTX101) has allowed tetrathiomolybdenate to be used successfully in clinical trials and initial results are promising. The data on long-term use are being gathered.[58] Other drugs such as methantobactin that have a high affinity for copper have been used successfully in animal models for WD but clinical trials in humans have not yet occurred.[59] Curcumin and 4-phenylbutyrate function as "chemical chaperones" and facilitate copper transport by relocating some of the mutant protein to its functional site in selected mutations of the *ATP7B* gene.[60]

Given that liver transplantation is effective in WD, cell-based therapies have been attempted in animal models. Healthy hepatocytes infused in Long-Evans Cinnamon rats with mutated ATP7B found improvement in copper metabolism, and the results improved with repeat infusions.[61] Gene therapy using an adenovirus vector to deliver ATP7B to hepatocytes of a mouse model of WD has been successful in demonstrating normalization of copper metabolism measured by urinary copper excretion and liver copper.[62] Clinical trials of gene therapy have recently started in adults.[63]

SUMMARY

WD, an autosomal recessively inherited disease of copper transport, has a wide spectrum of presentations. Animal models have been useful in understanding the pathways for copper metabolism and pathogenesis of WD. In the current era, after silver jubilee of the discovery of the mutation in *ATP7B* in WD, molecular diagnosis of WD has become the gold standard. In clinical practice, the time-honored measurement of liver copper more than 250 μg/g of liver tissue remains widely used to make a diagnosis of WD. Hepatic manifestations are seen more frequently in children, with identification as early as the newborn period in the course of genetic screening of family members after a new diagnosis of WD. Neuropsychiatric presentation is observed more commonly later in life, although both forms may be seen at any age. Scoring systems to aid diagnosis and prognosis are available. Chelating agents such as D-penicillamine and trientine remain the mainstay of therapy. Zinc is also very useful, acting synergistically with the chelators and often used alone in WD with neuropsychiatric manifestations. Liver transplantation becomes necessary when there is ALF and when medical therapy fails. Newborn screening has not included WD in the diseases screened—mainly because there does not seem to be a reliable biomarker. Earlier diagnosis and implementation of therapy can improve outcomes. Newer therapies are being explored and gene therapy is now in the horizon.

CLINICS CARE POINTS

- A low serum alkaline phosphatase in association with cholestasis and increased serum aminotransferases should prompt consideration of Wilson disease in the differential diagnosis.

- Kayser Fleischer rings are characteristically seen in neurologic Wilson disease, but can be a good diagnostic marker for Wilson disease, particularly in an acute liver failure setting.

- When initiating therapy with D-penicillamine the maxim is 'start low and go slow' , particularly as there may be paradoxical neurological deterioration associated with use of this medication. Trientene may be a safer alternative when possible.

- Important to administer Zinc and chelator at least two hours apart , so that the Zince is not chelated and rendered ineffective.

- In this era of molecular diagnosis, if the mutation in the proband is identified, then it is an excellent way of getting family members and siblings screened and also allow candidacy in gene replacement clinical trials.

DISCLOSURE

The authors have nothing to disclose.

REFERENCES

1. Tanner S: A History of Wilson Disease. In: Kerkar N, Roberts EA, eds Clinical and Translational Perspectives on Wilson Disease, Elsevier Publications: Academic press; London (UK): 2019; 1-11.

2. Stenson PD, Ball EV, Mort M, et al. The Human Gene Mutation Database (HGMD) and its exploitation in the fields of personalized genomics and molecular evolution. Curr Protoc Bioinformatics 2012. https://doi.org/10.1002/0471250953. bi0113s39. Chapter 1:Unit1 13.

3. Ala A, Walker AP, Ashkan K, et al. Wilson's disease. Lancet 2007;369:397–408.

4. Bull PC, Thomas GR, Rommens JM, et al. The Wilson disease gene is a putative copper transporting P-type ATPase similar to the Menkes gene. Nat Genet 1993; 5:327–37.

5. Petrukhin K, Fischer SG, Pirastu M, et al. Mapping, cloning and genetic characterization of the region containing the Wilson disease gene. Nat Genet 1993;5: 338–43.

6. Tanzi RE, Petrukhin K, Chernov I, et al. The Wilson disease gene is a copper transporting ATPase with homology to the Menkes disease gene. Nat Genet 1993;5:344–50.

7. Roberts EA, Schilsky ML, American Association for Study of Liver D. Diagnosis and treatment of Wilson disease: an update. Hepatology 2008;47:2089–111.

8. Olivares M, Uauy R. Limits of metabolic tolerance to copper and biological basis for present recommendations and regulations. Am J Clin Nutr 1996;63:846S–52S.

9. Sokol R, Silverman A: Copper metabolism and copper storage disorders in children. In: Suchy F, Sokol R, Balistreri W, Bezerra J, Mack C, Shneider B, eds Liver Disease in Children. 5th ed: Cambridge, 2021; 484-514.

10. Kaplan JH, Maryon EB. How mammalian cells acquire copper: an essential but potentially toxic metal. Biophys J 2016;110:7–13.

11. Czlonkowska A, Litwin T, Dusek P, et al. Wilson disease. Nat Rev Dis Primers 2018;4:21.

12. Berger SL, Kouzarides T, Shiekhattar R, et al. An operational definition of epigenetics. Genes Dev 2009;23:781–3.

13. Lin LJ, Wang DX, Ding NN, et al. Comprehensive analysis on clinical features of Wilson's disease: an experience over 28 years with 133 cases. Neurol Res 2014;36:157–63.

14. Saito T. Presenting symptoms and natural history of Wilson disease. Eur J Pediatr 1987;146:261–5.

15. Walshe JM. Wilson's disease presenting with features of hepatic dysfunction: a clinical analysis of eighty-seven patients. Q J Med 1989;70:253–63.

16. Oder W, Grimm G, Kollegger H, et al. Neurological and neuropsychiatric spectrum of Wilson's disease: a prospective study of 45 cases. J Neurol 1991;238:281–7.

17. Ferenci P, Czlonkowska A, Merle U, et al. Late-onset Wilson's disease. Gastroenterology 2007;132:1294–8.

18. Czlonkowska A, Litwin T, Chabik G. Wilson disease: neurologic features. Handb Clin Neurol 2017;142:101–19.

19. Lorincz MT. Neurologic Wilson's disease. Ann N Y Acad Sci 2010;1184:173–87.

20. European Association for Study of L. EASL clinical practice guidelines: Wilson's disease. J Hepatol 2012;56:671–85.

21. Ferenci P. Diagnosis of wilson disease. Handb Clin Neurol 2017;142:171–80.

22. Berman DH, Leventhal RI, Gavaler JS, et al. Clinical differentiation of fulminant Wilsonian hepatitis from other causes of hepatic failure. Gastroenterology 1991;100: 1129–34.

23. Tissieres P, Chevret L, Debray D, et al. Fulminant Wilson's disease in children: appraisal of a critical diagnosis. Pediatr Crit Care Med 2003;4:338–43.

24. Matsuda I, Pearson T, Holtzman NA. Determination of apoceruloplasmin by radioimmunoassay in nutritional copper deficiency, Menkes' kinky hair syndrome, Wilson's disease, and umbilical cord blood. Pediatr Res 1974;8:821–4.

25. Gitlin D, Janeway CA. Turnover of the copper and protein moieties of ceruloplasmin. Nature 1960;185:693.

26. Sternlieb I, Morell AG, Tucker WD, et al. The incorporation of copper into ceruloplasmin in Vivo: Studies with copper and copper. J Clin Invest 1961;40:1834–40.

27. Ferenci P, Steindl-Munda P, Vogel W, et al. Diagnostic value of quantitative hepatic copper determination in patients with Wilson's Disease. Clin Gastroenterol Hepatol 2005;3:811–8.

28. Roberts EA, Schilsky ML. Division of G, Nutrition HfSCTOC. A practice guideline on wilson disease. Hepatology 2003;37:1475–92.

29. Willeit J, Kiechl SG, Birbamer G, et al. [Wilson's disease with primary CNS manifestation–current status in diagnosis and therapy]. Fortschr Neurol Psychiatr 1992;60:237–45.

30. Koppikar S, Dhawan A. Evaluation of the scoring system for the diagnosis of Wilson's disease in children. Liver Int 2005;25:680–1.

31. Kyrana E, Sintusek P, Dhawan A: Role of Scoring Systems in Wilson Disease. In: Kerkar N, Roberts EA, editors. Clinical and Translational Perspectives on Wilson Disease, Elsevier Publications: Academic press; London(UK): 2019; 279-285.

32. Nazer H, Ede RJ, Mowat AP, et al. Wilson's disease: clinical presentation and use of prognostic index. Gut 1986;27:1377–81.

33. Dhawan A, Taylor RM, Cheeseman P, et al. Wilson's disease in children: 37-year experience and revised King's score for liver transplantation. Liver Transpl 2005;11:441–8.

34. Walshe JM. Treatment of Wilson's disease with penicillamine. Lancet 1960;1: 188–92.

35. Weiss KH, Thurik F, Gotthardt DN, et al. Efficacy and safety of oral chelators in treatment of patients with Wilson disease. Clin Gastroenterol Hepatol 2013;11:1028–35.e1-2.

36. Walshe JM. Penicillamine, a new oral therapy for Wilson's disease. Am J Med 1956;21:487–95.

37. Jan V, Callens A, Machet L, et al. [D-penicillamine-induced pemphigus, polymyositis and myasthenia]. Ann Dermatol Venereol 1999;126:153–6.

38. Brewer GJ. Penicillamine should not be used as initial therapy in Wilson's disease. Mov Disord 1999;14:551–4.

39. Kalita J, Kumar V, Chandra S, et al. Worsening of Wilson disease following penicillamine therapy. Eur Neurol 2014;71:126–31.

40. Litwin T, Dziezyc K, Karlinski M, et al. Early neurological worsening in patients with Wilson's disease. J Neurol Sci 2015;355:162–7.

41. Dziezyc K, Litwin T, Chabik G, et al. Measurement of urinary copper excretion after 48-h d-penicillamine cessation as a compliance assessment in Wilson's disease. Funct Neurol 2015;30:264–8.

42. Gibbs K, Walshe JM. Liver copper concentration in Wilson's disease: effect of treatment with 'anti-copper' agents. J Gastroenterol Hepatol 1990;5:420–4.

43. Iseki K, Kobayashi M, Ohba A, et al. Comparison of disposition behavior and decoppering effect of triethylenetetramine in animal model for Wilson's disease (Long-Evans Cinnamon rat) with normal Wistar rat. Biopharm Drug Dispos 1992;13:273–83.

44. Siegemund R, Lossner J, Gunther K, et al. Mode of action of triethylenetetramine dihydrochloride on copper metabolism in Wilson's disease. Acta Neurol Scand 1991;83:364–6.

45. Dubois RS, Rodgerson DO, Hambidge KM. Treatment of Wilson's disease with triethylene tetramine hydrochloride (Trientine). J Pediatr Gastroenterol Nutr 1990;10:77–81.

46. Mayr T, Ferenci P, Weiler M, et al. Optimized trientine-dihydrochloride therapy in pediatric patients with wilson disease: is weight-based dosing justified? J Pediatr Gastroenterol Nutr 2021;72:115–22.

47. Askari FK, Greenson J, Dick RD, et al. Treatment of Wilson's disease with zinc. XVIII. Initial treatment of the hepatic decompensation presentation with trientine and zinc. J Lab Clin Med 2003;142:385–90.

48. Kim B, Chung SJ, Shin HW. Trientine-induced neurological deterioration in a patient with Wilson's disease. J Clin Neurosci 2013;20:606–8.

49. Dathe K, Beck E, Schaefer C. Pregnancy outcome after chelation therapy in Wilson disease. Evaluation of the German Embryotox Database. Reprod Toxicol 2016;65:39–45.

50. Brewer GJ, Hill GM, Prasad AS, et al. Oral zinc therapy for Wilson's disease. Ann Intern Med 1983;99:314–9.

51. Wooton-Kee CR, Jain AK, Wagner M, et al. Elevated copper impairs hepatic nuclear receptor function in Wilson's disease. J Clin Invest 2015;125:3449–60.

52. Socha P, Janczyk W, Dhawan A, et al. Wilson's disease in children: a position paper by the Hepatology Committee of the European Society for Paediatric Gastroenterology, Hepatology and Nutrition. J Pediatr Gastroenterol Nutr 2018;66: 334–44.

53. Brewer GJ, Dick RD, Johnson VD, et al. Treatment of Wilson's disease with zinc XVI: treatment during the pediatric years. J Lab Clin Med 2001;137:191–8.

54. Brewer GJ, Askari FK. Wilson's disease: clinical management and therapy. J Hepatol 2005;42(Suppl):S13–21.

55. Arnon R, Annunziato R, Schilsky M, et al. Liver transplantation for children with Wilson disease: comparison of outcomes between children and adults. Clin Transplant 2011;25:E52–60.

56. Medici V, Mirante VG, Fassati LR, et al. Liver transplantation for Wilson's disease: the burden of neurological and psychiatric disorders. Liver Transpl 2005;11: 1056–63.

57. Brewer GJ, Askari F, Lorincz MT, et al. Treatment of Wilson disease with ammonium tetrathiomolybdate: IV. Comparison of tetrathiomolybdate and trientine in a double-blind study of treatment of the neurologic presentation of Wilson disease. Arch Neurol 2006;63:521–7.

58. Weiss KH, Askari FK, Czlonkowska A, et al. Bis-choline tetrathiomolybdate in patients with Wilson's disease: an open-label, multicentre, phase 2 study. Lancet Gastroenterol Hepatol 2017;2:869–76.

59. Lichtmannegger J, Leitzinger C, Wimmer R, et al. Methanobactin reverses acute liver failure in a rat model of Wilson disease. J Clin Invest 2016;126:2721–35.

60. van den Berghe PV, Stapelbroek JM, Krieger E, et al. Reduced expression of ATP7B affected by Wilson disease-causing mutations is rescued by pharmacological folding chaperones 4-phenylbutyrate and curcumin. Hepatology 2009; 50:1783–95.

61. Sauer V, Siaj R, Stoppeler S, et al. Repeated transplantation of hepatocytes prevents fulminant hepatitis in a rat model of Wilson's disease. Liver Transpl 2012;18: 248–59.

62. Murillo O, Luqui DM, Gazquez C, et al. Long-term metabolic correction of Wilson's disease in a murine model by gene therapy. J Hepatol 2016;64:419–26.

63. ClinicalTrials.gov. A Randomized, Double-Blind, Placebo-Controlled, Multicenter, Seamless, Adaptive, Safety, Dose-Finding, and Phase 3 Clinical Study of UX701 AAV-Mediated Gene Transfer for the Treatment of Wilson Disease. In; 2021.

Recent Insights into Pediatric Primary Sclerosing Cholangitis

James P. Stevens, MD, Nitika A. Gupta, MD, DCH, DNB, MRCPCH*

KEYWORDS

- Primary sclerosing cholangitis • Pediatric sclerosing cholangitis
- Autoimmune sclerosing cholangitis • Pediatric liver disease
- Immune-mediated liver disease

KEY POINTS

- The cause of primary sclerosing cholangitis (PSC) is unknown, although individual susceptibility is thought to be from a combination of genetic and environmental factors. Gut microbiome, gut-liver communication, bile acids, and subsequent hepatic immune-mediated response may all play interconnected roles in disease pathogenesis.
- Pediatric PSC has significant long-term morbidity and mortality. Progressive symptoms of portal hypertension and biliary complications lead to the need for liver transplantation in a subset of children. Disease recurrence is common, and hepatic or gastrointestinal malignancy can develop in adolescence and adulthood.
- Effective medical therapies for PSC are lacking. Pediatric data to support commonly used agents, such as ursodeoxycholic acid or oral vancomycin, are limited to retrospective observations or small, noncontrolled prospective studies.

DEFINITION AND EPIDEMIOLOGY

Primary sclerosing cholangitis (PSC) is a chronic, immune-mediated inflammatory liver disease of the intrahepatic and extrahepatic bile ducts. Patients may present asymptomatically with incidental findings on blood work or imaging, can have nonspecific complaints (fatigue, weight loss, abdominal pain, headache, pruritis), or may have signs of end-stage liver disease and portal hypertension.[1,2] Patients with PSC have abnormal liver enzymes with or without a cholestatic profile. Diagnosis requires either characteristic multifocal biliary strictures and dilatations on cholangiography (classically described as "beads on a string") or histologic findings on liver biopsy consistent with sclerosing cholangitis (such as concentric periductal fibrosis).[1,3] As the name

Department of Pediatrics, Division of Gastroenterology, Hepatology and Nutrition, 1760 Haygood Drive, Atlanta GA 30322, USA
* Corresponding author.
E-mail address: nitika.gupta@emory.edu

Clin Liver Dis 26 (2022) 489–519
https://doi.org/10.1016/j.cld.2022.03.009
1089-3261/22/© 2022 Elsevier Inc. All rights reserved.

liver.theclinics.com

suggests, PSC cannot be secondary to a different identified, primary underlying cause which have to be excluded (**Box 1**).

PSC is much less common in pediatrics than in adults, affecting between 0.2 and 1.5 per every 100,000 children (about one-fifth the prevalence of adults).[1,3,4] Those diagnosed in childhood are typically greater than 10 years of age, and boys are estimated to develop PSC around 1.5 times more frequently than girls.[3,5–7] Although individuals of all races can develop PSC, there is some evidence to suggest a higher prevalence in individuals of Northern European ancestry compared with other races.[8,9]

CAUSE AND PATHOGENESIS

Prior research on PSC pathogenesis is mostly limited to adult studies, with a paucity of data on juvenile PSC.[10] The underlying insult or series of events that activates PSC remains unknown and is likely multifactorial.[11] Susceptibility is recognized to be from a combination of genetic and environmental factors.[12] Based on currently available information, there are many hypotheses on the role of an inherited predisposition, gut microbiome, gut-liver communication, bile homeostasis, and downstream effects on the immune system, which lead to biliary inflammation and fibrosis.[12]

Genetic Background

Although there is not one "PSC gene" with Mendelian inheritance, it is known to run in families. Siblings of a patient with PSC are at between 9 and 39 times higher risk for developing it themselves compared with the general population.[2,13] Multiple HLA complex associations with PSC (on chromosome 6p21) are known, prominent among them being positive for HLA-DR3, HLA-DR6, HLA-B8, and HLA-DR13 haplotypes.[14,15] Interestingly, Bowlus and colleagues[16] showed HLA-DR3 association was present for European American and Hispanic patients but was not seen in African American patients, giving some insight into possible differences into the disease process in individuals of a given race.

Outside of HLA, a combination of pediatric and adult studies has identified more than 20 genes with possible risk loci for PSC.[12,17] Specifically, in a 2021 multicenter pediatric study by Haisma and colleagues,[17] whole-exome sequencing (WES) was performed on 29 patients and their parents (87 total samples) to assess for risk of early-onset PSC (defined as diagnosis before 12 years old; **Table 1**). Based on a pathogenicity algorithm and data on gene expression and function, 36 genes were identified in 22 patient-parent groups.[17] The genes of interest have a variety of roles in both innate and adaptive immunity, membrane transport, and supporting an epithelial barrier. These findings are in keeping with adult studies.[18–20]

Gut Microbiome

Overall, PSC susceptibility is currently estimated to be less than 10% genetic in origin, leading to the presumption of a strong environmental component.[10,12,16] Chief among these is the hypothesis of a disrupted gut microbiome potentially setting off or worsening a chronic inflammatory process.[21] Studies on fecal microbiota have found elevated levels of numerous species in patients with PSC compared with controls. Many of these studies suggest that microbial changes in PSC seem to be independent from associated colitis. In a Japanese pediatric study by Iwasawa and colleagues,[22] they obtained 27 stool samples from PSC patients, 16 from children with ulcerative colitis (UC), and 23 healthy controls. Analyzing 16S ribosomal (rRNA), they found that compared with healthy controls PSC was associated with decreased *Anaerostipes*

Box 1
Differential diagnosis for primary sclerosing cholangitis

Congenital/inherited (presenting at young age)
- Biliary atresia
- Neonatal sclerosing cholangitis (AR condition: DCDC2 gene)
- ABCB4 mutation (MDR3 deficiency, responsible for PFIC3, often presents as small-duct disease)

Anatomic/obstructive
- Choledocholithiasis
- Recurrent pancreatitis

Vascular
- Ischemic injury
- Portal biliopathy (2/2 portal vein thrombosis or other cause of portal hypertensive biliopathy)

Autoimmune
- Autoimmune pancreatitis/IgG4-positive sclerosing cholangitis
- Langerhans cell histiocytosis
- Autoimmune hepatitis/overlap disease

Allergic
- Eosinophilic cholangitis
- Mast cell cholangiopathy

Immunodeficiency
  Primary
    - Wiscott-Aldrich syndrome
    - Hyperimmunoglobulin M syndromes
  Secondary
    - AIDS-related cholangiopathy (2/2 *Cryptosporidium* infection)

Infectious
- Recurrent bacterial/pyogenic cholangitis
- 2/2 immunodeficiency as above

Systemic illness
- Cystic fibrosis
- Sickle cell disease
- Retroperitoneal fibrosis

Oncologic (less common in pediatrics):
- Cholangiocarcinoma
- Hepatic inflammatory pseudotumor
- Diffuse intrahepatic metastasis

Iatrogenic
- Intra-arterial chemotherapy
- Surgical trauma/complication

---

hadrus, *Blautia obeum*, and *Parabacteroides*, with increased *Enterococcus*, *Streptococcus*, and *Veillonella* species. Compared with UC, PSC had increased *Faecalibacterium*, *Roseburia*, and *Ruminococcus*. Consistent with adult studies, patients with PSC had decreased alpha diversity versus healthy controls (although increased compared with UC).[22–25] Cortez and colleagues[26] similarly found higher presence of *Streptococcus* in children with PSC, greater abundance of *Veillonella* in both PSC and PSC + UC, and greater *Escherichia*-Shigella in PSC + UC than controls. *Veillonella* was found to be more abundant in patients diagnosed under 10 years of age versus older children, whereas *Megasphaera* was only increased in patients diagnosed over 10 years of age. Interestingly, both genera correlated with "active" disease

Table 1
Relevant and recent articles in pediatric primary sclerosing cholangitis

First Author	Title	Area of PSC Focus (Pathogenesis, Natural History, Treatment, Prognosis/ Year Outcomes)	Research Aims and Methods	Prospective/ Retrospective	Study Size	Main Discoveries/ Conclusions	Strengths	Limitations
Clinical								
Gregorio	Autoimmune Hepatitis/Sclerosing Cholangitis Overlap Syndrome in Childhood: A 16-Year Prospective Study	2001 Treatment, Outcomes	To analyze the prevalence, presentation/ findings, treatment, and long-term outcomes of PSC-AIH among pediatric AIH patients	Prospective	55 patients: 28 AIH, 27 PSC-AIH	PSC-AIH and AIH present at similar rates and similar nonspecific symptoms. IBD is more common in overlap than AIH. Elevated IgG and positive p-ANCA are prevalent in overlap disease. Standard liver indices and AIH scoring systems cannot discriminate PSC-AIH from AIH. Most patients with overlap have biochemical and histologic improvement while on immunosuppression, although many PSC-AIH patients still have progressive biliary disease. PSC-AIH has lower transplant-free survival than AIH	One of the few prospective studies in pediatric PSC and the only major prospective study on PSC-AIH treatment/outcomes, has long-term follow-up	Observational, not randomized, does not include any patients with just PSC for comparison. Older data

Author	Title	Year	Category	Aim	Study Type	N	Results/Outcomes	Strengths	Weaknesses
Davies	Long-term Treatment of Primary Sclerosing Cholangitis in Children With Oral Vancomycin: An Immunomodulating Antibiotic	2008	Treatment	Describing trend in liver indices over time in children with PSC treated with OVT	Prospective	14	All patients had statistically significant improvement in ALT, GGT, ESR, and reported clinical symptoms while receiving OVT. Improvement was less evident in those patients who had already developed cirrhosis before initiating treatment. Authors conclude that vancomycin could thus be an effective treatment for pediatric PSC	First prospective study of OVT use in pediatric PSC, shows clear improvement in biochemistry in patients receiving OVT	Small cohort, all patients received treatment (no control group), variable treatment regimen/length, only analyzes biochemical outcomes not transplant-free survival
M. Deneau	The Natural History of Primary Sclerosing Cholangitis in 781 Children: A Multicenter, International Collaboration	2017	Natural History, Treatment, Prognosis/Outcomes	Use large, multisite consortium data to describe the disease phenotypes, laboratory findings, treatment, complications, and outcomes of pediatric PSC in different sites across the world	Retrospective	781	Phenotype: 1/3 of patients have concurrent AIH, 76% have IBD, 13% have small-duct PSC. Complications/outcomes: 10-y pHTN seen in 38% of patients, biliary complications in 25%. Each followed by transplant with median time 2.8 and 3.5 y and 14% of patients are transplanted. Cholangiocarcinoma occurs in 1%. Total event-free survival (pHTN, biliary complications, cholangiocarcinoma, liver transplantation, or liver-related death) 70% at 5 y, 53% at 10 y. Prognosis: Higher total bilirubin,	The PSC Consortium: Largest patient cohort ever described in pediatric PSC. Diverse patient population with a variety of clinical data (demographic, laboratory, imaging, histologic); long-term follow-up allows for a variety of powerful analyses	PSC Consortium: Retrospective, limited by what is directly provided in consortium patient forms, possibility of misclassification of some patients, inconsistent access to care, resources and follow-up between sites may skew data and outcomes

(continued on next page)

Table 1
(continued)

First Author	Title	Year	Area of PSC Focus (Pathogenesis, Natural History, Treatment, Prognosis/ Outcomes)	Research Aims and Methods	Prospective/ Retrospective	Study Size	Main Discoveries/ Conclusions	Strengths	Limitations
							GGT, APRI at diagnosis are associated with worse patient outcomes. IBD and small-duct phenotypes associated with better outcomes. Age, sex, and autoimmune hepatitis not associated with outcomes		
M. Deneau	Gamma Glutamyltransferase Reduction Is Associated With Favorable Outcomes in Pediatric Primary Sclerosing Cholangitis	2018	Treatment, Prognosis/ Outcomes	Assess trends in GGT for pediatric PSC patients over time and analyze concurrent long-term patient outcomes relative to GGT	Retrospective	287	Treatment: 81% of patients were treated with UDCA. UDCA-treated patients had a greater decrease in GGT compared with untreated ($P = .002$), but both groups had a significant decrease in GGT at 1 y compared with diagnosis. Prognosis/outcomes: GGT normalization at 1 y was associated with better 5-y event-free survival, regardless of treatment. GGT reduction >75% had better outcomes than GGT reduction <25% ($P = .005$). Overall, 5-y event-free survival was the same in treated and untreated groups. *Authors*	Strengths of pediatric PSC Consortium as above	No data on patient adherence with medication regimen

Author	Title	Year	Type	Aim	Design	Number	Results	Strengths	Limitations
Black	A Prospective Trial of Withdrawal and Reinstitution of Ursodeoxycholic Acid in Pediatric Primary Sclerosing Cholangitis	2019	Treatment	To trend biochemistry during a monitored withdrawal and reinstitution of UDCA in children with PSC	Prospective	27 (22 completed)	*conclude GGT is a useful prognostic marker for PSC* There was a statistically significant increase in GGT upon UDCA withdrawal ($P = .003$). Response to withdrawal was variable: although 7/22 patients had no increase in ALT or GGT, 8/22 had a "flare" of ALT or GGT >100, which responded to reintroduction of UDCA. Baseline GGT, IL-8, and TNF-alpha were higher in those that developed a flare. Bilirubin was not affected by UDCA withdrawal	Prospective, multisite, close monitoring	Small cohort, strict inclusion/exclusion criteria, short period of time off treatment, no control group. Primary biochemical outcomes may not correlate with long-term patient outcomes, such as transplant-free survival
M. Deneau	Oral Vancomycin, Ursodeoxycholic Acid, or No Therapy for Pediatric Primary Sclerosing Cholangitis: A Matched Analysis	2020	Treatment, Outcomes	Assess outcomes in propensity-matched patients treated with OVT, UDCA, or observation	Retrospective	264 (88 in each group)	Outcomes: Patients who received UDCA or OVT had lower median GGT than those untreated at 6 mo ($P<.05$), but this difference disappeared by 12 mo ($P = .657$). There was no difference in the percent of patients with GGT normalization at 1 y between groups ($P = NS$). Changes in liver	Strengths of pediatric PSC Consortium as previously listed. Ability to match patients on several factors	Retrospective data on treatment and patient outcomes are at risk for confounders and not sufficient to change clinical practice. Prospective, randomized controlled data are needed

(continued on next page)

Table 1
(continued)

First Author	Title	Year	Area of PSC Focus (Pathogenesis, Natural History, Treatment, Prognosis/ Outcomes)	Research Aims and Methods	Prospective/ Retrospective	Study Size	Main Discoveries/ Conclusions	Strengths	Limitations
							fibrosis over time were no different between groups. There was no significant difference in probability of being listed for liver transplantation at 5 y between either treatment group or observed patients *Authors conclude that UDCA and OVT in their cohort did not show improvement in outcomes and that placebo-controlled trials are needed for PSC treatment*		
M. Deneau	Assessing the Validity of Adult-derived Prognostic Models for Primary Sclerosing Cholangitis Outcomes in Children	2020	Prognosis	Analyze adult PSC prognostic tools (revised Mayo Clinic, Amsterdam-Oxford, and Boberg models) in children by comparing calculated/predicted vs observed transplant-free survival	Retrospective	781	Adult predictive s coring systems are able to risk-stratify children well at 1 y, although stratification is only fair at 10 y. Some adult modeling classifies children as higher risk and predicts worse outcomes than	Strengths of pediatric PSC Consortium as previously listed	Retrospective nature limits accurate classification. A subset of patients was missing some data

	Year	Type	Aim	Design	Sample	Results	Limitations
						their true transplant-free survival shows. Findings seen with concurrent autoimmune hepatitis (such as AST elevation) place patients in a higher-risk category, which may be the cause of discrepancy between predictive tools and actual outcomes *Authors conclude that the higher rate of AIH in pediatrics vs adults limits these tools and that a pediatric-specific model should be created*	No control group, not powered to assess long-term clinical outcomes, selection bias in those who requested to be included in treatment
Ali	2020	Treatment	Open-label prospective therapeutic clinical trials: oral vancomycin in children and adults with primary sclerosing cholangitis	Describing trend in liver indices over time in children and adults with PSC treated with OVT	Prospective	59 (30 enrolled, 29 off study protocol but received OVT)	Most patients treated with OVT had improvement in liver indices, with a minority having normalization of laboratory tests. No adverse events were reported with OVT use. 11/12 patients with small-duct PSC had improvement in inflammation on repeat biopsy, 26/34 with large-duct disease had improved MRCP, and none had progressive biliary disease *Authors conclude vancomycin was*	Prospective, larger than above study by Davies, long-term follow-up, reflects serologic improvement on vancomycin and reported tolerance/safety of medication

(continued on next page)

Table 1
(continued)

First Author	Title	Year	Area of PSC Focus (Pathogenesis, Natural History, Treatment, Prognosis/ Outcomes)	Research Aims and Methods	Prospective/ Retrospective	Study Size	Main Discoveries/ Conclusions	Strengths	Limitations
							well tolerated and associated with biochemical improvement in PSC		
M. Deneau	The Sclerosing Cholangitis Outcomes in Pediatrics (SCOPE) Index: A Prognostic Tool for Children	2021	Prognosis	Create and assess the strength of a pediatric-specific tool to predict PSC prognosis (primary: liver transplant or death; secondary: hepatobiliary complications)	Retrospective	1012	Tool was created using albumin, platelet count, total bilirubin, GGT, and cholangiography. Patients are stratified into low, medium, and high risk. Annual risk of death or transplant was <1%, 3%, and 9%, respectively, secondary complication rates of 2%, 6%, and 13% (*P*<.001) *Authors conclude this model is superior to adult scores for children and is shown to be independent predictor of patient response to PSC treatment initiation*	Strengths of pediatric PSC Consortium as previously listed	Limited long-term follow-up data before transition to adult care

Basic Science/Translational

Iwasawa	Characterisation of the Faecal Microbiota in Japanese Patients with Paediatric-Onset Primary Sclerosing Cholangitis	2017	Pathogenesis	Compare microbiome of stool samples in children with PSC, ulcerative colitis, and healthy controls analyzing 16S rRNA	Cross-sectional, translational	66 total: 27 PSC, 16 UC, 23 healthy controls	Numerous taxa are significantly enriched or depleted in PSC compared with in UC or in healthy patients. Alpha diversity is decreased in PSC vs healthy controls, further decreased in UC. Beta diversity is different between groups	The first significant study assessing gut microbiome via stool samples in pediatric PSC	Only Japanese children tested, small patient size, may limit generalizability of results
Cortez	Gut Microbiome of Children and Adolescents With Primary Sclerosing Cholangitis in Association With Ulcerative Colitis	2021	Pathogenesis	Compare microbiome of stool samples in children with PSC, PSC + UC, UC alone, and healthy controls analyzing 16S rRNA	Cross-sectional, translational	53 total: PSC = 11, UC = 12, PSC + UC = 723 healthy control	Greater abundance of multiple genera, such as Veillonella and Megasphaera, in PSC and PSC + UC. Genera seem to correlate with certain age groups and with patient biochemistry, suggesting that disease, disease activity, and age impact gut microbiome	One of only a handful of pediatric translational studies on PSC pathogenesis and the role of gut microbiome in PSC, has significant and possibly clinically relevant findings	Single hospital in Brazil, small cohort size for each subgroup

(continued on next page)

Table 1
(continued)

First Author	Title	Year	Area of PSC Focus (Pathogenesis, Natural History, Treatment, Prognosis/ Outcomes)	Research Aims and Methods	Prospective/ Retrospective	Study Size	Main Discoveries/ Conclusions	Strengths	Limitations
Haisma	Exome Sequencing in Patient-Parent Trios Suggests New Candidate Genes for Early-Onset Primary Sclerosing Cholangitis	2021	Pathogenesis	Analyze WES in children and their parents to search for genetic variants associated with pediatric PSC (diagnosed at <12 y old)	Translational	87 total (29 children and their parents)	54 rare variants were found in 36 potential genes, identified in 22 patient-parent groups. Eighteen of the genes were de novo variants. Twelve of the genes of interest have a variety of roles in innate and adaptive immunity, membrane transport, and maintaining an epithelial barrier. Authors conclude that there are many potential non-HLA genetic contributions to developing pediatric PSC but that further verification and analysis of the function of these genes are needed	First WES study identifying and analyzing rare genetic variants for pediatric PSC pathogenesis. Strengthened by analyzing children and their parent concurrently to determine inherited or de novo variants. Multicenter study strengthens diversity of population	Needs further replication; findings remain theoretic in relationship to disease at this time

Abbreviation: pHTN, portal hypertension.

severity based on gamma-glutamyl transferase (GGT) or total bilirubin.[26] This has been supported by animal studies showing increased susceptibility to hepatobiliary injury in germ-free mice who received fecal transplant from patients with PSC.[27,28] Data on microbiome based on gastrointestinal mucosal samples are less prevalent, with some showing no difference and others showing significant difference.[29–32] Together, these data have led some to use antibiotics, such as oral vancomycin (OVT), to treat PSC (see Current Treatment Modalities section).

Gut-Liver Communication

The exact communication between the gut and liver in PSC is unknown. Gastrointestinal dysbiosis and concurrent inflammatory bowel disease (IBD) in many patients with PSC may cause chronic gastrointestinal inflammation, which is hypothesized to lead to a "leaky gut barrier."[12,31] This can allow for translocation of bacteria to the liver through portal circulation. Microbes may also travel directly to the bile ducts in a retrograde fashion from the gastrointestinal tract.[21] Bacterial toxins can express pathogen-associated molecular patterns (PAMPs), which may be recognized by toll-like receptors (TLRs) and cause an immune response, leading to subsequent liver inflammation and fibrosis over time.[10,12] Bacterial gene expression in gut dysbiosis has also been suggested to bring gut-specific lymphocytes to the liver.[31] In a study previously mentioned, Nakamoto and colleagues[28] showed certain gut bacterial strains led to pore formation of intestinal epithelium using a human organoid model. Lichtman and colleagues[33,34] previously used rats to show how small bowel bacterial overgrowth could lead to hepatic changes consistent with PSC. A combined pediatric and adult study found elevated circulating markers of bacterial translocation (lipopolysaccharides) in patients with PSC.[35] High levels were associated with worse transplant-free survival. One of the identified PSC risk loci includes genes such as FUT2, which plays a role in protective mucosal barriers and assists with handling of translocated bacteria.[36]

Bile Acids

Some secondary bile acids (BA) created by specific gut microbes like *Clostridium* species are known to be anti-inflammatory and protect cholangiocytes via the BA receptor TGR5.[10,37,38] TGR5 is thought to help regulate the cystic fibrosis transmembrane conductance regulator, which is involved in forming a protective bicarbonate layer for cholangiocytes.[12] Gut dysbiosis in patients with PSC can affect BA production and thus prevent protection from bile toxicity.[12] This has led to the use of BA-based therapies for PSC.

Immune Response

As alluded to above, both innate immunity and adaptive immunity are thought to be involved in PSC. Bacterial PAMPs may cause an innate immune response via TLRs. HLA haplotypes associated with PSC suggest an adaptive immune role for T-cell receptor presentation.[12,14] Finally, the presence of positive autoantibodies in many patients with PSC (such as perinuclear antineutrophil cytoplasmic antibodies [p-ANCA], antinuclear antibody, or antiglycoprotein 2) means that B cells also likely play a role in the pathogenesis.[39,40] However, the inciting factors and complex interaction between immune cell types, which lead to progressive ductular fibrosis, have not been fully elicited.

Similar hepatic and gastrointestinal cell adhesion molecule profiles may allow for the gut-derived T cells to home to the liver despite being originally activated by antigens in the intestine.[12,41] Histologic evaluation of patients with PSC shows the presence of T cells near affected ducts in addition to neutrophils, macrophages, and other immune cells.[12] The ratio of CD4/CD8 cells has varied in prior studies, although may be from the normal distribution of CD4 cells to portal tracts and CD8 cells to lobules during times of inflammation.[42] A study of adult patients with PSC found that both CD4 and CD8 cells were more often CD28[-] compared with control tissue, with higher levels of TNF-alpha and interferon gamma versus CD28[+] cells.[43] Peripheral CD4[+] T cells in PSC have also been shown to have decreased apoptosis.[44] A study by Katt and colleagues[45] showed an increased Th17 response to stimulation by microbes in PSC versus healthy controls. Another adult study found peripheral CD4[+]CD25[+] regulatory T-cells level to be elevated in PSC-UC patients compared with those with only UC, although the impact of this difference is unclear.[46] Through studying mice intestine and livers simultaneously, Mathies and colleagues[47] were recently able to create a colitis model in which there was bacterial translocation, depleted regulatory T cells, and an increase of Th17 cells in the liver, with pathologic liver inflammation. This suggests that a Treg-Th17 imbalance may play a role in PSC pathogenesis. There is evidence that gamma-delta T cells may play a role in Th17 response.[48] Memory T cells have also been implicated in PSC's immune response, with cells of the same clonal origin found in paired gastrointestinal and liver samples in patients with PSC-IBD.[49] Cholangiocytes activated by T cells can secrete proteins that lead to inflammation, and patients with PSC have been shown to have different cytokine and chemokine profiles than controls or other immune-mediated liver diseases (such as elevation in CCL4, E3, E1, and decrease in CCL22 and IL-15).[50] WES-identified loci involve numerous genes for T- and B-cell activation, regulation, apoptosis, and many innate immune responses.[12] It is this conglomerate of communicating inflammatory cells, liver mesenchymal cells, and active cholangiocytes that form the ductular reaction of PSC.[11]

PATIENT PRESENTATION, DISEASE PHENOTYPES, AND DIAGNOSIS
Clinical Presentation and Laboratory Tests

Patients with PSC often present with nonspecific symptoms, such as abdominal pain and fatigue. Approximately 50% of patients will have an abnormal physical examination finding, such as jaundice.[1,2] Those individuals with a delay in diagnosis may have advanced or end-stage liver disease with evidence of portal hypertension, including hepatosplenomegaly, ascites, or gastrointestinal bleeding of varices.[2] Infectious cholangitis symptoms are rare at presentation except as a complication following endoscopic retrograde cholangiopancreatography (ERCP).[1]

Although adults rely on elevated serum alkaline phosphatase (ALP) as the most common presenting laboratory test abnormality in PSC, it can be elevated in children owing to nonhepatic causes, such as bone turnover and normal growth, and is thus less useful in pediatrics. Many patients have elevated GGT, alanine aminotransferase (ALT), and aspartate aminotransferase (AST). Transaminase elevation is often at least 2 to 3 times the normal range, although children can have much higher elevations in these laboratory tests than adults.[1] Bilirubin is normal or near-normal in most patients at time of diagnosis. Immunoglobulin G (IgG) and p-ANCA may be elevated in 50% or more of patients, although both are nonspecific, and thus, neither are typically used to diagnose PSC alone.[1,51]

Comorbidities and Disease Types

Much of the current clinical understanding of pediatric PSC comes from retrospective data from the Pediatric PSC Consortium, a large international patient cohort involving more than 50 sites across North America, Europe, the Middle East, and Asia. The PSC consortium has published several reports analyzing the presentation, management, and outcomes of pediatric PSC (see **Table 1**).[3,52–55] This cohort and its conclusions are inherently limited by its retrospective nature and by the level of detail provided from each individual site. However, given its large size and the lack of multisite prospective pediatric studies for pediatric PSC, it represents the strongest evidence currently available.

In the natural history study of pediatric PSC, 781 children were analyzed over 4277 person-years of follow-up.[3] This cohort had a median age of 12 years at diagnosis, and 61% was male children. Seventy-six percent of patients had concurrent IBD; 33% was diagnosed as having concurrent autoimmune hepatitis (AIH), and 7% of patients had at least one other immune-mediated process (such as thyroiditis, celiac disease, or type 1 diabetes mellitus). Finally, 13% of patients was diagnosed with "small duct" PSC, as defined by normal cholangiography despite expected clinical, serologic, and histologic features of PSC.[3] These major patient subgroups are each discussed in turn in later discussion.

Primary Sclerosing Cholangitis–Inflammatory Bowel Disease

The association with PSC and IBD is well known. In the PSC Consortium, 83% of PSC-IBD is UC or "indeterminate colitis," whereas the remaining 17% was diagnosed with Crohn.[3] This is consistent in multiple other pediatric and adult studies and equates to an estimated prevalence of PSC in between 2.5% and 7.5% of patients with UC.[1,56,57] The true prevalence may be underestimated given that not many patients with IBD routinely undergo cholangiography, may not have significant hepatic laboratory test abnormalities early in their disease course, or may not undergo routine screening with a GGT.[1,58] IBD is more often diagnosed first before PSC, although diagnoses can be concurrent or PSC can present first in one-fourth of patients.[1,56] PSC can also present after colectomy, or IBD can be diagnosed after a patient has already undergone liver transplant for PSC.[51,59]

In both children and adults, IBD-PSC has been shown to have a specific or classic phenotype. This often includes pancolitis with severe inflammation in the right colon (in both PSC-Crohn and PSC-UC, and as opposed to the worse left-sided colitis in typical UC), with backwash ileitis and typically with rectal sparing.[10,51,56,57,60] Patients are at increased risk of pouchitis after undergoing a colectomy. Despite this, patients with PSC can have discordantly mild clinical IBD symptoms.[61,62] Both prospective and retrospective pediatric data by Ricciuto and colleagues[57,63] found higher rates of reported clinical remission in PSC-IBD versus IBD alone. However, patient report of clinical remission was found to have poor correlation with endoscopic disease severity in PSC-IBD. Patients with PSC-IBD in clinical remission had lower rates of endoscopic remission than those in clinical remission with IBD alone. Pediatric patients with PSC-IBD overall have been shown to have lower rates of colectomy and biologic use,[64] although it is unclear if this is due to undertreatment given their underreported clinical symptoms. As they often have mild gastrointestinal symptoms and thus a poor reliability of subjective patient report, regular screening with objective data via fecal calprotectin is vital for timely IBD diagnosis and monitoring disease activity over time. Given the high risk for IBD development and increased risk of eventual colorectal cancer and mortality compared with IBD alone, colonoscopy should also be a consideration in patients with PSC. Societies such as the American Association for the Study of Liver Disease (AASLD), American College of Gastroenterology (ACG), European Crohn's and Colitis Organization, and European Association for the Study of the Liver (EASL) all recommend colonoscopy with biopsy in adult patients diagnosed with PSC, as well as screening colonoscopy every 1 to 2 years in adults with PSC-IBD.[1,51,65,66] Colonoscopy recommendations specific to pediatrics are more ambiguous, with adult society guidelines either not mentioning children or allowing flexibility for providers to determine when to perform endoscopy. Per prior AASLD guidelines, "it seems reasonable to consider" colonoscopy in all new diagnoses of pediatric PSC, and providers should have a "low threshold" to scope any patient with symptoms that could be consistent with IBD.[1] Although there is a dearth of data in the pediatric population, it may be reasonable to perform colonoscopies on teenagers with PSC-IBD every 1 to 2 years to screen for dysplasia as a precursor to colorectal cancer.

Retrospective data have shown that pediatric patients with PSC-IBD actually had less progression to cirrhosis with a longer transplant-free survival compared with PSC alone.[3] This is in contrast to patients with adult-onset PSC-UC who have worse prognosis of their liver disease than PSC alone.[67] PSC in Crohn has also been reported to have less severe disease than PSC with UC.[62] Hepatic disease has not been found to correlate with IBD disease severity or activity.[51,64]

Cholangiography and Large- Versus Small-Duct Disease

Several children have small-duct PSC, with normal cholangiographic findings (13%–36% in different studies).[3,68,69] About 1 in 4 children with small-duct PSC will eventually progress to large-duct disease as do many adults, which may suggest it to be an early presentation of large-duct disease in some.[70] The sensitivity and specificity of magnetic resonance cholangiopancreatography (MRCP) for pediatric PSC diagnosis are estimated as 81% to 89% and 84% to 100%, respectively, in prior studies.[71,72] Abdominal ultrasound is inadequate to diagnose PSC. ERCP is not a standard component of pediatric PSC diagnosis given the availability, accuracy, and safety of MRCP, which is the preferred modality for diagnosis of PSC in children. MRCP has the benefit of being noninvasive, without exposing patients to radiation and without the risk of complications, such as pancreatitis or infectious cholangitis. Although in adults ERCP has been used in some patients for early detection of subtle disease and allowing for sampling or intervention, biliary sampling is typically not indicated nor required at diagnosis in pediatric PSC.[1] Pediatric small-duct PSC had lower rates of long-term disease complications despite comparable disease progression at the time of diagnosis, leading to it being proposed as a prognostic marker in the recently created Sclerosing Cholangitis Outcomes in Pediatrics (SCOPE) Index (see Prognosis and Prognostic Tools in later discussion).[54]

Histologic Findings and Primary Sclerosing Cholangitis–Autoimmune Hepatitis Overlap

The classic histologic feature of PSC is the "onion skinning" appearance of periductal concentric fibrosis, formed through chronic injury via "cross-talk" between cholangiocytes and immune cells.[12] Onion skinning is an overall rare finding on histology though, as infrequent as 13.9% in one adult study.[73] Exact pediatric rates are not yet well documented but also suspected to be low, with a hypothesis that this is a feature that develops over time.[2] AASLD recommends against routine liver biopsy for diagnosis of PSC in adult patients who have MRCP/ERCP findings consistent with PSC. In cases whereby MRCP is equivocal, adult providers may consider repeating MRCP in the next few years or proceeding with a liver biopsy if there is high suspicion for small-duct PSC. Per 2021 recommendations from the International Primary Sclerosing Cholangitis Study Group (IPSCG), normal MRCP with elevated ALP or GGT and classic histologic findings, such as periductal fibrosis, lead to the diagnosis of a small-duct PSC, as does nonspecific compatible histologic findings with concurrent IBD.[74]

In contrast to adult practice, most pediatric hepatologists currently biopsy patients at PSC diagnosis given the increased reported concurrence of AIH.[1] More common than in adults, AIH was found as being at least "probable" in one-third of children with PSC and "definite" in 9% of the pediatric PSC Consortium.[3] In a large single-center pediatric study, 27% of children with PSC had AIH features.[69] In a different recent single-center study of pediatric PSC-IBD patients in the United Kingdom, as high as 72% was diagnosed as having AIH features.[75] Given the increased prevalence compared with adults, AASLD's 2010 guidelines recommended the use of liver biopsy in children to assess for AIH.[1] However, an ongoing gap in knowledge about definitive diagnostic criteria for overlap, or evidence of response to immunosuppression leading to a change in natural history of AIH-PSC, makes it increasingly challenging to provide definitive guidelines that are generalizable to the population at large. The decision to biopsy and/or treat should be made according to the clinical suspicion for AIH-PSC overlap, biochemical course, and response while taking into consideration the demographics of the population being served (eg, the incidence and prevalence of autoimmune diseases is higher in the black population).

When presenting together, this process has been called "PSC-AIH overlap," "overlap disease," "PSC with features of AIH," or autoimmune sclerosing cholangitis," although lack of clear diagnostic criteria precludes usage of specific terms, which may imply that this is a distinct clinical entity of its own.[74] It is not clear whether PSC-AIH overlap is a phenotype of PSC or 2 separate disease processes. Certain HLA profiles have been associated with pediatric overlap formation and disease severity.[76] In the authors' experience, although some patients are diagnosed with PSC-AIH overlap from initial biopsy, others can present first with AIH features, which on subsequent biopsies and imaging are more consistent with PSC-AIH overlap or PSC. This leads us to a proposed possible disease spectrum or continuum (**Fig. 1**). However, much work is still needed to further discern overlap predisposition, pathophysiology, presentation, and evolution.

There has only been one large prospective study analyzing PSC-AIH overlap among children. This 16-year longitudinal study by Gregorio and colleagues[77] followed 55 patients with autoantibody positivity consistent with AIH and estimated that 49% of them (27/55) actually had overlap disease based on cholangiography. Children with PSC-AIH and AIH presented at similar ages and with the same nonspecific symptoms. PSC-AIH overlap in children is thought to fall between PSC and AIH in terms of demographics (more likely female than PSC but less than AIH) and association with IBD (lower rates of IBD than PSC).[3,7,78] Patients with overlap had higher rates of other autoimmune processes, such as celiac disease.[1] Children with PSC-AIH can have

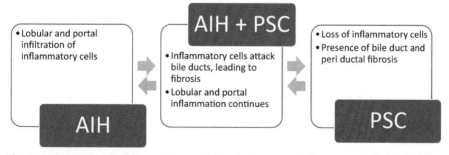

Fig. 1. A proposed possible continuum of PSC-AIH overlap. Inflammatory disease findings seen in patients with pediatric PSC, including those consistent with AIH. The presence and degree of AIH features of interface hepatitis and plasma cells can vary between patients and over time within an individual. Further research and standardized diagnostic criteria are needed to better understand and categorize these diseases or disease spectrum.

higher transaminases and higher IgG than PSC, whereas Gregorio and colleagues[77] did not find liver enzymes to be helpful in discriminating PSC-AIH from AIH.[1] IPSCG note that patients with PSC-AIH overlap can be more likely to have ALT that is greater than 5 times the upper limit of normal or IgG greater than 2 times upper limit of normal, which may be cutoffs for increased provider concern for PSC-AIH overlap and to better guide decisions for performing a biopsy.[74]

International AIH scoring systems have been used to identify overlap via clinical, histologic (lymphoplasmacytic inflammation and interface hepatitis), and serologic findings (positive autoantibodies and hypergammaglobulinemia).[79,80] Deneau and colleagues[3] and Gregorio and colleagues[77] both reported that 97% of children with PSC-AIH has type 1 AIH based on autoantibodies (smooth muscle antibody or antinuclear antibody–positive). However, AIH criteria are not able to differentiate pediatric PSC, AIH, and PSC-AIH overlap from one another owing to high autoantibody cutoffs and not incorporating cholangiographic findings.[2,6,77] A new pediatric scoring system was recently proposed that does include cholangiography at diagnosis, although is not yet formally validated.[6] Thus there remains no generally agreed-upon diagnostic criteria for PSC-AIH overlap.[6] Given this lack of standardization and subjectivity of pathologist reporting, there is expected variability in the management of PSC-AIH overlap. Prospective, multicenter studies are needed to better define overlap and determine pathogenic mechanisms for future, targeted therapies.

Secondary Sclerosing Cholangitis

When a patient presents with presumed PSC, careful consideration needs to be made as to whether anything in their past medical history could fit with their overall clinical picture and lead to the diagnosis of secondary sclerosing cholangitis (SSC). A list of potential causes of SSC is seen in **Table 1**.[1,2] For some conditions, serologic, imaging, and histologic findings can be similar in PSC and SSC. Atypical presentation, such as diagnosis in an infant or young child, recurrent infections or other history concerning for an immunodeficiency/immune dysregulation, history of recurrent pancreatitis, sickle cell disease, and so forth, should be investigated to find an underlying cause. The degree of workup to identify a primary cause is patient-specific, although for adult patients, AASLD recommends at minimum sending an IgG4 level on all patients with sclerosing cholangitis.[1]

NATURAL HISTORY, COMPLICATIONS, AND OUTCOMES
Natural History

PSC is typically a progressive inflammatory disorder. With ongoing biliary damage, pathologic repair, and deposited scar tissue, it will eventually lead to cirrhosis and complications of portal hypertension in most individuals. The average time from diagnosis until a person needs to undergo liver transplantation is 15 to 20 years.[1,38] There is some evidence that children have prolonged transplant-free survival versus adults. This may be due to differences in the disease process itself, fewer complicating comorbidities in children, or an earlier diagnosis causing lead-time bias.[3,11] The early course of PSC in children appears to be "waxing and waning," with spontaneous improvement in liver enzymes regardless of whether patients received any medications to treat PSC.[52,53] On average, there is a 60% reduction in GGT in untreated patients with PSC in the first year (mean decrease from 290 U/L at diagnosis to 115 U/L, with normalization in 29% of patients to less than 50 U/L as reported by Deneau and colleagues).[52] ALP can similarly vary in some adults in early stages, perhaps before the chronic unwavering cholestasis of adult PSC.[3,12] In untreated children with follow-up biopsy 1 year after diagnosis, 18% had improved fibrosis staging, whereas the majority (73%) was unchanged.[53] Children with PSC-AIH overlap were found to have similar rates of end-stage liver disease at diagnosis as patients with PSC, and prior adult data have shown PSC and PSC-AIH overlap to have similar rates of transplantation.[3,67]

Although historically PSC was studied in Caucasian populations, there is growing recognition of PSC affecting patients of all races. In an adult study by Bowlus and colleagues,[16] African American patients were found to develop PSC at a younger age than European American or Hispanic patients. They had lower rates of IBD and more advanced liver disease than other races, including higher risk for being listed for transplant and higher Model for End-Stage Liver Disease (MELD) scores.

Complications

Patients with PSC are at risk for various complications of progressive liver and biliary disease. In the first pediatric multicenter natural history report, Deneau and colleagues[3] defined outcomes by "event-free survival," with events including complications from portal hypertension (varices, ascites, hepatic encephalopathy); biliary complications (with a stricture requiring intervention); diagnosis of cholangiocarcinoma; need for liver transplantation; and death. Event-free survival was 70% at 5 years after diagnosis and 53% at 10 years. Among different PSC phenotypes, large-duct disease and the absence of IBD were both associated with lower rates of event-free survival, although IBD severity and severity of liver disease do not seem to correlate.[64] Patients with PSC-AIH had similar event-free survival and transplantation rates as PSC alone.[69]

Portal Hypertension

Although advanced fibrosis or cirrhosis can be seen in up to 40% or more of children with PSC at time of diagnosis, patients initially present with complications of portal hypertension only about 5% of the time.[3,69] Evidence of portal hypertension later develops in an estimated 38% of children by 10 years after diagnosis.[3] Although varices can be present in up to one-third of adults in the first year after diagnosis, they were found in only 13% to 15% of children.[3,69] Patients with concurrent IBD have a lower prevalence of portal complications than children with PSC alone. In the PSC Consortium, median transplant-free survival after developing complications of portal hypertension was 2.8 years.[3]

Biliary Complications

In the PSC Consortium, biliary strictures were present in 5% of patients at diagnosis and in 25% of patients at 10 years, with subsequent 3.5-year median transplant-free survival.[3] Adult PSC is often complicated by a "dominant stricture" with common bile duct diameter 1.5 mm or a hepatic duct diameter of only 1 mm.[1,81] Although most adults develop a dominant stricture by 5 years, only 1 in 6 children do.[3,81] Strictures can lead to choledocholithiasis and put patients at increased risk of bacterial cholangitis and disease progression. ERCP with dilation and with or without duct stenting is recommended in patients with worsening symptoms, concerning laboratory tests, or imaging suggestive of stricture development. In a large single-site study by Valentino and colleagues,[69] 18% of patients required ERCP over a median long-term follow-up period of 3.7 years. ERCP puts patients at risk of infection, pancreatitis, or bleeding. Percutaneous cholangiography with dilation is another option depending on ERCP success or candidacy, and surgical intervention is typically a last resort when other modalities have failed. Patients require antibiotics following manipulation of the bile ducts, and many with strictures and recurrent cholangitis benefit from long-term anti-microbial prophylaxis.[1,81]

Bone Disease

Chronic cholestasis can lead to osteodystrophy in patients, and AASLD recommends periodic measurement of markers of bone metabolism in children with PSC (vitamin D, parathyroid hormone, calcium, magnesium, phosphorus). Deficiencies should be treated and followed for improvement, and clinicians can perform periodic or targeted imaging to assess bone density.

Liver Transplantation and Disease Recurrence

PSC accounts for 2% of all pediatric liver transplants.[1–3] In the pediatric PSC Consortium, 14% of patients underwent liver transplantation at a median age of 15 years old, with a median follow-up of 4 years since diagnosis. This reflects 88% and 70% transplant-free survival at 5 and 10 years, respectively.[3] Valentino and colleagues[69] similarly found 89% 5-year childhood survival with native liver. Ten-year transplant-free survival is worse in adults, between 60% and 65%.[3,67] In a recent retrospective study of children with diagnosis of IBD-PSC, transplant-free survival was 100% at 5 years and 88% at 10 years after diagnosis.[75]

Indication for transplantation typically is for progressive complications of PSC, such as advanced liver disease with portal hypertension, biliary strictures not manageable with ERCP, recurrent cholangitis, or risk of cholangiocarcinoma.[82] Overall, patient and graft survival in pediatric PSC is similar to that of age-matched patients with other underlying primary liver diseases.[82] Disease recurrence in children is estimated to be in the range of 10% to 50%.[2,6,83] Recurrence in adults has been associated with several factors, such as male sex, history of acute cellular rejection, active IBD needing systemic steroids, or history of cholangiocarcinoma before transplant.[1] There is some evidence that colectomy may decrease the risk of PSC recurrence following transplantation, although further work is needed in this area of research.[62] Up to two-thirds of patients with recurrence will eventually need to be retransplanted.[84]

Cholangiocarcinoma and Colorectal Cancer

Cholangiocarcinoma is rare in children. There were only 8 cases (1%) within the pediatric PSC Consortium, all of whom were older than 15 years old.[3] Metastatic pediatric cases led to death (3/8), whereas localized disease was treated with surgical resection and chemotherapy (4/8), or transplantation (1/8). All but one patient was male. Cholangiocarcinoma is much more common in adults (between 7% and 9% 10-year incidence, overall lifetime risk of 10%–15%), as chronic immune activation of cholangiocytes can lead to malignant transformation over many years.[1,11,81,85] Cancer antigen 19-9 is a sensitive screening tool, which, along with imaging, can detect greater than 90% of adult cases. Increasing cholestasis, weight loss, or a progressive dominant stricture could be clues for developing cholangiocarcinoma. In adults, the European Society of Gastrointestinal Endoscopy and EASL recommend ductal sampling/brush cytology of biliary strictures during ERCP.[65] However, this is not routinely recommended in children because of the low incidence.[1]

Patients with PSC-IBD have up to a three- to four-fold greater risk of developing colorectal cancer than those with IBD alone, leading to the recommendations for screening colonoscopies discussed previously in the PSC-IBD section.[1,51,62,85]

Death

Death in pediatric PSC is overall rare (1%–2%) and follows several years of disease progression.[3,69] Malignancy, end-stage liver disease, and complications related to management following transplantation are common causes of mortality. As with any patient transplanted as a teenager, they are at high risk of death as a young adult, and successful transition to an adult provider is vital to their continued health and survival.[86]

CURRENT TREATMENT MODALITIES
Ursodeoxycholic Acid and Other Bile Acids

No medication has been conclusively proven effective for the treatment of PSC, although ursodeoxycholic acid (UDCA or ursodiol) is the most studied and most commonly prescribed. It is a secondary BA and theoretically works by protecting cells from the abnormal hydrophobic BA pool seen in PSC dysbiosis. It may have anti-inflammatory effects, while also stimulating protective hepatobiliary secretions. Eighty percent of children with PSC has been reported to be on UDCA at some point in time and often stay on treatment for several years.3 In a 2018 pediatric PSC Consortium paper, use of UDCA led to greater reduction in GGT at 1 year than untreated patients, with higher GGT normalization (53% vs 29%).[52] Similar improvements were seen in ALT and AST-to-platelet ratio index (APRI, an estimate of fibrosis). However, in subgroup analysis by risk of disease progression (based on APRI or GGT), GGT reduction was only better in patients with low-baseline risk. Patient event-free survival was no different in treated versus untreated patients at 5 years. In a prospective UDCA withdrawal and reinstitution pediatric study, Black and colleagues[87] found that withdrawal led to a biochemical "flare" (ALT or GGT >100) in only 8/22 children, without clear implications to patient outcome.

In a follow-up pediatric PSC Consortium study, 88 children who received either UDCA, Vancomycin, or no treatment (264 patients total) were matched based on disease phenotype, baseline characteristics, laboratory tests, and immunosuppression use.[53] Patients who received UDCA or Vancomycin had lower median GGT than those untreated at 6 months (52, 34, and 82 U/L, respectively; $P<.05$), although there was no difference by 1 year ($P = .657$). The same percent of patients had a normal GGT at 1 year (49%–53%; $P = $ NS). In those with follow-up biopsies, changes in liver fibrosis were no different between groups. Finally, there was not a significant difference in 5-year probability of being listed for liver transplant.

A Cochrane review showed UDCA improved biochemical measurements without any change in disease progression, as several adult studies have found that UDCA does not improve long-term patient outcomes.[88] This review noted several studies showing a good safety profile for UDCA. However, a notable adult randomized controlled trial (RCT) using high doses of UDCA (28–30 mg/kg/d) found an increased risk of death, liver transplantation, and serious adverse events in those who received UDCA, leading to an early ending of the study.[89] Thus, most pediatric providers use lower doses of no more than 20 mg/kg per day to avoid any potential adverse effects from higher dosing.[53,87] AASLD in 2010 recommended NOT using UDCA in adults with PSC.[1] ACG guidelines from 2015 do not directly recommend using or not using UDCA, but state that if it is used the dose should not be greater than 28 mg/kg per day.[66]

24-Norursodeoxycholic acid (norUDCA or norursodiol) is a homologue of UDCA whose mechanisms are thought to differ from UDCA. Mouse models have shown antifibrotic, anti-inflammatory (including CD8[+] T-cell modulation), and anticholestatic properties in norUDCA, with evidence it may be superior to UDCA.[90,91] An adult phase

2 RCT involving 38 centers found norUDCA to successfully reduce ALP, with a safety profile similar to patients receiving placebo.[91]

Vancomycin

OVT has historically been used in approximately 10% to 15% of children, to treat dysbiosis and modulate the immune response in PSC. It has typically been used chronically for an average of 4.3 years, as reported by the pediatric PSC Consortium.[3,53] There are no pediatric RCT data on this subject. Primary outcomes of most adult studies are of biochemical values rather than clinical outcomes. An adult RCT of 35 patients found both low-dose and high-dose OVT (125 and 250 mg 4 times per day) to decrease ALP, with lower dosing decreasing adult Mayo PSC Risk Score.[92] An Iranian RCT of 29 patients found no difference in combined OVT/UDCA versus UDCA alone.[93] In a small, prospective, noncontrolled trial by Davies and colleagues,[94] 14 children with PSC and IBD were all treated with OVT. All patients had statistically significant reduction in laboratory tests (ALT, GGT, erythrocyte sedimentation rate) and subjective improvement in symptoms. Patients with cirrhosis had less of a reduction in laboratory tests while on OVT. Stopping OVT during intermittent dosing practices was shown to lead to increased ALT, increased GGT, and worsening clinical symptoms, which all improved upon medication reinitiation. In a recent open-labeled study of 59 children and young adults, 57/59 experienced a reduction in GGT, with 50% of children having a normal GGT at 6 months and with similar reductions in ALP and ALT.[95] Deneau and colleagues[53] found no difference whether OVT was used as first treatment for PSC or as a "salvage" after trying UDCA. The potential risks of chronic OVT use in PSC have not been fully delineated.

Other antibiotics have been implicated and tried previously for PSC (such as rifaximin, tetracycline, or minocycline), although there is not great evidence for any of them. In the study by Tabibian and colleagues,[92] metronidazole was found to decrease Mayo PSC risk score, bilirubin, and patient complaints of pruritis. Similar to management of *Clostridium difficile* infections refractory to OVT, a small study of 10 patients with PSC-IBD receiving fecal microbiota transplantation showed the ability to decrease ALP and to increase bacterial diversity in some patients.[96]

Immunosuppression

Although immunosuppression is not used to treat PSC, for patients diagnosed with PSC-AIH, it is often the mainstay of therapy. In the prospective study of pediatric AIH and PSC-AIH by Gregorio and colleagues,[77] 23/27 patients with PSC-AIH received immunosuppression (typically 2 mg/kg per day prednisolone to a maximum dose of 60 mg $\pm$ 1 to 2 mg/kg per day azathioprine similar to standard treatment for AIH). Most patients who received treatment had normalization of liver enzymes (AST, 83%; bilirubin, 73%; GGT, 89%; ALP, 92%; albumin, 89%, international normalized ratio, 100%). Patients with PSC-AIH had faster serologic improvement than AIH, typically having normal laboratory tests within a few months. One-third of patients with PSC-AIH had a period of later biochemical relapse of increasing transaminases, which improved with starting higher steroid doses. These patients had statistically decreased inflammation on repeat liver biopsy compared with time of diagnosis. Other retrospective pediatric data likewise showed serologic improvements in AIH and PSC-AIH on immunosuppression.[97]

Despite these findings, 8/17 patients with PSC-AIH who had a repeat ERCP in the prospective study by Gregorio and colleagues[77] developed progression of bile duct disease during a follow-up period of 1 to 9 years. Overall 10-year transplant-free survival was estimated at only 65% in PSC-AIH versus 100% for AIH, nearing statistical significance (P = .053).[6,77] This study was not powered to compare treated versus untreated PSC-AIH, and no prospective RCTs exist on the subject.

In follow-up prospective data by the same group, patients resistant to first-line AIH therapy received mycophenolate mofetil. Transaminases improved in 16/18 (89%) children with AIH, but only 2/8 (25%) improved in PSC-AIH.[98] Likewise, there is no evidence that calcineurin inhibitors or other alternative immunosuppressants affect outcomes in PSC-AIH.[97] Together these findings suggest that PSC-AIH has a variable degree of currently untreatable cholangiopathy, which does not respond to immunosuppression. This may be the deciding factor for long-term patient outcomes. Per 2010 AASLD practice guidelines, "it is reasonable to attempt a trial of corticosteroids with or without azathioprine" in children if their histology, autoimmune markers, and IgG level are suggestive of PSC-AIH.[1] Given the inconsistent diagnostic criteria and variability in treatment protocols, interpretation of this guidance into daily practice should be dependent on clinical, biochemical course, and prevalence of autoimmunity in the population being served.

Farnesoid X Receptor Agonists

There is growing interest in agonists to Farnesoid X receptor (FXR), a nuclear receptor that regulates BA synthesis, conjugation, and transport. In a phase 2, adult RCT, obeticholic acid (a BA analogue and FXR agonist) and cilofexor (a small-molecule nonsteroidal FXR agonist) have both decreased ALP.[99,100] For all of these, further clinical trials and substantial pediatric data are needed.

PROGNOSIS AND PROGNOSTIC TOOLS

Large-duct disease and absence of prior IBD diagnosis are associated with worse outcomes, whereas the presence of PSC-AIH overlap features does not seem to change long-term outcome measures.[3,69] In the PSC Consortium, disease progression was not associated with patient characteristics such as sex or age at diagnosis.[3] Children with the higher total bilirubin, GGT, and APRI have been found to have worse outcomes with some studies reporting them as reliable prognostic markers.[52] GGT normalization to less than 50 U/L 1 year after diagnosis was associated with 5-year event-free survival (91% vs only 67% with persistently elevated GGT; P<.001). Regardless of normalization, greater than 75% reduction in GGT had improved outcomes compared with less than 25% reduction (88% vs 61% 5-year event free survival; P = .005).

Adult prognostic scoring systems exist for chronic liver disease, such as the Child-Pugh score, which predicts mortality in the setting of cirrhosis. However, this scoring system is not specific to PSC, and AASLD recommends against using prognostic models for patients with PSC.[1] A newer, PSC-specific tool called PSC Risk Estimate Tool incorporates 9 variables, including albumin, ALP, AST, bilirubin, hemoglobin, platelets, sodium, patient age, and years since diagnosis.[101] Although this performed well compared with MELD or Mayo risk score, this was only validated in adults to assess risk of hepatic decompensation. These adult scoring systems have been shown to lack reliability in the pediatric PSC population.[55]

To address this, Deneau and colleagues[54] used data from 1012 children at 40 centers to generate the SCOPE index. This uses patient albumin, platelet count, total bilirubin, GGT, and cholangiography to predict liver transplant or death, as well as secondary outcomes of hepatobiliary complications. Patients are scored 0 to 11 and stratified into low (0–3), medium (4–5), and high risk (6 or greater). Annual risk of progressing to death or needing transplant in these groups was determined to be less than 1%, 3%, and 9%, respectively, with secondary complication rates of 2%, 6%, and 13% annually ($P<.001$). This model was shown to be superior to adult scores by avoiding ALP or AST, which can vary in children from bone turnover or presence of AIH overlap. SCOPE was seen to be an independent predictor of patient response to PSC treatment initiation, although the management strategy itself did not make a significant difference within a given SCOPE risk category.[54]

SUMMARY

Pediatric PSC is a rare, poorly understood, chronic immune-mediated disease of the liver. Treatment options are limited, and those available have questionable efficacy in affecting long-term patient outcomes. Many individuals will progress to ESLD as an adolescent or young adult and require liver transplantation. Long term, patients are also at risk for colorectal or hepatobiliary malignancy. Prospective, multisite pediatric clinical data on PSC, PSC-AIH overlap, and PSC-IBD are severely lacking. Further translational work, meanwhile, is needed to create targeted therapies and improve patient outcomes. Pediatric studies will be particularly insightful to all patients with PSC given the lack of comorbidities and other confounding variables relative to adults. It remains an exciting area for future scientific discovery.

CLINICS CARE POINTS

- There are no medications available that have been prospectively shown to change clinical outcomes in pediatric primary sclerosing cholangitis. Ursodeoxycholic acid, and less commonly, oral vancomycin are used by many pediatric providers. At the appropriate dosing, these medications have been found to be safe for short-term use and have been associated with biochemical improvement in some patients over time. However, many patients also show spontaneous improvement in liver indices without treatment, and there is no evidence that biochemical improvement prevents or alters the natural history of primary sclerosing cholangitis progression. Further research is needed into ursodeoxycholic acid, oral vancomycin, as well as other medications regarding long-term disease outcomes.

- Many children with primary sclerosing cholangitis also have features of autoimmune hepatitis on liver biopsy (primary sclerosing cholangitis–autoimmune hepatitis overlap) and are often treated with systemic immunosuppression via steroids and azathioprine. Criteria for primary sclerosing cholangitis–autoimmune hepatitis overlap diagnosis and management guidelines are lacking. Limited pediatric data have shown a biochemical improvement and decrease in inflammation on liver biopsy in patients on immunosuppression, although there is evidence of progressive biliary disease on imaging, suggesting a degree of currently untreatable cholangiopathy. Given the side-effect profiles of these immunosuppressants, careful consideration should be made regarding treatment and monitoring. Prospective randomized controlled trials are greatly needed.

- Most patients with primary sclerosing cholangitis have concurrent inflammatory bowel disease, which can present with severe colonic inflammation and discordantly mild clinical symptoms. Patients with primary sclerosing cholangitis–inflammatory bowel disease are at increased risk of colonic and rectal dysplasia. Providers should maintain a high index of suspicion and use objective data (fecal calprotectin and endoscopy) to diagnose and monitor IBD in primary sclerosing cholangitis, although the frequency of endoscopic monitoring in pediatric patients is not yet well established.

- A pediatric-specific prognostic tool (Sclerosing Cholangitis Outcomes in Pediatrics) has been recently created that may help guide pediatric primary sclerosing cholangitis risk-stratification and monitoring practices for providers.

DISCLOSURE

The authors have no sources of funding to disclose.

CONFLICT OF INTEREST

The authors declare that they have no conflicts of interest relevant to this work.

REFERENCES

1. Chapman R, Fevery J, Kalloo A, et al. Diagnosis and management of primary sclerosing cholangitis. Review. Hepatology 2010;51(2):660–78.
2. Di Giorgio A, Vergani D, Mieli-Vergani G. Cutting edge issues in juvenile sclerosing cholangitis. review. Dig Liver Dis 2021. https://doi.org/10.1016/j.dld.2021.06.028.
3. Deneau MR, El-Matary W, Valentino PL, et al. The natural history of primary sclerosing cholangitis in 781 children: a multicenter, international collaboration. article. Hepatology 2017;66(2):518–27.
4. Deneau M, Jensen MK, Holmen J, et al. Primary sclerosing cholangitis, autoimmune hepatitis, and overlap in Utah children: epidemiology and natural history. article. Hepatology 2013;58(4):1392–400.
5. Lazaridis KN, LaRusso NF. Primary sclerosing cholangitis. review. N Engl J Med 2016;375(12):1161–70.
6. Mieli-Vergani G, Vergani D, Baumann U, et al. Diagnosis and management of pediatric autoimmune liver disease: ESPGHAN hepatology committee position statement. article. J Pediatr Gastroenterol Nutr 2018;66(2):345–60.
7. Smolka V, Karaskova E, Tkachyk O, et al. Long-term follow-up of children and adolescents with primary sclerosing cholangitis and autoimmune sclerosing cholangitis. Article. Hepatobiliary Pancreat Dis Int 2016;15(4):412–8.
8. Toy E, Balasubramanian S, Selmi C, et al. The prevalence, incidence and natural history of primary sclerosing cholangitis in an ethnically diverse population. article. BMC Gastroenterol 2011;1183. https://doi.org/10.1186/1471-230X-11-83.
9. Trivedi PJ, Hirschfield GM. Recent advances in clinical practice: epidemiology of autoimmune liver diseases. article. Gut 2021. https://doi.org/10.1136/gutjnl-2020-322362.
10. Little R, Wine E, Kamath BM, et al. Gut microbiome in primary sclerosing cholangitis: a review. review. World J Gastroenterol 2020;26(21):2768–80.
11. Banales JM, Huebert RC, Karlsen T, et al. Cholangiocyte pathobiology. review. Nat Rev Gastroenterol Hepatol 2019;16(5):269–81.
12. Karlsen TH, Folseraas T, Thorburn D, et al. Primary sclerosing cholangitis – a comprehensive review. review. J Hepatol 2017;67(6):1298–323.
13. Bergquist A, Montgomery SM, Bahmanyar S, et al. Increased risk of primary sclerosing cholangitis and ulcerative colitis in first-degree relatives of patients with primary sclerosing cholangitis. article. Clin Gastroenterol Hepatol 2008;6(8):939–43.
14. Karlsen TH, Boberg KM, Vatn M, et al. Different HLA class II associations in ulcerative colitis patients with and without primary sclerosing cholangitis. article. Genes Immun 2007;8(3):275–8.
15. Wiencke K, Karlsen TH, Boberg KM, et al. Primary sclerosing cholangitis is associated with extended HLA-DR3 and HLA-DR6 haplotypes. article. Tissue Antigens 2007;69(2):161–9.

16. Bowlus CL, Li CS, Karlsen TH, et al. Primary sclerosing cholangitis in genetically diverse populations listed for liver transplantation: unique clinical and human leukocyte antigen associations. article. Liver Transplant 2010;16(11):1324–30.

17. Haisma SM, Weersma RK, Joosse ME, et al. Exome sequencing in patient-parent trios suggests new candidate genes for early-onset primary sclerosing cholangitis. article. Liver Int 2021;41(5):1044–57.

18. Folseraas T, Melum E, Rausch P, et al. Extended analysis of a genome-wide association study in primary sclerosing cholangitis detects multiple novel risk loci. article. J Hepatol 2012;57(2):366–75.

19. Liu JZ, Hov JR, Folseraas T, et al. Dense genotyping of immune-related disease regions identifies nine new risk loci for primary sclerosing cholangitis. article. Nat Genet 2013;45(6):670–5.

20. Melum E, Franke A, Schramm C, et al. Genome-wide association analysis in primary sclerosing cholangitis identifies two non-HLA susceptibility loci. article. Nat Genet 2011;43(1):17–9, 8.

21. O'Hara SP, LaRusso NF. The gut-liver axis in primary sclerosing cholangitis: are pathobionts the missing link? Note. Hepatology 2019;70(3):1058–60.

22. Iwasawa K, Suda W, Tsunoda T, et al. Characterisation of the faecal microbiota in Japanese patients with paediatric-onset primary sclerosing cholangitis. letter. Gut 2017;66(7):1344–6.

23. Kummen M, Holm K, Anmarkrud JA, et al. The gut microbial profile in patients with primary sclerosing cholangitis is distinct from patients with ulcerative colitis without biliary disease and healthy controls. article. Gut 2017;66(4):611–9.

24. Rühlemann M, Liwinski T, Heinsen FA, et al. Consistent alterations in faecal microbiomes of patients with primary sclerosing cholangitis independent of associated colitis. Article. Aliment Pharmacol Ther 2019;50(5):580–9.

25. Sabino J, Vieira-Silva S, Machiels K, et al. Primary sclerosing cholangitis is characterised by intestinal dysbiosis independent from IBD. Article. Gut 2016; 65(10):1681–9.

26. Cortez RV, Moreira LN, Padilha M, et al. Gut microbiome of children and adolescents with primary sclerosing cholangitis in association with ulcerative colitis. article. Front Immunol 2021;11:598152.

27. Liao L, Schneider KM, Galvez EJC, et al. Intestinal dysbiosis augments liver disease progression via NLRP3 in a murine model of primary sclerosing cholangitis. Article. Gut 2019;68(8):1477–92.

28. Nakamoto N, Sasaki N, Aoki R, et al. Gut pathobionts underlie intestinal barrier dysfunction and liver T helper 17 cell immune response in primary sclerosing cholangitis. article. Nat Microbiol 2019;4(3):492–503.

29. Kevans D, Tyler AD, Holm K, et al. Characterization of intestinal microbiota in ulcerative colitis patients with and without primary sclerosing cholangitis. article. J Crohn's Colitis 2016;10(3):330–7.

30. Quraishi MN, Acharjee A, Beggs AD, et al. A pilot integrative analysis of colonic gene expression, gut microbiota, and immune infiltration in primary sclerosing cholangitis-inflammatory bowel disease: association of disease with bile acid pathways. article. J Crohn's Colitis 2020;14(7):935–47.

31. Quraishi MN, Sergeant M, Kay G, et al. The gut-adherent microbiota of PSC-IBD is distinct to that of IBD. Letter. Gut 2017;66(2):386–8.

32. Rossen NG, Fuentes S, Boonstra K, et al. The mucosa-associated microbiota of PSC patients is characterized by low diversity and low abundance of uncultured clostridiales II. article. J Crohn's Colitis 2015;9(4):342–8.

33. Lichtman SN, Keku J, Clark RL, et al. Biliary tract disease in rats with experimental small bowel bacterial overgrowth. Article. Hepatology 1991;13(4): 766–72.

34. Lichtman SN, Sartor RB, Keku J, et al. Hepatic inflammation in rats with experimental small intestinal bacterial overgrowth. Article. Gastroenterology 1990; 98(2):414–23.

35. Dhillon AK, Kummen M, Trøseid M, et al. Circulating markers of gut barrier function associated with disease severity in primary sclerosing cholangitis. article. Liver Int 2019;39(2):371–81.

36. Jiang X, Karlsen TH. Genetics of primary sclerosing cholangitis and pathophysiological implications. review. Nat Rev Gastroenterol Hepatol 2017;14(5): 279–95.

37. Högenauer K, Arista L, Schmiedeberg N, et al. G-protein-coupled bile acid receptor 1 (GPBAR1, TGR5) agonists reduce the production of proinflammatory cytokines and stabilize the alternative macrophage phenotype. article. J Med Chem 2014;57(24):10343–54.

38. Tabibian JH, Bowlus CL. Primary sclerosing cholangitis: a review and update. review. Liver Res 2017;1(4):221–30.

39. Hov JR, Boberg KM, Karlsen TH. Autoantibodies in primary sclerosing cholangitis. editorial. World J Gastroenterol 2008;14(24):3781–91.

40. Sebode M, Weiler-Normann C, Liwinski T, et al. Autoantibodies in autoimmune liver disease-clinical and diagnostic relevance. review. Front Immunol 2018; 9(MAR):609.

41. Trivedi PJ, Adams DH. Mucosal immunity in liver autoimmunity: a comprehensive review. review. J Autoimmun 2013;46:97–111.

42. Pollheimer MJ, Halilbasic E, Fickert P, et al. Pathogenesis of primary sclerosing cholangitis. article. Best Pract Res Clin Gastroenterol 2011;25(6):727–39.

43. Liaskou E, Jeffery LE, Trivedi PJ, et al. Loss of CD28 expression by liver-infiltrating T cells contributes to pathogenesis of primary sclerosing cholangitis. article. Gastroenterology 2014;147(1):221–32, e7.

44. Schoknecht T, Schwinge D, Stein S, et al. CD4+ T cells from patients with primary sclerosing cholangitis exhibit reduced apoptosis and down-regulation of proapoptotic Bim in peripheral blood. Article. J Leukoc Biol 2017;101(2): 589–97.

45. Katt J, Schwinge D, Schoknecht T, et al. Increased T helper type 17 response to pathogen stimulation in patients with primary sclerosing cholangitis. article. Hepatology 2013;58(3):1084–93.

46. Kekilli M, Tunc B, Beyazit Y, et al. Circulating CD4+CD25+ regulatory T cells in the pathobiology of ulcerative colitis and concurrent primary sclerosing cholangitis. article. Dig Dis Sci 2013;58(5):1250–5.

47. Mathies F, Steffens N, Kleinschmidt D, et al. Colitis promotes a pathological condition of the liver in the absence of Foxp3 + regulatory T cells. article. J Immunol 2018;201(12):3558–68.

48. Tedesco D, Thapa M, Chin CY, et al. Alterations in intestinal microbiota lead to production of interleukin 17 by intrahepatic γδ T-cell receptor–positive cells and pathogenesis of cholestatic liver disease. article. Gastroenterology 2018;154(8): 2178–93.

49. Henriksen EKK, Jørgensen KK, Kaveh F, et al. Gut and liver T-cells of common clonal origin in primary sclerosing cholangitis-inflammatory bowel disease. article. J Hepatol 2017;66(1):116–22.

50. Landi A, Weismuller TJ, Lankisch TO, et al. Differential serum levels of eosinophilic eotaxins in primary sclerosing cholangitis, primary biliary cirrhosis, and autoimmune hepatitis. article. J Interferon Cytokine Res 2014;34(3):204–14.

51. Mertz A, Nguyen NA, Katsanos KH, et al. Primary sclerosing cholangitis and inflammatory bowel disease comorbidity: an update of the evidence. Review. Ann Gastroenterol 2019;32(2):124–33.

52. Deneau MR, Mack C, Abdou R, et al. Gamma glutamyltransferase reduction is associated with favorable outcomes in pediatric primary sclerosing cholangitis. article. Hepatol Commun 2018;2(11):1369–78.

53. Deneau MR, Mack C, Mogul D, et al. Oral vancomycin, ursodeoxycholic acid, or no therapy for pediatric primary sclerosing cholangitis: a matched analysis. article. Hepatology 2021;73(3):1061–73.

54. Deneau MR, Mack C, Perito ER, et al. The sclerosing cholangitis outcomes in pediatrics (SCOPE) index: a prognostic tool for children. article. Hepatology 2021;73(3):1074–87.

55. Deneau MR, Valentino PL, Mack C, et al. Assessing the validity of adult-derived prognostic models for primary sclerosing cholangitis outcomes in children. article. J Pediatr Gastroenterol Nutr 2020;70(1):E12–7.

56. Loftus EV Jr, Harewood GC, Loftus CG, et al. PSC-IBD: a unique form of inflammatory bowel disease associated with primary sclerosing cholangitis. article. Gut 2005;54(1):91–6.

57. Ricciuto A, Hansen BE, Ngo B, et al. Primary sclerosing cholangitis in children with inflammatory bowel diseases is associated with milder clinical activity but more frequent subclinical inflammation and growth impairment. article. Clin Gastroenterol Hepatol 2020;18(7):1509–17, e7.

58. Fausa O, Schrumpf E, Elgjo K. Relationship of inflammatory bowel disease and primary sclerosing cholangitis. article. Semin Liver Dis 1991;11(1):31–9.

59. Verdonk RC, Dijkstra G, Haagsma EB, et al. Inflammatory bowel disease after liver transplantation: risk factors for recurrence and de novo disease. article. Am J Transplant 2006;6(6):1422–9.

60. Rasmussen HH, Fallingborg JF, Mortensen PB, et al. Hepatobiliary dysfunction and primary sclerosing cholangitis in patients with Crohn's disease. article. Scand J Gastroenterol 1997;32(6):604–10.

61. Faubion WA Jr, Loftus EV, Sandborn WJ, et al. Pediatric "PSC-IBD": a descriptive report of associated inflammatory bowel disease among pediatric patients with PSC. article. J Pediatr Gastroenterol Nutr 2001;33(3):296–300.

62. Ricciuto A, Kamath BM, Griffiths AM. The IBD and PSC phenotypes of PSC-IBD. Review. Curr Gastroenterol Rep 2018;20(4):16.

63. Ricciuto A, Fish J, Carman N, et al. Symptoms do not correlate with findings from colonoscopy in children with inflammatory bowel disease and primary sclerosing cholangitis. article. Clin Gastroenterol Hepatol 2018;16(7):1098–105, e1.

64. Shiau H, Ihekweazu FD, Amin M, et al. Unique inflammatory bowel disease phenotype of pediatric primary sclerosing cholangitis: a single-center study. article. J Pediatr Gastroenterol Nutr 2017;65(4):404–9.

65. Aabakken L, Karlsen TH, Albert J, et al. Role of endoscopy in primary sclerosing cholangitis: European Society of Gastrointestinal Endoscopy (ESGE) and European Association for the Study of the Liver (EASL) clinical guideline. review. Endoscopy 2017;49(6):588–608.

66. Lindor KD, Kowdley KV, Harrison ME. ACG clinical guideline: primary sclerosing cholangitis. article. Am J Gastroenterol 2015;110(5):646–59.
67. Weismüller TJ, Strassburg CP, Trivedi PJ, et al. Patient age, sex, and inflammatory bowel disease phenotype associate with course of primary sclerosing cholangitis. article. Gastroenterology 2017;152(8):1975–84, e8.
68. Kerkar N, Miloh T. Sclerosing cholangitis: pediatric perspective. review. Curr Gastroenterol Rep 2010;12(3):195–202.
69. Valentino PL, Wiggins S, Harney S, et al. The natural history of primary sclerosing cholangitis in children: a large single-center longitudinal cohort study. article. J Pediatr Gastroenterol Nutr 2016;63(6):603–9.
70. Björnsson E, Olsson R, Bergquist A, et al. The natural history of small-duct primary sclerosing cholangitis. article. Gastroenterology 2008;134(4): 975–80.
71. Chavhan GB, Roberts E, Moineddin R, et al. Primary sclerosing cholangitis in children: utility of magnetic resonance cholangiopancreatography. article. Pediatr Radiol 2008;38(8):868–73.
72. Ferrara C, Valeri G, Salvolini L, et al. Magnetic resonance cholangiopancreatography in primary sclerosing cholangitis in children. article. Pediatr Radiol 2002; 32(6):413–7.
73. Burak KW, Angulo P, Lindor KD. Is there a role for liver biopsy in primary sclerosing cholangitis? article. Am J Gastroenterol 2003;98(5):1155–8.
74. Ponsioen C, Assis D, Boberg K, et al. Defining primary sclerosing cholangitis: results from an international primary sclerosing cholangitis study group consensus process. Gastroenterology 2021. Epub ahead of printdoi:10.1053.
75. Hensel KO, Kyrana E, Hadzic N, et al. Sclerosing cholangitis in pediatric inflammatory bowel disease: early diagnosis and management affect clinical outcome. Article. J Pediatr 2021. https://doi.org/10.1016/j.jpeds.2021.07.047.
76. Ma Y, Su H, Yuksel M, et al. Human leukocyte antigen profile predicts severity of autoimmune liver disease in children of European ancestry. Article. Hepatology 2021. https://doi.org/10.1002/hep.31893.
77. Gregorio GV, Portmann B, Karani J, et al. Autoimmune hepatitis/sclerosing cholangitis overlap syndrome in childhood: a 16-year prospective study. article. Hepatology 2001;33(3):544–53.
78. Nayagam J, Miquel R, Joshi D. Overlap syndrome with autoimmune hepatitis and primary sclerosing cholangitis. EMJ Hepatol 2019;7(1):95–104.
79. Hennes EM, Zeniya M, Czaja AJ, et al. Simplified criteria for the diagnosis of autoimmune hepatitis. article. Hepatology 2008;48(1):169–76.
80. Mileti E, Rosenthal P, Peters MG. Validation and modification of simplified diagnostic criteria for autoimmune hepatitis in children. article. Clin Gastroenterol Hepatol 2012;10(4):417–21, e2.
81. Chapman MH, Webster GJM, Bannoo S, et al. Cholangiocarcinoma and dominant strictures in patients with primary sclerosing cholangitis: a 25-year single-centre experience. review. Eur J Gastroenterol Hepatol 2012;24(9): 1051–8.
82. Squires RH, Ng V, Romero R, et al. Evaluation of the pediatric patient for liver transplantation: 2014 practice guideline by the American Association for the Study of Liver Diseases, American Society of Transplantation and the North American Society for Pediatric Gastroenterology, Hepatology and Nutrition. article. Hepatology 2014;60(1):362–98.

83. Feldstein AE, Perrault J, El-Youssif M, et al. Primary sclerosing cholangitis in children: a long-term follow-up study. Article. Hepatology 2003;38(1):210–7.

84. Scalori A, Heneghan M, Hadzic N, et al. Outcome and survival in childhood onset autoimmune sclerosing cholangitis and autoimmune hepatitis: a 13-year follow up study. Hepatology 2007;46 (supp) 555A.

85. Khaderi SA, Sussman NL. Screening for malignancy in primary sclerosing cholangitis (PSC). review. Curr Gastroenterol Rep 2015;17(4). https://doi.org/10.1007/s11894-015-0438-0.

86. Katz M, Gillespie S, Stevens JP, et al. African American pediatric liver transplant recipients have an increased risk of death after transferring to adult healthcare. article. J Pediatr 2021;233:119–25, e1.

87. Black DD, Mack C, Kerkar N, et al. A prospective trial of withdrawal and reinstitution of ursodeoxycholic acid in pediatric primary sclerosing cholangitis. article. Hepatol Commun 2019;3(11):1482–95.

88. Poropat G, Giljaca V, Stimac D, et al. Bile acids for primary sclerosing cholangitis. review. Cochrane database Syst Rev (Online) 2011;1.

89. Lindor KD, Kowdley KV, Luketic VAC, et al. High-dose ursodeoxycholic acid for the treatment of primary sclerosing cholangitis. article. Hepatol 2009;50(3):808–14.

90. Björnsson ES, Kalaitzakis E. Recent advances in the treatment of primary sclerosing cholangitis. review. Expert Rev Gastroenterol Hepatol 2021;15(4):413–25.

91. Fickert P, Hirschfield GM, Denk G, et al. norUrsodeoxycholic acid improves cholestasis in primary sclerosing cholangitis. article. J Hepatol 2017;67(3):549–58.

92. Tabibian JH, Weeding E, Jorgensen RA, et al. Randomised clinical trial: vancomycin or metronidazole in patients with primary sclerosing cholangitis - a pilot study. article. Aliment Pharmacol Ther 2013;37(6):604–12.

93. Rahimpour S, Nasiri-Toosi M, Khalili H, et al. A triple blinded, randomized, placebo-controlled clinical trial to evaluate the efficacy and safety of oral vancomycin in primary sclerosing cholangitis: a pilot study. article. J Gastrointest Liver Dis 2016;25(4):457–64.

94. Davies YK, Cox KM, Abdullah BA, et al. Long-term treatment of primary sclerosing cholangitis in children with oral vancomycin: an immunomodulating antibiotic. article. J Pediatr Gastroenterol Nutr 2008;47(1):61–7.

95. Ali AH, Damman J, Shah SB, et al. Open-label prospective therapeutic clinical trials: oral vancomycin in children and adults with primary sclerosing cholangitis. article. Scand J Gastroenterol 2020;55(8):941–50.

96. Allegretti JR, Kassam Z, Carrellas M, et al. Fecal microbiota transplantation in patients with primary sclerosing cholangitis: a pilot clinical trial. article. Am J Gastroenterol 2019;114(7):1071–9.

97. Di Giorgio A, Hadzic N, Dhawan A, et al. Seamless management of juvenile autoimmune liver disease: long-term medical and social outcome. article. J Pediatr 2020;218:121–9, e3.

98. Aw MM, Dhawan A, Samyn M, et al. Mycophenolate mofetil as rescue treatment for autoimmune liver disease in children: a 5-year follow-up. Article. J Hepatol 2009;51(1):156–60.

99. Kowdley KV, Vuppalanchi R, Levy C, et al. A randomized, placebo-controlled, phase II study of obeticholic acid for primary sclerosing cholangitis. Article. J Hepatol 2020;73(1):94–101.

100. Trauner M, Gulamhusein A, Hameed B, et al. The nonsteroidal farnesoid X receptor agonist cilofexor (GS-9674) improves markers of cholestasis and liver injury in patients with primary sclerosing cholangitis. article. Hepatology 2019; 70(3):788–801.
101. Eaton JE, Vesterhus M, McCauley BM, et al. Primary sclerosing cholangitis risk estimate tool (PREsTo) predicts outcomes of the disease: a derivation and validation study using machine learning. Hepatology 2020;71(1):214–24.

Pediatric Liver Transplantation

Sara Kathryn Smith, MD[a],*, Tamir Miloh, MD[b]

KEYWORDS

- Pediatric liver transplant • Liver failure • End stage liver disease
- Immunosuppression • Split liver transplant • Living donor transplant • Liver rejection

KEY POINTS

- Advances in surgical techniques, improved postoperative management, and immunosuppression optimization have made liver transplant an important lifesaving operation in children with acute or chronic liver disease, hepatic tumors, and select metabolic and genetic diseases.
- Because of donor scarcity, there has been an increased use of split hepatic grafts and other variant techniques with outcomes as those pediatric patients receiving whole hepatic grafts.
- Optimal outcomes require multidisciplinary care of patients, including, but not limited to, transplant surgeons, transplant hepatologists, intensivists, nutritionists, social workers, and transplant coordinators.

INTRODUCTION

In 1967, Dr Starzl and his team performed the first successful pediatric liver transplant in a patient with biliary atresia. Now approximately 600 children receive a liver transplant each year in the United States and in 2019 alone, and 686 new candidates were added to the waiting list. Pediatric liver transplants account for about 6% of total number of liver transplants performed in the United States (Scientific Registry of Transplant Recipients [SRTR] data). Improvement in pretransplant care, patient selection, surgical techniques, organ preservation, immunosuppression management, and post-transplant follow-up has led to outstanding results in patient and graft survival and quality of life (QoL). Liver transplantation (LT) is the treatment of choice for children with acute and chronic end-stage liver disease, selected liver tumors, and certain metabolic disorders. The indications for LT in children are different than in adults,

[a] Department of Pediatric Gastroenterology, Hepatology, and Nutrition, Johns Hopkins School of Medicine, 600 N Wolfe Street, Baltimore, MD 21287, USA; [b] Department of Pediatric Gastroenterology, Hepatology, and Nutrition, University of Miami, Highland Professional Building, 1801 Northwest 9th Avenue, Miami, FL 33136, USA
* Corresponding author.
E-mail address: ssmit403@jhmi.edu

Clin Liver Dis 26 (2022) 521–535
https://doi.org/10.1016/j.cld.2022.03.010
1089-3261/22/© 2022 Elsevier Inc. All rights reserved.

liver.theclinics.com

with cholestatic biliary atresia as the leading cause of liver failure in children. Organs are allocated according to clinical need based on scoring using the Pediatric End-Stage Liver Disease (PELD) score for patients younger than 12 years and Model of End-Stage Liver Disease (MELD) score for patients older than 12 years. In 2019, 60% of all children listed for LT in 2019 were aged 5 years or younger (SRTR). More children are now receiving split grafts, with 20.3% of all pediatric liver transplant recipients receiving split liver grafts in 2019 compared with 24.4% a decade ago (SRTR). The scarcity of cadaveric donors has led to increased use of living donor grafts, with 14.3% of children undergoing living donor liver transplants in 2019 (SRTR).[1]

Immunosuppression management has evolved over the years and remains one of the most important aspects of long-term posttransplant care. Tailoring the immunosuppressant regimen to the individual patient is pertinent, on one hand, for prevention of acute cellular, chronic, and antibody-mediated rejection and, on the other hand, for avoiding significant morbidities such as infection, posttransplant lymphoproliferative disease (PTLD), and medication side effects.[2] Patients need close laboratory monitoring to follow-up liver enzymes, liver function, immunosuppressant levels, and viral levels (specifically cytomegalovirus and Epstein-Barr virus).

Adherence with lifelong medication is vital to successful long-term outcomes and can be challenging, especially in the adolescent population. Nonadherence is associated with rejection and graft loss, and measures should be taken to ensure patients have the tools and resources necessary to enhance adherence to recommended regimens. The true ceiling for patient survival and graft longevity in pediatric LT recipients remains unknown. Many centers now perform surveillance liver biopsies to increase understanding and management of immunosuppression management. Interestingly, surveillance biopsies have shown an increased frequency of hepatitis and fibrosis despite normal serum transaminases in many patients, suggesting that we still have a lot to learn regarding long-term management strategies.[3] Some centers have demonstrated that select children develop operational tolerance and may be weaned off immunosuppressants, although studies are ongoing.

INDICATIONS FOR LIVER TRANSPLANT

The goal of LT in children is to increase life expectancy and/or QoL. The indications for LT in children include end-stage liver disease with significant synthetic dysfunction (acute or chronic); intractable portal hypertension evidenced by refractory ascites, coagulopathy, encephalopathy, or variceal bleeds; recurrent life-threatening episodes of cholangitis; spontaneous bacterial peritonitis; refractory pruritus; deforming xanthomas; failure to thrive despite maximal nutritional support; unresectable select hepatic tumors; and certain metabolic diseases. The common disease processes leading to LT evaluation are listed in **Table 1**. The SRTR data show that the most common indication for pediatric LT continues to be biliary atresia across all ages. In infants up to age 1 year, common indications for LT include biliary atresia, metabolic disease, acute liver failure, and other cholestatic diseases. In children age 1 to 5 years, malignant liver tumors become the fourth indication for LT. In children age 11 to 17 years, noncholestatic cirrhosis is the most common cause for LT, followed by acute liver failure, metabolic disease, biliary atresia, and cholestatic cirrhosis.

Biliary atresia remains the leading cause of liver failure in children despite improved screening, diagnosis, and Kasai portoenterostomy. Only 16% of children with biliary atresia survive up to 2 years with their native liver when the total serum bilirubin measured 3 months following Kasai procedure is greater than 6 mg/dL, compared with 84% for children with a total bilirubin less than 2 mg/dL.[4] Parenteral nutrition–

Table 1
Indications for liver transplantation in children

Cholestatic Conditions	• Biliary atresia • Sclerosing cholangitis • Parenteral nutrition–associated cholestasis • Alagille syndrome • Progressive familial intrahepatic cholestasis • Langerhans cell histiocytosis
Hepatitis	• Hepatitis B • Hepatitis C • Autoimmune hepatitis
Metabolic Disease	• Alpha 1 antitrypsin deficiency • Cystic fibrosis • Crigler-Najjar syndrome • Urea cycle defects • Organic academia • Maple syrup urine disease • Tyrosinemia • Wilson disease • Primary hyperoxaluria • Glycogen storages disorders • Hemophilia • Familial hypercholesterolemia • Certain mitochondrial disorders
Tumors	• Hepatoblastoma • Hemangioendothelioma • Hepatocellular carcinoma • Sarcoma
Other	• Cryptogenic cirrhosis • Gestational alloimmune liver disease • Budd-Chiari syndrome • Congenial hepatic fibrosis • Caroli disease • Drug induced • Hepatopulmonary syndrome
Acute Liver Failure	—

associated liver disease has decreased as an indication for LT, likely due to improved chronic total parenteral nutrition management and intestinal rehabilitation.[5] Some metabolic diseases can present with acute liver failure, whereas others can present later with cirrhosis and even liver tumors such as, alpha 1 antitrypsin deficiency, tyrosinemia, and Wilson disease. There are other metabolic diseases (urea cycle defects, organic acidemias, Crigler-Najjar syndrome type 1) in which transplanting the liver works to replace the associated defective enzyme that leads to decreased morbidity. In some metabolic diseases, such as maple syrup urine disease, LT only corrects the enzyme deficiency in the liver that is sufficient to improve QoL and decrease extrahepatic complications. There are some diseases in which an LT is needed to prevent progression of extrahepatic disease, such as primary hyperoxaluria type 1 and organic acidemias.[6] In certain circumstances, a combined liver kidney transplant (hyperoxaluria, methyl malonic acidemia) or combined liver lung transplant (cystic fibrosis) is required. LT can be beneficial in selected patients with secondary hemophagocytic lymphohistiocytosis. Nonalcoholic fatty liver disease has become one of the leading causes of LT in adults and young adolescents, in the setting of a nationwide obesity epidemic.[7,8]

Current contraindications to liver transplant in children include nonresectable extrahepatic malignant tumors, multisystem organ failure with concomitant end-stage organ failure that cannot be corrected by a combined transplant, uncontrolled sepsis, irreversible serious neurologic damage, and uncorrectable life-limiting defects in critical organs (heart, lungs, kidneys).

Relative contraindications include inadequate social support; however, this requires careful evaluation and consideration in pediatrics with multidisciplinary involvement of social work, case management, and child protective services, if needed.

ALLOCATION

Liver transplant candidates younger than 18 years at the time of registration may be assigned any of the following:

- Pediatric status 1A
- Pediatric status 1B
- Calculated MELD or PELD score
- Exception MELD or PELD score
- Inactive status (status 7)

Requirements to be listed in Status 1A include one of the following:

- Fulminant liver failure without preexisting liver disease; defined as the onset of hepatic encephalopathy within 56 days of the first signs and symptoms of liver disease with at least one of the following criteria: ventilator dependent, dialysis, or international normalized ratio (INR) greater than 2
- Primary nonfunction of a transplanted liver within 7 days of liver transplant
- Hepatic artery thrombosis (HAT) in a transplanted liver within 14 days of transplant
- Acute decompensated Wilson disease

Requirements to be listed in Status 1B include the following:

- Hepatoblastoma without evidence of metastatic disease
- Organic acidemia or urea cycle defect (after being listed for 30 days with PELD score of 30 without offers)
- Chronic liver disease with a calculated PELD or MELD score greater than 25 and at least one of the following criteria: mechanical ventilator, gastrointestinal bleeding requiring greater than 30 mL/kg of red blood cell transfusion within previous 24 hours, dialysis, or Glasgow coma score less than 10 within 48 hours

The PELD scoring system was implemented in 2002 and was developed to provide a numerical assessment of the risk of death in patients younger than 12 years and includes age, INR, albumin, total bilirubin, and the presence or absence of growth failure. However, the PELD score has been criticized for ineffectively predicting mortality of children on the liver transplant wait list.[9] Other scores, such as the pCLIF-SOFA scores, have been recommended as better prognosticators of 28-day mortality.[10] The MELD score is used for children who are 12 years of age and older and includes creatinine, bilirubin, INR, sodium, and absence or presence of dialysis. Candidates meeting specific standardized MELD/PELD exceptions can be found on the OPTN Web site and include patients with cardiac failure (CF), hepatocellular carcinoma, cholangiocarcinoma, hepatopulmonary syndrome, portopulmonary hypertension, and hyperoxaluria. As both calculated PELD and MELD often do not reflect the risk of mortality on the wait list, nonstandard exceptions appeals are requested in 44% of children awaiting liver transplant. The proportion of pediatric candidates with exception scores on the waitlist increased from 13.9% in 2009 to 27.6% in 2019 (SRTR). Common reasons for appeal include severe failure to thrive with requirement of parenteral nutrition, intractable ascites despite maximal doses of intravenous diuretic therapy, pathologic bone fractures, refractory pruritus, and hemorrhage due to complications associated with portal hypertension. For children aged 2 to 18 years at listing, exception denials increased the risk of waitlist and post-LT mortality.[11] In May 2019, the National Liver Review Board was established with a specific pediatric committee to address widespread regional variations in exception acceptance and disparity in use of exception scoring.[12]

Once an organ becomes available, the allocation priority is based on the pediatric versus adult recipient, age of donor, geographic location of the donor and recipient (within acuity circles), and recipient–donor blood type match (identical vs compatible). There is a difference in pediatric organ allocation policies across the world. Some countries such as Brazil triple the calculated PELD score to prioritize children. In the United States, 20 to 30 children die on the wait list every year, of which close to 50% received no offers. Pediatric prioritization in the allocation of organs with development of improved risk stratification systems continues to be a focus to reduce waitlist mortality among children.[13]

LIVER TRANSPLANT EVALUATION

Referral for consideration of LT depends on the child's clinical circumstances: emergent, such as acute liver failure or acute decompensation; urgent, such as progressive liver disease; or anticipatory, such as hepatoblastoma and other tumors. In some metabolic diseases, early referral may offer the benefit of avoiding multisystemic complications and irreversible organ damage.[14] The primary goal of the evaluation process is to identify appropriate candidates for LT and establish a peritransplantation plan. Children are different from adults and as such, have distinct diseases, clinical susceptibilities, physiologic responses, as well as unique neurocognitive and neurodevelopmental features. Optimal care of pediatric liver transplant patients requires a multidisciplinary team. Members of this team include transplant surgeons, hepatologist/gastroenterologists with expertise in pediatric liver disease, transplant coordinators, social workers, dieticians, transplant pharmacists, anesthesiologists, and financial counselors. In select patients, other members are necessary, including infectious disease specialists, transplant immunologists, critical care specialists, psychologist/neuropsychologist/child development specialists, psychiatrists, child life specialists, cardiologists, nephrologists, neurologists, genetic/metabolic specialists, oncologists, pulmonologists, radiologists (diagnostic or interventional), dentists, and ethics specialists.

The purpose of the evaluation process is to confirm the indication for transplantation, discuss alternative treatments, exclude contraindications, and optimize pretransplant medical therapy. Completion of all age-appropriate vaccinations, for the child and family members, should occur before transplantation on an accelerated schedule. Inactivated influenza vaccination should be given to patients and their family members. Nutritional status has been proved to be linked to outcomes in pediatric LT, with aggressive nutritional support for children with failure to thrive pretransplant. Nasogastric tube feedings and parenteral nutrition may be needed in some circumstances.[15,16] Neurocognitive testing is suggested in children awaiting LT to identify areas warranting early intervention to minimize later cognitive difficulties. Renal function should also be screened during the evaluation for liver transplant. Serum creatinine alone should not be used to assess renal function; either cystatin C or the revised Schwartz Formula should be used to estimate the glomerular filtration rate in children with chronic liver disease.[14] Required imaging studies for a comprehensive evaluation include chest radiograph, ultrasound of the liver with Doppler study, electrocardiogram, and echocardiogram. Transplant surgeons often request cross-sectional imaging of the abdomen for surgical planning. In children with hepatic tumors, chest or other body imaging should be considered. Obtaining informed consent from parents includes discussing indication, contraindications, alternative for transplant, organ availability and option of living donors, increased risk donors, right to refuse transplant, and posttransplant complications. Case managers and social workers should work closely with families to establish a plan of action for when an organ becomes available. Other important components include obtaining prior records, assessing disease severity and urgency/timing of LT, and consideration of live donors. It is vital during the evaluation stage that effort is made to develop a strong and trusting therapeutic relationship between the child, family, and transplant team.

Elements of liver transplant evaluation are specific to the underlying disease process. For example, with Alagille syndrome, there is a risk for cerebral vascular malformations and as such, brain imaging should be considered.[17] Children with portal hypertension and end-stage liver disease are at risk for development of hepatopulmonary syndrome and portopulmonary hypertension, in which oxygen saturations and/or heart catheterization should be performed, as these patients are prioritized on the wait list. In patients with CF, pulmonary function tests, including forced expiratory volume in 1 second and forced vital capacity, should be performed.[14] In some cases, multiorgan transplant should be considered.

SURGICAL TECHNIQUES AND VARIANT TRANSPLANTS

Children younger than 1 year (29.9%) and 1 to 5 years (29.9%) account for the largest number of candidates on the wait list for liver transplant (SRTR). The number of pediatric candidates exceeds the number of small-sized pediatric donors of similar weight. As a result, pretransplant mortality is highest for candidates younger than 1 year on the waitlist.[18,19] Because of scarcity of donors and better size matching between graft and recipients, most of the pediatric LTs in recent practice consist of variant techniques instead of whole LTs. The first variant techniques for LT consisted of graft reduction of cadaveric livers, which aimed to improve size matching. Early data from large series show that life expectancy of children who receive a reduced graft including living related donor and split grafts, have the added benefit of increasing the donor pool.[20] These techniques require precise knowledge of the internal anatomy of the liver, which is divided into lobes and segments that have their own separated vascular and biliary network. The split technique allows a cadaveric liver to be divided into 2 functional segments, thus increasing the total number of organs available for transplant. The larger right lobe is typically transplanted into an adult recipient and the left lateral segment or left lobe transplanted into a child.[21] The first split was made in 1988 by Pichlmayr and colleagues,[22,23] with early reports showing inferior patient and graft survival rates compared with conventional transplants. However, progressive technical improvements have led to results such as those of standard transplantations.[24] In living donor LT, the donor undergoes removal of the left lateral segment, which represents between 15% and 20% of the total liver mass, or the full left lobe, which represents 30% to 35%, depending on the weight of the potential recipient.

The remaining liver mass quickly regenerates without functional sequelae.[25–31] The first successful living related donor transplant (LRDT) was performed in 1989 by Strong in Brisbane. Multiple studies have shown that long-term outcomes are comparable between LRDT and cadaveric hepatic transplantation.[32–34]

More recent meta-analysis suggests that now technical variant grafts are comparable with whole liver grafts in terms of outcomes with no significant difference in 5-year graft survival rate between the 2 groups. The incidence of portal vein thrombosis and biliary complications were significantly lower in the whole LT group, whereas the incidence of HAT was comparable between the 2 groups.[35] Because variant techniques are essential to increase the donor pool in pediatric LT, continued focus on improving outcomes in split and living donor transplantation is necessary.

Regarding postoperative complications, biliary complications are the most frequent (14%–15%) with hepatic artery thrombosis, portal vein thrombosis, and suprahepatic stenosis much less common. Vascular complications are more frequent in younger children due to the small size of the vessels.[34] With living donor transplantation, there is a potential risk of mortality and morbidity to the donor, especially in cases of left lateral segment donation or full left hepatectomy.[32]

MEDICATIONS

Controlling host cellular responses while minimizing infection are key in reducing morbidity and mortality associated with LT. Success in pediatric solid organ transplantation has resulted in large part from improved prevention and control of T-cell–mediated acute rejection episodes. The incidence of acute cellular rejection and chronic rejection in pediatric LTs has been reported to be as high as 49.7% and 9%, respectively.[2] The use of increasingly potent T-cell–directed immunosuppressants has led to a reduction in graft loss from acute cellular rejection.[36]

Most immunosuppression protocols from pediatric LT programs include tacrolimus (calcineurin inhibitor) corticosteroids, mycophenolate mofetil (MMF), and sirolimus (mTOR inhibitor). Typically, patients are placed on 2 or more immunosuppressants postoperatively as induction, with most centers using a combination of tacrolimus, mycophenolate mofetil, and steroids or tacrolimus and steroids. Tacrolimus (Prograf) has become the preferred calcineurin inhibitor due to reduction in steroid-resistant acute rejection, improved graft survival, and reduced rates of nephrotoxicity compared with cyclosporine. Drug levels and dosing must be monitored closely with all immunosuppressants. Dosages and target therapeutic drug levels vary depending on the time since transplantation, history of rejection episodes, and side effects and should be personalized to the individual patient. Some children may require more immunosuppression and some may require intentional dose reduction (ie, after Epstein-Barr virus seroconversion). Care must be taken in balancing risk of overimmunosuppression (nephrotoxicity, infection, PTLD, and so forth) and underimmunosuppression (rejection).

Commonly used immunosuppressive agents, dosing, side effects, and administration considerations in pediatric LT are outlined in **Table 2**.[37]

OUTCOMES AND COMPLICATIONS

According to recent US Organ Procurement and Transplantation Network and Studies in Pediatric Liver Transplantation (SPLIT), patient survival rates at 1 and 5 years after a pediatric LT are now 91% to 91.4% and 84% to 86.5%.[2,38,39]

Large pediatric series have shown better survival rates in patients with less than 25 PELD points, the graft weight to body weight ratios (GWBWR) less than 3%, and

Table 2
Commonly used immunosuppressive agents, dosing, and side effects in pediatric liver transplantation

Medication	Dose	Side Effects
Tacrolimus	0.15–0.2 mg/kg/d po divided q12 h	Alopecia, pruritus, photosensitivity, constipation, diarrhea, nausea, vomiting, anemia, leukocytosis, thrombocytopenia, headache, insomnia, paresthesia, tremor, seizure, leukoencephalopathy (rare), nephrotoxicity, hypertension, cardiomyopathy, prolonged QT interval, diabetes mellitus, hypercholesterolemia, lymphoproliferative disease, hypomagnesaemia, hyperkalemia, hypophosphatemia
Cyclosporine	15 mg/kg/d po divided q12 h for 2 wk posttransplant, then 4–12 mg/kg/d po divided bid	Nephrotoxicity, hypertension, edema, arrhythmia, hirsutism, gingival hyperplasia, gynecomastia, diarrhea, leukopenia, hypomagnesaemia, hyperkalemia, hyperuricemia hyperglycemia, hyperlipidemia, tremor, paresthesia, leg cramps, weakness, encephalopathy, progressive multifocal leukoencephalopathy, seizure
Sirolimus	Loading dose: 3 mg/m^2 on day 1 Maintenance dose: 1 mg/m^2/d divided q12 h or given daily	Hyperlipidemia, proteinuria, myelosuppression, pneumonitis, hypersensitivity reactions, hepatic artery thrombosis, poor wound healing, mouth ulcers, acne, edema, anemia, thrombocytopenia, arthralgia, headache, increased serum creatinine, fever, pain, progressive multifocal leukoencephalopathy

(continued on next page)

Table 2 (continued)		
Medication	**Dose**	**Side Effects**
Mycophenolate	10–15 mg/kg/dose po BID mofetil (max 1 g/dose)	Diarrhea, abdominal pain, constipation, nausea, teratogenic, neutropenia, anemia, thrombocytopenia, constipation, nausea, hypertension, edema, opportunistic infections, hyperglycemia, hypocalcemia, hypokalemia, hypomagnesaemia, hypercholesterolemia, pleural effusion, lymphoma, progressive multifocal leukoencephalopathy
Corticosteroids	Induction with high-dose methylprednisolone IV 20 mg/kg/dose (max 1 g) Taper over 5 d to maintenance prednisone or prednisolone (approximately 0.2–0.3 mg/kg/dose po daily)	Hypertension, impaired wound healing, gastrointestinal ulcers, diabetes mellitus, fluid retention, adrenal insufficiency, depression, mood swings, insomnia, cataracts, weight gain, osteopenia, pancreatitis, cosmetic (acne, Cushing, striae), decreased growth
Basiliximab	Wt <35 kg: 10 mg IV × 2 Wt ≤35 kg: 20 mg IV × 2 First dose given within 2 h of transplant, second dose on day 4	Hypersensitivity reaction, abdominal pain, vomiting, asthenia, dizziness, insomnia, edema, hypertension, anemia, dysuria, cough, dyspnea, fever
Antithymocyte globulin (rabbit)	1.5 mg/kg/d administered by IV infusion for 7–14 d	Cytokine-release storm, serum sickness, thrombocytopenia, leukopenia, neutropenia, hypertension, peripheral edema, posttransplant, lymphoproliferative disease, hyperkalemia

From Miloh T, Barton A, Wheeler J, et al. Immunosuppression in pediatric liver transplant recipients: unique aspects. Liver Transpl 2017;23(2):244–56; with permission.

recipient weight more than 7 kg. HAT remains a significant cause of graft loss after an LT in children, with incidence ranging from 5.7% to 8.4%.[40] Microsurgical techniques with an operational microscope have been used in hepatic arterial anastomosis reconstruction to lower the risk of HAT.[41]

Portal vein thrombosis, another significant complication in pediatric LT, reportedly affects approximately 5% to 10% of pediatric recipients. In children with portal hypertension, the diameter of the portal vein tends to decrease because of reduced flow and in children with biliary atresia, the inflammation can extend to the portal vein.[42,43] Optimizing the GWBWR and technical skills to avoid redundancy, kinking, or stretching of the portal vein can help to prevent portal vein thrombosis. Doppler ultrasound is routinely performed after reperfusion to ensure vascular flow in the hepatic artery before closing the abdomen.

The SPLIT group reported the overall incidence of early biliary complications were more frequent in segmental LTs (21.8%) than in whole LTs (5.8%).[40] Kanmaz and colleagues recommend Roux-en-Y hepaticojejunostomy as the first choice for left lateral segment LT.

SPLIT registry data indicate that infection contributed to mortality in nearly half of all patients (46%), typically through multisystem organ failure or cardiopulmonary failure. Malignancy accounted for an additional 5.1% of posttransplant mortality. Rejection contributed directly or indirectly, by necessitating retransplantation in 4.7%. Infants were at highest risk to develop infection and at lowest risk to experience rejection.

Sepsis/infection, multisystem organ failure, and PTLD, as complications of immunosuppression, accounted for 41% of late deaths in pediatric LT. Chronic rejection accounted for rare deaths but was the dominant cause, along with acute rejection, for graft loss, accounting for half of the cases.[39,40] The morbidity from PTLD was reduced by early detection of EBV infection, decreasing the dosage of immunosuppressive medication and continuing intravenous ganciclovir.

LONG-TERM MANAGEMENT

As more and more recipients enter adulthood, more attention is paid to the potential harm of chronic immunosuppressive therapy itself, with side effects including renal insufficiency, cardiovascular disease, diabetes mellitus, PTLD, and osteopenia. Opportunistic infection and PTLD account for 30% of late mortality in pediatric LT recipients.[39,44,45]

As a result of the concern for potential side-effect morbidities, there is an increase in interest in immunosuppression minimization and withdrawal. It is estimated that 20% to 25% of pediatric LT recipients will be operationally tolerant without immunosuppression.[46,47]

Abnormal liver enzymes are common among long-term pediatric LT survivors, with up to one-third with abnormal transaminases and almost half with abnormal gamma-glutamyltransferase 5 years post-LT.[48] Furthermore, chronic hepatitis, liver fibrosis, or both have been described in 40% to 50% of otherwise asymptomatic 5-year survivors with normal liver function tests, supporting the need for protocol biopsies and further investigation.[3,49–52]

ADHERENCE AND TRANSITION

The long-term outcomes after LT strongly depend on adherence to lifelong immunosuppression and close medical follow-up. The most common cause of late graft loss is chronic and late rejection.[39] Nonadherence is estimated to occur in 35% to 50% of adolescents and is the most common cause of late acute rejection in children who receive an LT.[53] Nonadherence is associated with graft loss, increased expenditures on care, and ultimately death.[54,55] As children get older, the medication intake responsibility shifts from caregiver (usually parent) to child. By 9 years of age, 30% of children are expected to be responsible for taking their medication, which is a vulnerable time for nonadherence.[53] Pediatric LT recipients' medical and psychosocial needs change over time as they transition from childhood to adolescence and early adulthood.[56,57]

Nonadherence can be challenging to identify. Subjective methods, such as patient reports, are unreliable, and pill counts, refills, and electronic monitoring impose additional burden on the patient. It is crucial to identify high-risk populations, improve detection methods, and intervene early. A 2004 study showed the most reported barrier to adherence in children is forgetfulness and vomiting (70%), followed by bad taste and interruptions in routine (60%), anxiety, depression, and posttraumatic stress disorder.[58] A systematic review of immunosuppressant adherence interventions in transplant recipients revealed only a few successful interventions, including counseling, increased clinic visits, mobile devices with automated reminders, and telemonitoring.[59] It is important to address adolescent psychosocial health issues with the patients and their families and provide counseling on smoking, illicit drug use, alcohol use, birth control, and sexually transmitted disease. Female LT patients who are of childbearing age on MMF should use methods of birth control due to the known teratogenicity of this immunosuppressive agent. Adolescents may lose insurance coverage into adulthood, which may restrict care. The medication regimen should be as clear and simple as possible. Addressing these topics early and repeatedly is important in improving adherence and thereby maximizing long-term outcome.

As patients mature into young adulthood, a process of transition has to take place to allow safe and effective transfer of care from a pediatric facility to the care of adult providers. In the absence of a transfer process, patients may experience anxiety, confusion, distress, inability to manage the requirements of the new setting, increased risk of nonadherence, rejection, and even mortality.[60] There are various potential barriers to transitioning and ultimately transferring care. These barriers arise at the level of the patient, parent/family, and the pediatric and adult provider. In adult settings, patients are expected to display behaviors consistent with self-management for instance, independently discussing one's illness and concerns with the treatment team, scheduling and attending appointments, and so on. However, when patients endorse more responsibility for their care too early, clinical outcomes are worse, indicating that indiscriminate promotion of self-management by adolescents may not be advisable.[61] Assessment of adolescent executive function skills may help guide the development of individualized transition readiness guidelines to promote successful gains in self-management abilities as well as eventual transfer to adult medical services. There are a few transition readiness questionnaires available, such as The Readiness for Transition Questionnaire, and the process can start as early as 11 to 12 years of age.[62] A 2014 technical review by the Agency for Healthcare Research and Quality emphasized the importance of transition programs, transition coordinator, a special clinic for young adults in transition, and provision of educational materials.[63] A multidisciplinary approach aiming at fostering adherence should be used. Parents should be supported to move from a "managerial" to a "supervisory" role during transition to help young people engage independently with the health care team.

CLINICS CARE POINTS

- Pediatric liver transplantation is a successful intervention for many pediatric liver diseases.
- It is important to know the indications and contraindications for pediatric liver transplant.
- While pediatric liver transplant is lifesaving, it requires a specialized team and routine lifelong monitoring.

DISCLOSURE

Neither author has any direct financial interest in subject matter or materials discussed in article or with a company making a competing product.

REFERENCES

1. Mogul DB, Luo X, Bowring MG, et al. Fifteen-year trends in pediatric liver transplants: split, whole deceased, and living donor grafts. J Pediatr 2018;196: 148–53.e2.
2. Ng VL, Alonso EM, Bucuvalas JC, et al. Health status of children alive 10 years after pediatric liver transplantation performed in the US and Canada: report of the studies of pediatric liver transplantation experience. J Pediatr 2012;160(5): 820–6.e3.
3. Scheenstra R, Peeters PM, Verkade HJ, et al. Graft fibrosis after pediatric liver transplantation: ten years of follow-up. Hepatology 2009;49(3):880–6.
4. Shneider BL, Brown MB, Haber B, et al. A multicenter study of the outcome of biliary atresia in the United States, 1997 to 2000. J Pediatr 2006;148(4):467–74.
5. Nandivada P, Fell GL, Gura KM, et al. Lipid emulsions in the treatment and prevention of parenteral nutrition-associated liver disease in infants and children. Am J Clin Nutr 2016;103(2):629S–34S.
6. Mazariegos G, Shneider B, Burton B, et al. Liver transplantation for pediatric metabolic disease. Mol Genet Metab 2014;111(4):418–27.
7. Alkhouri N, Hanouneh IA, Zein NN, et al. Liver transplantation for nonalcoholic steatohepatitis in young patients. Transpl Int 2016;29(4):418–24.
8. Amir AZ, Ling SC, Naqvi A, et al. Liver transplantation for children with acute liver failure associated with secondary hemophagocytic lymphohistiocytosis. Liver Transpl 2016;22(9):1245–53.
9. Shneider BL, Neimark E, Frankenberg T, et al. Critical analysis of the pediatric end-stage liver disease scoring system: a single center experience. Liver Transpl 2005;11(7):788–95.
10. Bolia R, Srivastava A, Yachha SK, et al. Pediatric CLIF-SOFA score is the best predictor of 28-day mortality in children with decompensated chronic liver disease. J Hepatol 2018;68(3):449–55.
11. Braun HJ, Perito ER, Dodge JL, et al. Nonstandard exception requests impact outcomes for pediatric liver transplant candidates. Am J Transplant 2016; 16(11):3181–91.
12. Hsu EK, Shaffer M, Bradford M, et al. Heterogeneity and disparities in the use of exception scores in pediatric liver allocation. Am J Transplant 2015;15(2):436–44.
13. Hsu EK, Shaffer ML, Gao L, et al. Analysis of liver offers to pediatric candidates on the transplant wait list. Gastroenterology 2017;153(4):988–95.
14. Squires RH, Ng V, Romero R, et al. Evaluation of the pediatric patient for liver transplantation: 2014 practice guideline by the American Association for the Study of Liver Diseases, American Society of Transplantation and the North American Society for Pediatric Gastroenterology, Hepatology and Nutrition. Hepatology 2014;60(1):362–98.
15. Carter-Kent C, Radhakrishnan K, Feldstein AE. Increasing calories, decreasing morbidity and mortality: is improved nutrition the answer to better outcomes in patients with biliary atresia? Hepatology 2007;46(5):1329–31.
16. Carpenter CD, Linscott LL, Leach JL, et al. Spectrum of cerebral arterial and venous abnormalities in Alagille syndrome. Pediatr Radiol 2018;48(4):602–8.

17. Squires JE. Protecting the allograft following liver transplantation for PFIC1. Pediatr Transplant 2016;20(7):882–3.
18. Busuttil RW, Colonna JO 2nd, Hiatt JR, et al. The first 100 liver transplants at UCLA. Ann Surg 1987;206(4):387–402.
19. Otte JB, de Ville de Goyet J, Reding R, et al. Pediatric liver transplantation: from the full-size liver graft to reduced, split, and living related liver transplantation. Pediatr Surg Int 1998;13(5–6):308–18.
20. Otte JB, de Ville de Goyet J, Sokal E, et al. Size reduction of the donor liver is a safe way to alleviate the shortage of size-matched organs in pediatric liver transplantation. Ann Surg 1990;211(2):146–57.
21. Otte JB, de Ville de Goyet J, Alberti D, et al. The concept and technique of the split liver in clinical transplantation. Surgery 1990;107(6):605–12.
22. Pichlmayr R, Ringe B, Gubernatis G, et al. Transplantation of a donor liver to 2 recipients (splitting transplantation)–a new method in the further development of segmental liver transplantation. Langenbecks Arch Chir 1988;373(2):127–30 [in German].
23. Broelsch CE, Emond JC, Whitington PF, et al. Application of reduced-size liver transplants as split grafts, auxiliary orthotopic grafts, and living related segmental transplants. Ann Surg 1990;212(3):368–75 [discussion: 375–7].
24. Rogiers X, Malago M, Gawad K, et al. In situ splitting of cadaveric livers. The ultimate expansion of a limited donor pool. Ann Surg 1996;224(3):331–9 [discussion: 339–41].
25. Iwatsuki S, Shaw BW Jr, Starzl TE. Experience with 150 liver resections. Ann Surg 1983;197(3):247–53.
26. Nagao T, Inoue S, Mizuta T, et al. One hundred hepatic resections. Indications and operative results. Ann Surg 1985;202(1):42–9.
27. Raia S, Nery JR, Mies S. Liver transplantation from live donors. Lancet 1989; 2(8661):497.
28. Singer PA, Siegler M, Lantos JD, et al. The ethical assessment of innovative therapies: liver transplantation using living donors. Theor Med 1990;11(2):87–94.
29. Strong RW, Lynch SV, Ong TH, et al. Successful liver transplantation from a living donor to her son. N Engl J Med 1990;322(21):1505–7.
30. Kiuchi T, Inomata Y, Uemoto S, et al. Living-donor liver transplantation in Kyoto, 1997. Clin Transplant 1997;191–8.
31. Tanaka K, Ogura Y, Kiuchi T, et al. Living donor liver transplantation: Eastern experiences. HPB (Oxford) 2004;6(2):88–94.
32. Burgos L, Hernández F, Barrena S, et al. Variant techniques for liver transplantation in pediatric programs. Eur J Pediatr Surg 2008;18(6):372–4.
33. Otte JB. Paediatric liver transplantation–a review based on 20 years of personal experience. Transpl Int 2004;17(10):562–73.
34. Tanaka K, Uemoto S, Tokunaga Y, et al. Surgical techniques and innovations in living related liver transplantation. Ann Surg 1993;217(1):82–91.
35. Ye H, Zhao Q, Wang Y, et al. Outcomes of technical variant liver transplantation versus whole liver transplantation for pediatric patients: a meta-analysis. PLoS One 2015;10(9):e0138202.
36. Meier-Kriesche HU, Schold JD, Kaplan B. Long-term renal allograft survival: have we made significant progress or is it time to rethink our analytic and therapeutic strategies? Am J Transplant 2004;4(8):1289–95.
37. Miloh T, Barton A, Wheeler J, et al. Immunosuppression in pediatric liver transplant recipients: unique aspects. Liver Transpl 2017;23(2):244–56.

38. McDiarmid SV, Anand R, Martz K, et al. A multivariate analysis of pre-, peri-, and post-transplant factors affecting outcome after pediatric liver transplantation. Ann Surg 2011;254(1):145–54.

39. Soltys KA, Mazariegos GV, Squires RH, et al. Late graft loss or death in pediatric liver transplantation: an analysis of the SPLIT database. Am J Transplant 2007; 7(9):2165–71.

40. Diamond IR, Fecteau A, Millis JM, et al. Impact of graft type on outcome in pediatric liver transplantation: a report from Studies of Pediatric Liver Transplantation (SPLIT). Ann Surg 2007;246(2):301–10.

41. Kanmaz T, Yankol Y, Mecit N, et al. Pediatric liver transplant: a single-center study of 100 consecutive patients. Exp Clin Transplant 2014;12(1):41–5.

42. Takahashi Y, Nishimoto Y, Matsuura T, et al. Surgical complications after living donor liver transplantation in patients with biliary atresia: a relatively high incidence of portal vein complications. Pediatr Surg Int 2009;25(9):745–51.

43. Venick RS, Farmer DG, Soto JR, et al. One thousand pediatric liver transplants during thirty years: lessons learned. J Am Coll Surg 2018;226(4):355–66.

44. Mohammad S, Hormaza L, Neighbors K, et al. Health status in young adults two decades after pediatric liver transplantation. Am J Transplant 2012;12(6): 1486–95.

45. Duffy JP, Kao K, Ko CY, et al. Long-term patient outcome and quality of life after liver transplantation: analysis of 20-year survivors. Ann Surg 2010;252(4):652–61.

46. Feng S, Ekong UD, Lobritto SJ, et al. Complete immunosuppression withdrawal and subsequent allograft function among pediatric recipients of parental living donor liver transplants. JAMA 2012;307(3):283–93.

47. Porrett P, Shaked A. The failure of immunosuppression withdrawal: patient benefit is not detectable, inducible, or reproducible. Liver Transpl 2011;17(Suppl 3): S66–8.

48. Ng VL, Fecteau A, Shepherd R, et al. Outcomes of 5-year survivors of pediatric liver transplantation: report on 461 children from a North American multicenter registry. Pediatrics 2008;122(6):e1128–35.

49. Ekong UD, Melin-Aldana H, Seshadri R, et al. Graft histology characteristics in long-term survivors of pediatric liver transplantation. Liver Transpl 2008;14(11): 1582–7.

50. Evans HM, Kelly DA, McKiernan PJ, et al. Progressive histological damage in liver allografts following pediatric liver transplantation. Hepatology 2006;43(5): 1109–17.

51. Fouquet V, Alves A, Branchereau S, et al. Long-term outcome of pediatric liver transplantation for biliary atresia: a 10-year follow-up in a single center. Liver Transpl 2005;11(2):152–60.

52. Herzog D, Soglio DB, Fournet JC, et al. Interface hepatitis is associated with a high incidence of late graft fibrosis in a group of tightly monitored pediatric orthotopic liver transplantation patients. Liver Transpl 2008;14(7):946–55.

53. McDiarmid SV. Adolescence: challenges and responses. Liver Transpl 2013; 19(Suppl 2):S35–9.

54. Fredericks EM, Lopez MJ, Magee JC, et al. Psychological functioning, nonadherence and health outcomes after pediatric liver transplantation. Am J Transplant 2007;7(8):1974–83.

55. Shemesh E, Shneider BL, Savitzky JK, et al. Medication adherence in pediatric and adolescent liver transplant recipients. Pediatrics 2004;113(4):825–32.

56. Alonso EM, Neighbors K, Barton FB, et al. Health-related quality of life and family function following pediatric liver transplantation. Liver Transpl 2008;14(4):460–8.

57. Shemesh E, Bucuvalas JC, Anand R, et al. The medication level variability index (MLVI) predicts poor liver transplant outcomes: a prospective multi-site study. Am J Transplant 2017;17(10):2668–78.
58. Shemesh E. Non-adherence to medications following pediatric liver transplantation. Pediatr Transplant 2004;8(6):600–5.
59. Duncan S, Annunziato RA, Dunphy C, et al. A systematic review of immunosuppressant adherence interventions in transplant recipients: decoding the streetlight effect. Pediatr Transplant 2018;22(1). https://doi.org/10.1111/petr.13086.
60. Annunziato RA, Emre S, Shneider B, et al. Adherence and medical outcomes in pediatric liver transplant recipients who transition to adult services. Pediatr Transplant 2007;11(6):608–14.
61. Annunziato RA, Bucuvalas JC, Yin W, et al. Self-management measurement and prediction of clinical outcomes in pediatric transplant. J Pediatr 2018;193:128–33.e2.
62. Fredericks EM. Transition readiness assessment: the importance of the adolescent perspective. Pediatr Transplant 2017;21(3). https://doi.org/10.1111/petr.12921.
63. Davis AM, Brown RF, Taylor JL, et al. Transition care for children with special health care needs. Pediatrics 2014;134(5):900–8.

Fat Soluble Vitamin Assessment and Supplementation in Cholestasis

Binita M. Kamath, MBBChir, MRCP, MTR[a,b,]*, Estella M. Alonso, MD[c],
James E. Heubi, MD[d], Saul J. Karpen, MD, PhD[e],
Shikha S. Sundaram, MD, MSCI[f], Benjamin L. Shneider, MD[g],
Ronald J. Sokol, MD[h]

KEYWORDS

- Nutrition • Liver • Children • Biliary atresia

KEY POINTS

- Fat soluble vitamin (FSV) deficiencies are an integral feature of cholestatic children.
- Surveillance for FSV deficiency in a cholestatic infant is required as soon as cholestasis is established and should continue on a monthly basis.
- The use of a multivitamin preparation specifically designed for cholestasis (eg, DEKAs Essential liquid) is, in the authors' experience, the preferred supplementation strategy.

---

[a] Division of Gastroenterology, Hepatology and Nutrition, The Hospital for Sick Children, 555 University Avenue, Toronto, Ontario M5G 1X8, Canada; [b] University of Toronto, Canada; [c] Division of Gastroenterology, Hepatology and Nutrition, Siragusa Transplant Center, Ann & Robert H. Lurie Children's Hospital of Chicago, Northwestern University Feinberg School of Medicine, 225 East Chicago Avenue Box 57, Chicago, IL 60611, USA; [d] Division of Gastroenterology, Hepatology and Nutrition, Center for Clinical and Translational Science and Training, University of Cincinnati/Cincinnati Children's Hospital Medical Center, 3333 Burnet Avenue, Cincinnati, OH 45229-3039, USA; [e] Pediatric Gastroenterology, Hepatology and Nutrition, Emory University School of Medicine, Children's Healthcare of Atlanta, 1760 Haygood Drive Northeast, HSRB E204, Atlanta, GA 30322, USA; [f] Pediatric Liver Transplant Program, Section of Pediatric Gastroenterology, Hepatology and Nutrition, The Digestive Health Institute, University of Colorado School of Medicine, Children's Hospital Colorado, Box B290, 13123 East 16th Avenue, Aurora, CO 80045, USA; [g] Gastroenterology, Hepatology and Nutrition, Baylor College of Medicine, Texas Children's Hospital; [h] Section of Pediatric Gastroenterology, Hepatology and Nutrition, Colorado Clinical and Translational Sciences Institute, University of Colorado Denver, University of Colorado School of Medicine, Children's Hospital Colorado, Box B290, 13123 East 16th Avenue, Aurora, CO 80045, USA
* Corresponding author.
E-mail address: binita.kamath@sickkids.ca
Twitter: @BinitaKamath (B.M.K.)

Clin Liver Dis 26 (2022) 537–553
https://doi.org/10.1016/j.cld.2022.03.011
1089-3261/22/© 2022 Elsevier Inc. All rights reserved.

liver.theclinics.com

INTRODUCTION

Malnutrition in children with chronic cholestasis is a prevalent issue and a major risk factor for adverse outcomes. In a large study of 755 children with biliary atresia (BA) listed for liver transplantation, 30% of the overall deaths occurred in children waiting for LT.[1] Growth failure was found to be an independent risk factor for pre-transplant mortality, post-transplant mortality, and graft failure in this cohort. Fat soluble vitamin (FSV) deficiency is an integral feature of cholestatic disease in children, often occurring within the first months of life in those with neonatal cholestasis. Even in specialized care centers, FSV deficiency frequently occurs and persists in children with chronic cholestasis. In a prospective multicenter study of 92 infants with BA, FSV deficiency was common at all assessed time points for all vitamins.[2] In this study, infants were receiving AquADEKs and supplemental vitamin K three times per week and this was inadequate for most infants, especially for those with a total serum bilirubin >2 mg/dL. Thus, there is an unmet need for optimizing the approach to FSV supplementation in cholestasis. A "one size fits all" algorithm does not work as important factors such as cost to families and availability of various FSV preparations at different centers require consideration. This review focuses on FSVs in cholestasis with particular emphasis on a practical approach to surveillance and supplementation that includes options taking into account local resources. In this review the term deficiency will refer to biochemical deficiency, meaning below the recommended serum level for a particular vitamin. The overarching strategy suggested is to closely monitor and aggressively replete FSV in infants and children with cholestasis in order to avoid long periods of inadequate levels and clinical sequalae.

VITAMIN A
Metabolism

Vitamin A (also generally referred to as retinol) is an essential nutrient as it cannot be synthesized by humans. It is available in various precursor dietary sources and is metabolized to biologically active molecules like retinaldehyde (critical for rhodopsin and vision) and retinoic acid (with a myriad of potential targets for transcriptional regulation). As a fat-soluble molecule, vitamin A, must be micellized by bile acids in the intestine to permit passage through the unstirred water layer at the brush border of enterocytes. Retinol can be taken up directly at the intestinal brush border, while retinyl esters must be hydrolyzed by brush border or pancreatic enzymes prior to absorption of the esterified retinol by enterocytes (**Fig. 1**). Vitamin A is also released by enterocyte cleavage of absorbed dietary beta-carotene. Once within the enterocyte, retinol associates with retinol binding protein-2, is re-esterified, and then packaged into chylomicrons which can be secreted into the intestinal lymphatic system. Chylomicrons containing vitamin A are processed with the inclusion of apolipoprotein E, which facilitates uptake by hepatocytes. The liver clears about 70% of chylomicron-based vitamin A, while the rest may be stored in peripheral tissues. In the liver, endosomal processes extract retinol from chylomicron remnants, permitting retinol association with retinol binding protein 4 (RBP4). Hepatocyte based retinol is then transferred to stellate cells for storage via mechanisms that are not well understood. A substantial amount of stored vitamin A in the liver is found within stellate cells. The exact mechanisms by which vitamin A needs are "sensed" leading to release of vitamin A by stellate cells are also not well understood nor the relevance of peripheral stores of vitamin A.[3]

Effects of Deficiency

Worldwide, vitamin A deficiency is a leading cause of blindness. Hemeralopia, or reduced visual acuity in bright lights, may be the first sign of deficiency. With

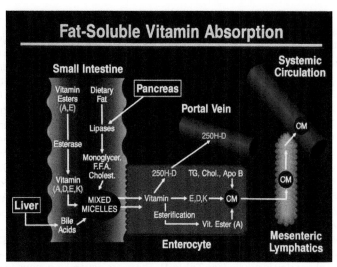

Fig. 1. Pathways of Fat-soluble vitamin absorption. 25OH-D, 25-hydroxyvitamin D; Apo B, apolipoprotein B; chol, cholesterol; CM, chylomicrons; FFA, free fatty acids; monoglycer, monoglycerides; TG, triglycerides.

progressive retinol deficiency, the time for regeneration of rhodopsin increases, with delays in the adaptation to darkness and "night blindness".[4,5] A more significant ocular manifestation of vitamin A deficiency is epithelial ocular disease involving the conjunctiva and cornea, xeropthalmia.[6] Patients develop dryness of the conjunctiva, atrophy and even Bitot's spots (white or yellow spots that occur because of bacterial gas production from Corynebacterium). Later, corneal lesions may appear with corneal xerosis, keratomalacia with softening and then deformation and ulceration of the cornea that eventually leads to eye destruction and blindness.[7]

Vitamin A deficiency may also cause follicular keratosis with atrophy of the sebaceous and sweat glands along with dry skin. Retinoids are important for growth and differentiation of several cell types in the skin. This activity is mediated though NR1B and NR2B subgroups of the nuclear receptor superfamily—also known as RARs and RXRs, respectively.[8] These nuclear receptors bind and activate distinct response elements of genes required for differentiation and proliferation of epithelial tissue. Deficiency of vitamin A can lead to delayed skin epithelialization, wound healing and wound closure along with poor collagen synthesis.[9]

Vitamin A also modulates the immune response through RAR and RXR heterodimers.[9] Experimental studies have suggested that retinoic acid, the active vitamin A metabolite, is important for modulation of the immune system, maturation of dendritic cells, and T and B cells in the intestine.[10] Neonatal vitamin A supplementation may enhance the mucosal targeting of T regulatory cells in low birthweight infants.[11]

Evaluation and Monitoring of Vitamin A Status in Cholestasis

Studies in healthy children and adults have demonstrated that serum retinol and RBP should be used to screen for potential vitamin A deficiency and correlate well with liver stores.[12,13] A serum retinol level less than 0.7 umol/L (<20 ug/dL) is considered deficient (**Table 1**). A fasting serum RBP is abnormal if < 1.0 mg/dL.[14] The retinol/RBP molar ratio (retinol [ug/dL]/RBP [mg/dL] X 0.0734) is often used in clinical practice, with abnormal being considered less than 0.8 mol/mol. Both retinol and RBP are influenced by inflammation and concentrations may transiently decrease during an acute phase response.[15] Thus, assessing vitamin A status during an acute infection may lead to inaccurate results. In addition, the serum retinol level can decrease if the RBP is low, as occurs with iron and zinc deficiency.[16,17]

Vitamin A Supplementation

Vitamin A can be derived from both animal and plant-based sources. The liver stores and therefore is rich in vitamin A. Meats such as chicken, duck and veal liver are all excellent sources of vitamin A, as is cod liver oil. Some dairy foods are also high in vitamin A, such as butter, cheese and whole milk. Lower amounts are found in eggs and fish, such as trout and salmon. Plant based foods high in carotenoids, primarily beta-carotene, are also excellent sources of vitamin A. These typically include yellow and orange fruits and vegetables such as yams, pumpkin, carrots, apricots, and dark green leafy vegetables, such as spinach, broccoli, and brussels sprouts.[5]

Vitamin A exists in a number of pharmacologic formulations for oral or intramuscular/intravenous administration. The recommended daily allowance is age dependent increasing from $\sim$ 1000 units (300 μg) of retinol per day in infants to 10,000 units (3000 μg) per day in adults (see **Table 1**). There are several regimens for addressing vitamin A deficiency including large oral or intramuscular doses (eg,100,000 units intramuscular for 3 consecutive days followed by 50,000 units per day for 2 weeks followed by oral therapy, or 200,000 units orally each day for 2 days). A great deal of the experience in treatment of vitamin A deficiency comes from experiences in low-income countries.[18] Vitamin A supplementation regimens have been described for cholestasis associated with biliary atresia[2] and include stepwise increases in oral dosing from 5000 up to 50,000 units (1500 up to 15,000 μg) per day. In severe cholestasis, intramuscular administration may be more effective, although its use is more limited due to decreased acceptance of this approach by patients and physicians. Hepatic toxicity in the form of stellate cell-related fibrosis/cirrhosis is a concern in long-term high dose vitamin A supplementation and argues for continued monitoring of vitamin A levels in patients receiving supplementation.

VITAMIN E
Metabolism

The term vitamin E refers to a group of eight compounds called tocopherols and tocotrienols. Alpha-tocopherol has the highest biologic activity and predominates in foods, except for vegetable oils that contain large amounts of γ-tocopherol. The recommended daily intake of α-tocopherol is 15 mg per day in adults and 4 to 11 mg per day in children.[19] Ingested vitamin E requires solubilization by bile acids into mixed micelles, and if present as a vitamin E ester, hydrolysis by pancreatic or intestinal esterases prior to absorption into enterocytes (see **Fig. 1**). Absorbed α- and γ-tocopherols are then incorporated into chylomicrons and VLDL and are secreted into the mesenteric lymphatics, finally reaching the systemic circulation via the thoracic duct. Vitamin E is primarily transported in blood in LDL and HDL. When chylomicron remnants are taken up by the hepatocyte, the RRR(D-)-stereoisomer of α-tocopherol is preferentially re-secreted within hepatocyte derived VLDL. The hepatic tocopherol transfer protein plays a critical role in the hepatocyte differentiation process by which D-α-tocopherol is preferentially incorporated into lipoproteins and other forms of vitamin E are not. Vitamin E is then delivered to peripheral tissues through hydrolysis of chylomicrons and LDL binding to receptors. In cholestasis, the impaired secretion of bile acids and the resulting insufficient intraluminal bile acid concentrations for micellar

Table 1
Fat soluble vitamin supplementation

Vitamin	Serum Marker	Target Range[a]	Supplementation Doses[b,c]
A	Retinol	>0.7 mmol/L (>20ug/dL)	1000 IU (300 μg)/kg/d <10 kg start at 5000 IU/day >10 kg start at 10,000 IU/day [IM: 50,000 IU]
D	25-OH Vitamin D	20–60 ng/mL (75–150 nmol/L) Toxicity: > 150 ng/mL (>375 nmol/L)	2000 IU/day as cholecalciferol (D3) Increase in 2000 IU per day increments according to level Severe deficiency (<20 ng/mL) consider 50,000 IU po weekly [IM: 50,000–100,000 IU]
E	Alpha-tocopherol	Serum Vitamin E: Total Lipid ratio: > 0.6 mg/gm for < 1 year old >0.8 mg/gm for ≥1 year old	25 IU/kg/d (16.6 mg/kg/d) as TPGS 50–200 IU/kg/d (22.5–90 mg/kg/d) as D-alpha tocopherol [IM 10 mg/kg]
K	INR	≤1.2	>1.2 and ≤1.5 2–5 mg po daily (re-check INR: 7–10 d) >1.5–2.0 5 mg po daily AND consider single dose of 5 mg IM, SQ or IV (10 mg if > 20 kg). If bleeding or bruising, follow recommendations for > 2.0. >2.5 Consider admission for IM or IV Vitamin K dose and or Fresh Frozen Plasma (if bleeding) and expedient follow-up to assess response to therapy[d]

[a] See text for recommended frequency for monitoring of levels.
[b] It is strongly recommended that that individual vitamins are administered orally mixed with a TPGS based solution.
[c] Frequency of IM supplementation based on periodic assessments.
[d] Admission should also be considered for any bruising, bleeding or anemia, regardless of INR.

formation, leads to malabsorption of this, the most hydrophobic of the FSV. Absorption of vitamin E during an oral tolerance test was directly related to intraluminal bile acid concentrations and the extent of steatorrhea.[20] Vitamin E deficiency has been noted in 49% to 77% of children with cholestasis despite routine vitamin supplementation.[19]

Effects of Deficiency

Vitamin E is the predominant fat-soluble antioxidant in the human body. It maintains the structure and function of the developing human nervous system and skeletal muscle; thus vitamin E deficiency primarily affects these systems. Involved regions include the spinocerebellar tracts, cranial nerve nuclei II and IV, large caliber myelinated axons in peripheral nerves, posterior columns of the spinal cord, gracillus and cuneatus nuclei in the brainstem, skeletal muscle, and the ocular retina. Hyporeflexia may occur as early as 6 to 12 months in deficient infants, followed by truncal and limb ataxia, decreased vibratory and position sensation, peripheral neuropathy, ophthalmoplegia, weakness and retinopathy.[21] Cognitive and behavioral alterations have also been described. The CNS lesions may become irreversible if vitamin E deficiency remains prolonged, resulting in debilitating cerebellar ataxia. However, reversal of vitamin E deficiency before ages 3 to 4 years old has been shown to prevent or reverse neuromuscular features of vitamin E deficiency.

Evaluation and Monitoring of Vitamin E Status in Cholestasis

In general, normal serum vitamin E levels are 3 to 15 μg/mL in infants and 5 to 20 μg/mL in older children and adults. Because of its lipid solubility, α-tocopherol is carried almost exclusively in serum lipoproteins, resulting in a direct relationship of serum vitamin E to total serum lipid concentrations (sum of cholesterol, triglycerides, and phospholipids) as well as a less strong relationship with total serum cholesterol levels. Thus, children with cholestasis and hyperlipidemia (which is common in cholestasis) have been described with normal serum α-tocopherol levels despite having profound vitamin E deficiency, however their vitamin E: total serum lipid ratio was low.[22] A vitamin E: total lipid ratio is considered in the deficient range if < 0.6 mg/gm for those less than 1 year of age and less than 0.8 mg/gm for those age 1 year and older[23] (see **Table 1**). Monitoring should be instituted each 3 months during the first year of life for infants with any cholestatic condition, and more frequently if dose adjustments are needed to ensure correction of deficiency, and at least each 6 months thereafter. Serum E: total lipid ratios greater than 3.0 mg/gm should be considered excessive, and doses of vitamin E reduced. Some recommend monitoring the vitamin E: total cholesterol ratio instead, however it is not as accurate a predictor of vitamin E deficiency during cholestasis.[22] Since hyporeflexia and truncal ataxia are early signs of vitamin E deficiency, deep tendon reflexes, gait and limb ataxia should be assessed at each clinical visit.

Vitamin E Supplementation

To prevent vitamin E deficiency, routine supplementation with vitamin E should be instituted in all infants and children with cholestasis. Newly diagnosed infants with cholestasis should be treated with 25 IU/kg per day of standard forms of vitamin E (D-α-tocopherol, α-tocopheryl acetate, succinate, or nicotinate) or, more preferably, 20 to 25 IU/kg/d (16.6mg/kg/d) of the water-soluble form D-α-tocopheryl polyethylene glycol-1000 succinate (TPGS; tocophersolen).[24] The latter is almost always absorbed, even in the context of severe cholestasis,[24,25] and is present in some of the multiple vitamin preparations designed for infants with cholestasis (see below). Vitamin E should be ideally given in a single dose with breakfast (or the morning feed for infants) when bile flow is maximal, and 2 hours apart from any medication that could interfere with its absorption (eg, iron or bile acid binding resins). If forms other than TPGS are used, the dose can be increased by 25 to 50 IU/Kg/d increments up to 100 to 200 IU/Kg/d (45-90mg/kg/d) guided by serum vitamin E: total serum lipid ratio measurements.[19] One of the additional benefits of TPGS, is that is can solubilize and enhance the absorption of other FSVs when administered concurrently, either orally as concurrent separate vitamin preparations or as a single high-dose multiple vitamin preparation that contains TPGS (see below). Currently there is no FDA approved parenteral form of vitamin E for IM or IV administration, other than the small dose found in multiple vitamin preparations designed for parenteral nutrition. Neurologic status should be monitored as above during correction of vitamin E deficiency. Because up to 3% to 4% of the PEG in the TPGS is absorbed and could theoretically lead to a hyperosmolar state, caution should be exercised in children with renal failure or dehydration.[20] Toxicity of excess vitamin E includes exacerbation of vitamin K-deficiency coagulopathy, inhibition of neutrophil oxidative burst and risk for infection, and necrotizing enterocolitis in preterm infants.

VITAMIN D
Metabolism

Vitamin D is present in 2 forms, ergocalciferol (vitamin D_2) which derives from plant sources and cholecalciferol (vitamin D_3) which may be synthesized by the skin or delivered in foods. Vitamin D is a provitamin synthesized by the skin from ultraviolet exposure B radiation. Seasonal variations, skin pigmentation and the geographic latitude where patients reside affect serum 25-OH Vitamin D (25-OHD) levels due to sunlight exposure.[26,27] In the skin, 7-dehydrocholesterol is converted by UVB to provitamin D_3 to vitamin D_3 (cholecalciferol). However, North Americans, including children who spend significant time indoors, reduce their sunlight exposure and thus this does not provide a reliable source of vitamin D.

Vitamin D_2 and D_3 is provided in the diet in fortified foods like milk, egg yolks or fish oils or as a supplement, which for infants is present in commercial formulas, but needs to be supplemented in exclusively breast-fed infants. After oral intake, vitamin D is emulsified in the stomach and in the proximal small intestine, incorporated into micelles by bile acids, which renders it water soluble facilitating entry in the enterocyte. Within the enterocyte, vitamin D_2 and D_3 is incorporated into chylomicrons and transported to the liver via the lymphatics (see **Fig. 1**). In the liver, vitamin D_2 and D_3 are metabolized to 25-OHD_2 and D_3 by separate pathways within hepatocytes and thereafter converted to 1,25-$(OH)_2$ vitamin D_2 and D_3 forms within the kidney via a parathyroid hormone stimulated process. In serum, vitamin D and its metabolites bind to D-binding protein, a protein highly expressed in hepatocytes and related to albumin.[26] The active form of vitamin D is known to impact bone and muscle and immune function. It is now recognized that 1,25-$(OH)_2$ vitamin D_3 is bound intracellularly by a single member of the nuclear receptor superfamily, the Vitamin D Receptor (VDR; NR1I1), present in nearly all organs in the body including the liver, gastrointestinal tract, pancreas, and placenta.[27] From a teleologic basis, the goal of the parathyroid-VDR-vitamin D axis is to maintain serum calcium in the physiologic range through stimulating intestinal absorption and bone resorption, hence in Vitamin D deficiency, the profound ramifications of rickets (see below) become apparent. How intracellular vitamin D metabolism is affected in cholestasis is not well understood, but there are likely contributing roles of elevated intracellular levels of bile acids that are themselves ligands (eg, lithocholic acid) of the VDR.[28,29]

Vitamin D absorption is strictly dependent upon micellar solubilization by bile acids. In cholestasis, especially evident in neonates, intraluminal bile acids fall below the critical micellar concentration and vitamin D absorption is markedly reduced.[30,31] There is minimal absorption of vitamin D in cholestatic infants, especially newborns with genetic causes where bile acids are not properly synthesized or transported (eg, bile acid synthesis gene defects or BSEP deficiencies) or obstructive (eg, BA). The essential need for hydrophobic bile acids to solubilize dietary vitamin D can be evident as soon as 4 to 6 weeks of age in these cholestatic infants whose intestinal lumen lacks bile acids, indicating a clinical need to investigate and address vitamin D deficiency often alongside the first diagnostic evaluations in cholestasis.

Effects of Vitamin D Deficiency

In infants and children with cholestasis, due to the lack of intraluminal bile acids, dietary vitamin D deficiency can develop very early, leading to rickets, bone dystrophy and reduced muscle strength.[32] Clinically, infants and children may have swelling at the metaphyseal-epiphyseal junctions in their arms and legs, a rachitic rosary manifest as costochondral junction swellings, and softening bones with increased fracture risk. If prolonged, Vitamin D deficiency leads to stunted growth and bowed upper and lower extremities. In BA, rickets has been shown to develop by 7 months with associated fractures in childhood or adolescence. Clearance of jaundice before 3 months was inversely related to rickets.[33] In a study of cholestatic children in Egypt, 28 of 50 (mean age 6 years) had rickets, while 7 had one or more fractures and 30% of those had serum 25-OHD levels less than 20 ng/ml.[34] In addition to rickets and fractures, cholestatic patients are at risk for reduced bone mass as assessed by quantitative measures such as dual x-ray absorptiometry (DXA). Osteopenia and fractures are reported in children with cholestatic liver disease including Alagille Syndrome (ALGS), progressive familial intrahepatic cholestasis (PFIC) and BA. There have been no observed differences in fracture rates based upon DXA measurements or serum 25-OHD levels between patients with ALGS and other childhood cholestatic diseases.[32] Vitamin D deficiency in animal models and some adult cholestatic disorders has been associated with increased fibrosis and impaired immune defenses.[35,36]

Evaluation and Monitoring of Vitamin D Status in Cholestasis

Vitamin D status is assessed by measuring serum 25-OHD and several groups have provided normal ranges for children and adults.[37–40] There is no benefit to measuring $1,25\text{-}(OH)_2$ D since the levels are variable even when rickets is present. The Institute of Medicine and the American Association of Pediatrics have recommended that serum 25-OHD exceed 20 ng/mL with a normal range of 20 to 80 ng/mL at any age, while the Endocrine Society has recommended that levels should exceed 30 ng/mL based upon studies showing that PTH levels rise when 25 OH vitamin D levels fall below 30 ng/ml.[39–41] Conflicting data exists whether this inflection point for PTH is observed in adolescents and no supporting evidence for this idea exists for infants and younger children.[41] In patients with cholestasis requiring large doses of vitamin D to overcome impaired absorption, it is important to remember that serum 25-OHD should be monitored for excess (100 ng/ml or 250 nmol/L) and intoxication (150 ng/mL or >375 nmol/L).[39] Taken together, using adult and pediatric guidelines, the targeted range for 25-OHD is 20 to 60 ng/mL (75–150 nmol/L), with less than 20 ng/mL (50 nmol/L) considered deficient (see **Table 1**).

Vitamin D deficiency is common in cholestatic infants, especially notable in BA, present as early as the time of evaluation prior to hepatoportoenterostomy (HPE). Among 92 U.S. and Canadian patients with BA post HPE, 21% to 37% had vitamin D deficiency (defined as serum 25-OHD <15 ng/mL). Vitamin D deficiency was seen after HPE at 1 month in 36%, 3 months in 21% and 6 months in 30% of this cohort. Cholestatic infants with serum bilirubin levels $\geq$ 2 mg/dL having a much higher frequency of vitamin D deficiency than those with serum total bilirubin less than 2 mg/dl[2]. Serum 25-OHD was negatively correlated with serum total bilirubin, which presumably correlates with intraluminal bile acid concentrations. Serum total bilirubin has been demonstrated to be a better predictor of 25-(OH) vitamin D levels in BA compared to serum bile acids.[42] although these studies have not been performed prospectively. In a cohort of 266 Chinese infants and children with BA, 88% were vitamin D deficient (<10 ng/mL) before HPE and 94%, 92%, 49%, and 54% at 2 weeks and 1, 3, and

6 months after surgery. Serum 25-OHD was negatively correlated with total bilirubin (Dong R). Patients with PFIC treated with partial external biliary diversion are at particular risk for vitamin D deficiency and require similar or higher vitamin D doses after compared to before diversion.[43] Prior to liver transplantation, vitamin D deficiency was slightly more common in Egyptian cholestatic patients (37.6%) versus non-cholestatic (30.8%) patients suggesting that all infants and children with liver disease are at risk.[44] In a small study of Polish children prior to liver transplantation, ½ have had serum 25-OHD levels less than 20 ng/ml.[45] Taken together, it is imperative to evaluate serum 25-OHD early in the lives of infants with cholestasis, to identify those who are at risk of complications and initiate adequate supplementation.

Even with resolution of hyperbilirubinemia, cholestatic infants and children can still be vitamin D deficient and warrant scheduled monitoring. In infants, serum 25-OHD should be checked at the diagnostic evaluation, and if deficient, undergo supplementation (see below) and monitored monthly until evidence of sufficiency (>30 ng/mL) is established (see **Table 1**). Often, vitamin D levels are the most labile of the FSVs in cholestasis, especially in infants, thus close monitoring of serum levels of this FSV, when sufficient, can serve as a bellwether for the other FSVs.

Vitamin D Supplementation and Therapeutic Monitoring

Without adequate intraluminal bile acids, supplemental dosing of oral vitamin D will have minimal capability of physiologic replenishment, thus requiring alternate and early applied approaches. One successful means is to utilize the properties of micellar solubilization of vitamin D with D-alpha-tocopheryl polyethylene glycol-1000 succinate (TPGS). Use of TPGS solutions mixed with oral vitamin D preparations has been shown to improve vitamin D absorption in cholestasis.[46] Additional studies demonstrated that the more polar metabolite, 25-OH D was better absorbed than vitamin D in cholestatic children but still reduced compared to control children[47] and 1,25-$(OH)_2$ vitamin D may be effective in treating rickets.[48]

Vitamin D supplementation for cholestatic infants and children may be provided from a variety of sources. Initially, it is recommended that all patients with BA receive a multivitamin such as TPGS-based AquADEKs (vitamin D_3 600 IU/mL) or TPGS-based DEKAs Essential liquid (2000 U/ml of Vitamin D) (**Table 2**). Patients with BA who have total serum bilirubin less than 2 mg/dL will likely be adequately supplemented with this regimen, but do require periodic monitoring, ~3 months in infancy, after sufficiency has been established (see **Table 1**). Infants with persistent jaundice will require adjustments in dosing which can be made after assessing serum 25-OHD. If there is inadequate restoration of normal serum 25-OH D levels with a TPGS based vitamin D containing multivitamin, supplementing with additional oral Vitamin D (1000 IU/kg/d) may be necessary for those profoundly cholestatic infants with some institutions giving doses ≥ 50,000 IU weekly, especially those with clinical consequences such as rickets. It is also worth noting that vitamin D deficiency can occur even after resolution of direct hyperbilirubinemia in BA post-HPE and other cholestatic disorders such as ALGS and PFIC, since metabolism and transport of bile acids and bilirubin are distinct and impairments in bile acid flux often continues even in the presence of resolution of direct hyperbilirubinemia. Thus, periodic monitoring of serum 25-OHD is recommended in all pediatric patients at risk for consequences of cholestasis.

In older children, supplementation with vitamin D as D2 and D3 are available in liquid and tablet form in the US and Canada. Older patients with cholestasis who can swallow pills could receive AquADEKs chewable with 600 IU vitamin D3 or soft gels with1200 IU vitamin D3. Alternative preparations include DEKAs plus in soft gels

Table 2 Multivitamin preparations				
Multivitamin (per 1 mL)	**A**	**D**	**E**	**K**
DEKAs Essential liquid	750mcg	50mcg	50 mg	2000mcg
[also available as capsules)	2500 IU	2000 IU	75 IU	
DEKAs Plus liquid	1727mcg	18.8mcg	33.6 mg	500mcg
[also available as softgels, capsules, chewable]	5751 IU	750 IU	50 IU	
AquADEKs	5751 IU	400 IU	50 IU	400mcg
Polyvisol/Trivisol	750 IU	400 IU		

Note: all vitamin E in DEKAs Essential liquid is TPGS.

with 3000IU vitamin D3, DEKAs plus chewable with 2000 IU vitamin D3, or DEKAs Essential capsules with 2000 IU vitamin D3. Adjustments in dosing should be made when supplementation is started based upon responses to serum 25-OH vitamin D monthly until the level is greater than 30 ng/mL and which point less frequent monitoring at every 3 months or longer intervals may occur (see **Table 1**).

VITAMIN K
Metabolism

Vitamin K is an FSV which serves as an essential co-factor required for post-translational gamma-carboxylation of glutamic acid residues and subsequent activation of coagulation factors, II, VII, IX, X, Protein S and Protein C.[49] Depletion of body stores results in hypo-carboxylated clotting proteins, ineffective coagulation, and significant risk of spontaneous bleeding. There are two dietary forms of the vitamin, K_1 (phylloquinone) primarily found in plants, especially green leafy vegetables, and K_2 (menaquinones) which are mainly found in animal foods, including liver and fermented dairy products. Menaquinones are also synthesized by colonic bacteria, but the dietary contribution of this source is not significant. Both forms require solubilization by bile salts to facilitate small intestinal absorption and cholestatic liver disease is an important risk factor for deficiency.[49]

In the setting of normal liver function, K_1 is solubilized by bile salts and absorbed in the jejunum and ileum (see **Fig. 1**). It is then transported in chylomicrons through the lymphatic system. The majority of K_1 is utilized in the liver in clotting factor synthesis, but a small fraction is also transported in very-low-density lipoproteins to extra hepatic tissues. This fraction has been demonstrated to have a role in both bone and cardiovascular health by modulating activity of other gamma-carboxylated proteins that regulate calcium deposition in vessels and bone matrix.[50,51] Dietary requirements are not well documented, but deficiency can result within days to weeks when vitamin K is eliminated from the diet. The current recommended adequate intake (AI) in healthy adults 19 years and older, is 120 μg (mcg) daily for men and 90 mcg for women. This would be equivalent to approximately a $1/4$ cup serving of kale or spinach or a 2 ounce serving of hard cheese.[52] The AI for infants is based on the vitamin K content of mature human milk (2.5 mg/L of phylloquinone) and the estimated daily milk intake for this age range. An AI of 2.0 mcg per day is recommended for infants age 0 to 6 months, but this amount is well below the usual intake of infants receiving formula feeds which contain 50 to 100 mg/L. Recommendations for older children range from 30 mcg per day for ages 1 to 3 years to 60 to 75 mcg per day in pre-adolescents.

Patients with interrupted bile flow have diminished absorption of dietary sources and frequently require K supplementation to maintain body stores. Malabsorption due to small intestinal injury is also a common cause of vitamin K deficiency that may not be adequately addressed with oral supplementation. Other risk factors such as prolonged hospitalization, critical illness and inflammatory states may further compromise absorption, even without gut injury, and patients with these exposures are at particular risk of becoming deficient.[53]

Effects of Vitamin K Deficiency

Hepatic vitamin K stores will maintain carboxylation of coagulation factors during short term depletion, but carboxylation of other proteins will be compromised. Vitamin K insufficiency can progress silently as the first indications are manifest only as stores drop below what is required for adequate coagulation factor synthesis. Patients can present with bleeding secondary to profound derangement in clotting function. Screening with periodic measurement of PT/INR can identify patients who require supplementation before this progression. However, the impact of more prolonged subtle deficiencies on bone and cardiovascular health are not well established.

Evaluation and Monitoring of Vitamin K Status in Cholestasis

The most practical way to measure vitamin K deficiency in clinical practice is by assessing vitamin K dependent clotting factor activity through the prothrombin time (PT) and its derived value International Normalized Ratio, INR.[51] Measurement of plasma vitamin K_1 levels fluctuate widely related to variations in daily intake since the vitamin has a relatively short half-life of 1 to 3 hours. Vitamin K_2 levels have been rarely studied as they are highly dependent upon intake of very specific foods, not frequently found in a Western diet. Overall vitamin K status can be estimated by measuring the uncarboxylated fractions of the vitamin K dependent proteins such as osteocalcin or matrix gla protein, but threshold concentrations for optimal function have not been established. PIVKA-II, proteins induced by vitamin K absence factor II, have also been explored as a biomarker of vitamin K sufficiency. These proteins are biologically inactive, under gamma-carboxylated vitamin K dependent clotting factors, which become detectable in deficiency states and in patients treated with warfarin. However, commercially available assays are not sensitive enough to detect variations in a healthy population and PIVKA measurement has not been widely adopted as a biomarker of deficiency in at risk patients. Thus, measurement of PT/INR remains the accepted measure of vitamin K status, even though vitamin levels must be decreased by at least 50% before measurements fall outside the normal range. This may explain why the PT/INR measurement can increase briskly in follow-up once any alteration is observed. Direct measurement of Factor VII levels in the context of Factor V levels (which are vitamin K independent) may also be helpful in determining sufficiency, but specific clotting factor assays may not be as broadly available as standard clotting assays.

Vitamin K Supplementation

Deficiency states can be treated either parenterally or orally depending upon the degree of alteration in clotting function and underlying co-morbidities. In chronic cholestatic liver disease, oral vitamin K supplementation may not be effective in treating deficiency unless dissolved in a micellar vehicle like TPGS (see below), and parenteral administration may be necessary. The parenteral formulation can be administered either by intravenous or intramuscular route. However, both intramuscular and intravenous administration have been associated with a small, but measurable risk of anaphylaxis.[54] This reaction is likely related to a dispersant in the drug vehicle, as vitamin K itself is not considered to be an allergenic compound. Cremophor, in particular, has been implicated as other drugs suspended in this vehicle have likewise induced severe allergic responses. Newer preparations of parenteral vitamin K, that avoid such vehicles, may not pose this same risk. Significantly coagulopathy may correct with a single dose of intramuscular vitamin K, especially in the newborn with newly identified neonatal cholestasis. There are several oral preparations available. For older children, tablets are a well-tolerated formulation that can be administered on alternated days or daily depending upon response. Infants and younger children can receive either crushed tablets or liquid formulations, many of which include solubilizing agents such as TPGS (see **Table 1**). In children with chronic cholestasis, DEKAs (Callion Pharma) has become the formulation of choice because of the combination with TPGS. Even in older children, absorption of the tablet formulation may be augmented by co-administration with other vitamin solutions that include TPGS, such as Liqui-E. In patients that cannot tolerate enteral nutrition and supplements, vitamin K can be administered in TPN solutions.[53] The primary source of vitamin K in parenteral feeding regimens is in the lipid emulsion. The concentration of phylloquinone varies by oil source with the highest levels in soybean oil and the lowest levels in safflower oil. In patients receiving exclusive parenteral nutrition with low K_1 content lipid sources for greater than 2 weeks, the risk of PT prolongation is significantly higher, but this risk may not lead to clinically relevant change in coagulation. US FDA regulations stipulate that adult parenteral multivitamin solutions should provide at least 150 µg of K_1 per day in addition to what is included in lipid solutions.

PRACTICAL APPROACH TO MANAGEMENT OF FAT-SOLUBLE VITAMIN DEFICIENCY IN CHOLESTASIS

The typical scenario in which FSV deficiency is encountered is the cholestatic infant or toddler with BA, PFIC, or ALGS and the approach outlined here is largely fashioned for those patient populations. However, the principles described are applicable to most children with chronic cholestasis and specific special situations are addressed separately below.

Surveillance for Fat-Soluble Vitamin Deficiency

Surveillance for FSV deficiency in a cholestatic infant is generally required as soon as cholestasis is established and should continue monthly. Serum levels of retinol, 25-OH D and vitamin E/total lipids along with INR should be checked monthly to bimonthly, initially, and once these levels have stabilized and are in the target range, the frequency of monitoring can be reduced to every 3 to 6 months. If there are limitations to the volume of blood that can be drawn on a small infant, it is appropriate to prioritize 25-OH D and INR as the two that are likely to have the earliest clinical sequelae in the setting of deficiency.

Supplementation of Fat-Soluble Vitamins

The approach selected for supplementing FSV is dependent on multiple factors including availability of multivitamin preparations at a given institution, tolerability and cost to families as these supplements are typically not covered by insurance in North America. There are 3 approaches that are generally employed: (1) use of a high-dose multivitamin preparation designed for cholestasis (2) supplementation with large doses of each individual vitamin (orally and/or intramuscularly) and (3) use of a standard multivitamin preparation with additional individual vitamin supplements.

1. The *use of a multivitamin preparation specifically designed for cholestasis* is, in the authors' experience, the preferred supplementation strategy. To our knowledge, the only formulation of this kind is DEKAs Essential and the components are described in **Table 2**. One milliliter of DEKAs Essential contains appropriate amounts and ratios of FSVs for most infants with cholestasis, including adequate amounts of vitamin K, and the dose can be doubled if vitamin levels fail to correct. Occasionally additional oral vitamin D supplementation is required with DEKAs Essential and should be administered according to levels. Overall, this is the most efficacious and cost-effective strategy for FSV supplementation in cholestasis.
2. *Supplementation of individual vitamins* based on the levels is feasible but has limitations. Doses for individual supplementation are provided in **Table 1**. The drawbacks to this approach are limited tolerance for the volume and taste of liquid vitamin preparations in infants and small children and the cost to families of multiple individual vitamin preparations. If this approach is adopted, it is important to ensure that the TPGS formulation of vitamin E is used as this enhances the absorption of the other FSVs, as discussed above in the section on Vitamin E. Without the use of a TPGS-based solution, the success of concurrent administration of individual FSV supplements is often ineffective.
3. *The use of a standard multivitamin preparations with individual supplementation can be used.* Several multivitamin preparations exist that contain increased levels of FSV, however, these have been developed for supplementation in other diseases characterized by fat malabsorption, such as cystic fibrosis. Commonly used preparations are listed in **Table 2**. A comparison with DEKAs Essential highlights the limited benefit of these other preparations in cholestasis. As noted earlier, AquADEKs (with supplemental vitamin K) has been studied in infants with BA and was found to be inadequate to address FSV deficiencies in most infants who remained cholestatic. However, if DEKAS Essential is unavailable, of the available standard multivitamin strategies, AquADEKs likely remains the preferred option. Use of AquADEKs will likely require additional supplementation with individual vitamins. It is imperative to ensure close monitoring of vitamin levels in infants supplemented with AquADEKs and other similar formulations; in infants with cholestasis, it is advisable to supplement with daily vitamin D (2000 IU) and K (2.5 mg) at initiation of AquADEKs even without baseline vitamin levels. A drawback of this approach remains the financial burden of multiple vitamin preparations to families.

Special Circumstances

A few circumstances are worthy of special consideration. Cholestatic children requiring parenteral nutrition require close surveillance and supplementation as guided by levels of vitamins and other nutrients. It is important not to disregard the need for surveillance of FSV levels when nutrition is being provided parenterally. This is also true of children in the first few months following liver transplantation when it cannot be assumed that all FSV deficiencies have been corrected immediately following transplant surgery. Certain therapeutic interventions greatly increase the risk of FSV deficiency and the need for close monitoring and supplementation should be anticipated and addressed proactively. Such scenarios include those in which the enterohepatic circulation of bile acids is interrupted, such as following surgical biliary diversion and potentially with the use of ileal bile acid transporter (IBAT) inhibitors or bile acid binding resins such as cholestyramine and colesevelam. In some children with biliary diversion and in those receiving colesevelam, free intraluminal bile acid concentrations may be markedly reduced and the risk for vitamin deficiency, including potentially lethal vitamin K deficiency, warrants close monitoring and aggressive supplementation.

SUMMARY

FSV deficiency in cholestasis is a prevalent issue, even in specialized centers. Early and frequent monitoring are essential followed by aggressive supplementation and ongoing monitoring. Although local resources will impact supplementation strategies, we recommend the use of multivitamin preparations designed for cholestasis, if available. In addition to availability, the cost of vitamin and multivitamin preparations poses a significant burden to families, especially in North America where there is a strong need for advocacy to establish coverage for nutritional supplements.

ACKNOWLEDGMENTS

The authors dedicate this article to our friend and colleague, the late James (Jim) Heubi, MD who inspired and developed many of the concepts covered in this report that are crucial to the care of children and adults with cholestatic liver disorders.

DISCLOSURE

B.M. Kamath: Mirum (Consultant, Unrestricted Educational Grant); Albireo (Consultant, Unrestricted Educational Grant); Astellas, Third Rock Ventures. S.J. Karpen: Consultant for Albireo, Intercept, Mirum, Vertex. S.S. Sundaram: Consultant for Mirum. R.J. Sokol: Consultant for Albireo, Mirum, Alexion.

REFERENCES

1. Utterson EC, Shepherd RW, Sokol RJ, et al. Biliary atresia: clinical profiles, risk factors, and outcomes of 755 patients listed for liver transplantation. J Pediatr 2005;147(2):180–5.
2. Shneider BL, Magee JC, Bezerra JA, et al. Efficacy of fat-soluble vitamin supplementation in infants with biliary atresia. Pediatrics 2012;130(3):e607–14.
3. Blaner WS, Li Y, Brun PJ, et al. Vitamin A absorption, storage and mobilization. Subcell Biochem 2016;81:95–125.
4. Norsa L, Zazzeron L, Cuomo M, et al. Night blindness in cystic fibrosis: the key role of Vitamin A in the digestive system. Nutrients 2019;11(8):1876.
5. Vidailhet M, Rieu D, Feillet F, et al. Vitamin A in pediatrics: an update from the nutrition committee of the French society of pediatrics. Arch Pediatr 2017;24(3): 288–97.
6. Chiu M, Dillon A, Watson S. Vitamin A deficiency and xerophthalmia in children of a developed country. J Paediatr Child Health 2016;52(7):699–703.
7. Ferrari G, Vigano M. Images in clinical medicine. Bitot's spot in vitamin A deficiency. N Engl J Med 2013;368(22):e29.
8. Evans RM, Mangelsdorf DJ. Nuclear receptors, RXR, and the big bang. Cell 2014;157(1):255–66.
9. Polcz ME, Barbul A. The role of vitamin A in wound healing. Nutr Clin Pract 2019; 34(5):695–700.
10. Ross AC. Vitamin A and retinoic acid in T cell-related immunity. Am J Clin Nutr 2012;96(5):1166S-72S.
11. Ahmad SM, Huda MN, Raqib R, et al. High-dose neonatal vitamin A supplementation to Bangladeshi infants increases the percentage of CCR9-positive treg cells in infants with lower birthweight in early infancy, and decreases plasma

sCD14 concentration and the prevalence of vitamin A deficiency at two years of age. J Nutr 2020;150(11):3005–12.

12. Flores H, Azevedo MN, Campos FA, et al. Serum vitamin A distribution curve for children aged 2-6 y known to have adequate vitamin A status: a reference population. Am J Clin Nutr 1991;54(4):707–11.

13. Underwood BA. Methods for assessment of vitamin A status. J Nutr 1990; 120(Suppl 11):1459–63.

14. Feranchak AP, Gralla J, King R, et al. Comparison of indices of vitamin A status in children with chronic liver disease. Hepatology 2005;42(4):782–92.

15. Larson LM, Guo J, Williams AM, et al. Approaches to assess vitamin A status in settings of inflammation: biomarkers reflecting inflammation and nutritional determinants of anemia (BRINDA) project. Nutrients 2018;10(8):1100.

16. Oliveira JM, Michelazzo FB, Stefanello J, et al. Influence of iron on vitamin A nutritional status. Nutr Rev 2008;66(3):141–7.

17. Christian P, West KP Jr. Interactions between zinc and vitamin A: an update. Am J Clin Nutr 1998;68(2 Suppl):435S–41S.

18. Stevens GA, Bennett JE, Hennocq Q, et al. Trends and mortality effects of vitamin A deficiency in children in 138 low-income and middle-income countries between 1991 and 2013: a pooled analysis of population-based surveys. Lancet Glob Health 2015;3(9):e528–36.

19. Suchy FJ, Sokol RJ. Chapter 9. Medical and nutritional management of choestasis in infants and children. In: Suchy FJ, Sokol RJ, Balistreri WF, et al, editors. Liver disease in children. Cambridge University Press; 2021. p. 116–46.

20. Sokol RJ, Heubi JE, Iannaccone S, et al. Mechanism causing vitamin E deficiency during chronic childhood cholestasis. Gastroenterology 1983;85(5):1172–82.

21. Sokol RJ, Guggenheim MA, Heubi JE, et al. Frequency and clinical progression of the vitamin E deficiency neurologic disorder in children with prolonged neonatal cholestasis. Am J Dis Child 1985;139(12):1211–5.

22. Sokol RJ, Heubi JE, Iannaccone ST, et al. Vitamin E deficiency with normal serum vitamin E concentrations in children with chronic cholestasis. N Engl J Med 1984; 310(19):1209–12.

23. Sokol RJ. Assessing vitamin E status in childhood cholestasis. J Pediatr Gastroenterol Nutr 1987;6(1):10–3.

24. Sokol RJ, Butler-Simon N, Conner C, et al. Multicenter trial of d-alpha-tocopheryl polyethylene glycol 1000 succinate for treatment of vitamin E deficiency in children with chronic cholestasis. Gastroenterology 1993;104(6):1727–35.

25. Thebaut A, Nemeth A, Le Mouhaer J, et al. Oral tocofersolan corrects or prevents Vitamin E deficiency in children with chronic cholestasis. J Pediatr Gastroenterol Nutr 2016;63(6):610–5.

26. Chun RF. New perspectives on the vitamin D binding protein. Cell Biochem Funct 2012;30(6):445–56.

27. Christakos S, Dhawan P, Verstuyf A, et al. Vitamin D: metabolism, molecular mechanism of action, and pleiotropic effects. Physiol Rev 2016;96(1):365–408.

28. Karpen SJ, Trauner M. The new therapeutic frontier–nuclear receptors and the liver. J Hepatol 2010;52(3):455–62.

29. Makishima M, Lu TT, Xie W, et al. Vitamin D receptor as an intestinal bile acid sensor. Science 2002;296(5571):1313–6.

30. Heubi JE, Hollis BW, Specker B, et al. Bone disease in chronic childhood cholestasis. I. Vitamin D absorption and metabolism. Hepatology 1989;9(2):258–64.

31. Lo CW, Paris PW, Clemens TL, et al. Vitamin D absorption in healthy subjects and in patients with intestinal malabsorption syndromes. Am J Clin Nutr 1985;42(4): 644–9.

32. Loomes KM, Spino C, Goodrich NP, et al. Bone density in children with chronic liver disease correlates with growth and cholestasis. Hepatology 2019;69(1): 245–57.

33. Ruuska S, Laakso S, Leskinen O, et al. Impaired bone health in children with biliary atresia. J Pediatr Gastroenterol Nutr 2020;71(6):707–12.

34. Samra NM, Emad El Abrak S, El Dash HH, et al. Evaluation of vitamin D status bone mineral density and dental health in children with cholestasis. Clin Res Hepatol Gastroenterol 2018;42(4):368–77.

35. Ding N, Yu RT, Subramaniam N, et al. A vitamin D receptor/SMAD genomic circuit gates hepatic fibrotic response. Cell 2013;153(3):601–13.

36. Udomsinprasert W, Jittikoon J. Vitamin D and liver fibrosis: molecular mechanisms and clinical studies. Biomed Pharmacother 2019;109:1351–60.

37. Weydert JA. Vitamin D in children's health. Children (Basel) 2014;1(2):208–26.

38. Holick MF. Vitamin D deficiency. N Engl J Med 2007;357(3):266–81.

39. Misra M, Pacaud D, Petryk A, et al. Vitamin D deficiency in children and its management: review of current knowledge and recommendations. Pediatrics 2008; 122(2):398–417.

40. Ross AC, Manson JE, Abrams SA, et al. The 2011 report on dietary reference intakes for calcium and vitamin D from the Institute of Medicine: what clinicians need to know. J Clin Endocrinol Metab 2011;96(1):53–8.

41. Hill KM, McCabe GP, McCabe LD, et al. An inflection point of serum 25-hydroxyvitamin D for maximal suppression of parathyroid hormone is not evident from multi-site pooled data in children and adolescents. J Nutr 2010;140(11):1983–8.

42. Venkat VL, Shneider BL, Magee JC, et al. Total serum bilirubin predicts fat-soluble vitamin deficiency better than serum bile acids in infants with biliary atresia. J Pediatr Gastroenterol Nutr 2014;59(6):702–7.

43. Squires JE, Celik N, Morris A, et al. Clinical variability after partial external biliary diversion in familial intrahepatic cholestasis 1 deficiency. J Pediatr Gastroenterol Nutr 2017;64(3):425–30.

44. Veraldi S, Pietrobattista A, Liccardo D, et al. Fat soluble vitamins deficiency in pediatric chronic liver disease: the impact of liver transplantation. Dig Liver Dis 2020;52(3):308–13.

45. Kryskiewicz E, Pawlowska J, Pludowski P, et al. Bone metabolism in cholestatic children before and after living-related liver transplantation–a long-term prospective study. J Clin Densitom 2012;15(2):233–40.

46. Argao EA, Heubi JE, Hollis BW, et al. d-Alpha-tocopheryl polyethylene glycol-1000 succinate enhances the absorption of vitamin D in chronic cholestatic liver disease of infancy and childhood. Pediatr Res 1992;31(2):146–50.

47. Heubi JE, Hollis BW, Tsang RC. Bone disease in chronic childhood cholestasis. II. Better absorption of 25-OH vitamin D than vitamin D in extrahepatic biliary atresia. Pediatr Res 1990;27(1):26–31.

48. Heubi JE, Tsang RC, Steichen JJ, et al. 1,25-Dihydroxyvitamin D3 in childhood hepatic osteodystrophy. J Pediatr 1979;94(6):977–82.

49. Amitrano L, Guardascione MA, Brancaccio V, et al. Coagulation disorders in liver disease. Review. Semin Liver Dis 2002;22(1):83–96.

50. Rodriguez-Olleros Rodriguez C, Diaz Curiel M. Vitamin K and bone health: a review on the effects of vitamin K deficiency and supplementation and the effect of

non-vitamin K antagonist oral anticoagulants on different bone parameters. Rev J Osteoporos 2019;2019:2069176.
51. van Ballegooijen AJ, Beulens JW. The role of vitamin K status in cardiovascular health: evidence from observational and clinical studies. Review. Curr Nutr Rep 2017;6(3):197–205.
52. Micronutrients IoMUPo. Dietary reference intakes for vitamin A, vitamin K, arsenic, boron, chromium, copper, iodine, iron, manganese, molybdenum, nickel, silicon, vanadium, and zinc. National Academies Press (US; 2001.
53. Shearer MJ. Vitamin K in parenteral nutrition. Review. Gastroenterology 2009; 137(5 Suppl):S105–18.
54. Fiore LD, Scola MA, Cantillon CE, et al. Anaphylactoid reactions to vitamin K. Research support, non-U.S. Gov't review. J Thromb Thrombolysis 2001;11(2): 175–83.

Moving?

Make sure your subscription moves with you!

To notify us of your new address, find your **Clinics Account Number** (located on your mailing label above your name), and contact customer service at:

Email: journalscustomerservice-usa@elsevier.com

800-654-2452 (subscribers in the U.S. & Canada)
314-447-8871 (subscribers outside of the U.S. & Canada)

Fax number: 314-447-8029

Elsevier Health Sciences Division
Subscription Customer Service
3251 Riverport Lane
Maryland Heights, MO 63043

ELSEVIER

Printed and bound by CPI Group (UK) Ltd, Croydon, CR0 4YY

03/10/2024

01040476-0004